Decision Making in Spinal Care

Second Edition

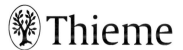

Decision Making in Spinal Care

Second Edition

D. Greg Anderson, MD
Professor
Departments of Orthopaedic Surgery and Neurological Surgery
Clinical Director, Spine Section
The Orthopaedic Research Laboratory
Thomas Jefferson University
The Rothman Institute
Philadelphia, Pennsylvania

Alexander R. Vaccaro, MD, PhD
The Everrett J. and Marion Gordon Professor of Orthopaedic Surgery
Professor of Neurosurgery
Co-Director, Delaware Valley Spinal Cord Injury Center
Co-Chief, Spine Surgery
Co-Director, Spine Fellowship Program
Thomas Jefferson University
The Rothman Institute
Philadelphia, Pennsylvania

Contributing Editor
Gregory Gebauer, MD, MS
Orthopedic Spine Surgeon
Advanced Orthopedic Center
Port Charlotte, Florida

Thieme
New York · Stuttgart

Thieme Medical Publishers, Inc.
333 Seventh Ave.
New York, NY 10001

Executive Editor: Kay Conerly
Managing Editor: Judith Tomat
Editorial Director, Clinical Reference:
  Michael Wachinger
Production Editor: Kenneth L. Chumbley
International Production Director:
  Andreas Schabert

Senior Vice President, International
  Marketing and Sales: Cornelia Schulze
Vice President, Finance and Accounts:
  Sarah Vanderbilt
President: Brian D. Scanlan
Compositor: Prairie Papers Inc.
Spine bullet illustration by Karl Wesker
Printer: Sheridan Books, Inc.

Library of Congress Cataloging-in-Publication Data

Decision making in spinal care / [edited by] D. Greg Anderson, Alexander R. Vaccaro.—2nd ed.
  p. ; cm.
  Includes bibliographical references.
  ISBN 978-1-60406-417-9 (alk. paper)—ISBN 978-1-60406-418-6 (e-ISBN)
  I. Anderson, D. Greg. II. Vaccaro, Alexander R.
  [DNLM: 1. Spinal Diseases—therapy. 2. Decision Making. 3. Orthopedic Procedures.
4. Spinal Injuries—therapy. WE 725]

  616.7′3—dc23

                                                                          2012016862

Important note: Medical knowledge is ever-changing. As new research and clinical experience broaden our knowledge, changes in treatment and drug therapy may be required. The authors and editors of the material herein have consulted sources believed to be reliable in their efforts to provide information that is complete and in accord with the standards accepted at the time of publication. However, in view of the possibility of human error by the authors, editors, or publisher of the work herein or changes in medical knowledge, neither the authors, editors, nor publisher, nor any other party who has been involved in the preparation of this work, warrants that the information contained herein is in every respect accurate or complete, and they are not responsible for any errors or omissions or for the results obtained from use of such information. Readers are encouraged to confirm the information contained herein with other sources. For example, readers are advised to check the product information sheet included in the package of each drug they plan to administer to be certain that the information contained in this publication is accurate and that changes have not been made in the recommended dose or in the contraindications for administration. This recommendation is of particular importance in connection with new or infrequently used drugs.

Some of the product names, patents, and registered designs referred to in this book are in fact registered trademarks or proprietary names even though specific reference to this fact is not always made in the text. Therefore, the appearance of a name without designation as proprietary is not to be construed as a representation by the publisher that it is in the public domain.

Printed in the United States of America

5 4 3 2 1

ISBN 978-1-60406-417-9
eISBN 978-1-60406-418-6

I dedicate this book to my son Bradley, whose vast inner potential motivates me to pursue excellence.

D. Greg Anderson, MD

This book is dedicated to the staff of Thieme, whose vision, expertise, guidance, and talent allow medical care professionals the privilege of educating the students of spinal science.

Alexander R. Vaccaro, MD, PhD

I dedicate this book to my wonderful wife, who has supported me every step of the way and who has given us three beautiful children.

Gregory Gebauer, MD, MS

.

Contents

II Thoracolumbar Trauma

III Cervical Degenerative/Metabolic Disease

XIV Spinal Imaging

XV Spinal Monitoring

XVI Miscellaneous Topics

Preface

Spinal medicine has emerged as a mature and semi-independent specialty of medicine. Spinal problems are complex and often require a detailed workup and decision-making process. This second edition of *Decision Making in Spinal Care* is designed to focus on this crucial process. We have strived to include a wide spectrum of both common and relatively specialized topics that might be encountered by those treating spinal patients.

The first edition of this text brought favorable feedback, as well as helpful suggestions that have been incorporated into the current edition. This text will be a valuable resource for an array of medical readers, from students to practicing physicians, who have the need for a quick and concise reference covering the broad spectrum of spinal medicine. We have again elicited the help of a wide range of experts in writing chapters for this text along with including useful figures, diagrams, flow charts, and references that are designed to simplify the learning process.

Included in these pages is pertinent "must know" information that will affect clinical decision making. The text remains organized according to diagnosis (topic) and anatomic region and covers various pathologies, including spinal trauma, metabolic, degenerative, and deformity-related spinal conditions. The contemporary topic section has been expanded to address the growth in new spinal technologies. We believe that this text will make a substantial impact on a reader's understanding of spinal conditions in a concise and efficient manner, and we dedicate this effort to those who strive to provide the highest quality care to patients with spinal conditions.

Contributors

Todd J. Albert, MD
Richard H. Rothman Professor and
    Chairman
Department of Orthopaedic Surgery
Professor of Neurosurgery
Thomas Jefferson University and
    Hospitals
President
The Rothman Institute
Philadelphia, Pennsylvania

David T. Anderson, MD
Resident
Jefferson Medical College
Philadelphia, Pennsylvania

D. Greg Anderson, MD
Professor
Departments of Orthopaedic Surgery
    and Neurological Surgery
Clinical Director, Spine Section
The Orthopaedic Research Laboratory
Thomas Jefferson University
The Rothman Institute
Philadelphia, Pennsylvania

Vincent Arlet, MD
Professor
Department of Orthopaedic Surgery
University of Pennsylvania
Philadelphia, Pennsylvania

Eli M. Baron, MD
Attending Neurosurgeon
Spine Surgeon
Cedars-Sinai Spine Center
Department of Neurosurgery
Los Angeles, California

Rahul Basho, MD
Clinical Instructor of Spine Surgery
Department of Orthopaedic Surgery
Riverside County Regional Medical
    Center
Moreno Valley, California

John M. Beiner, MD
Connecticut Orthopedic Specialists
Clinical Instructor and Attending
    Surgeon
Department of Orthopedics,
Yale–New Haven Hospital and
    Hospital of St. Raphaels
New Haven, Connecticut

Vidya M. Bhalodia, MA, DABNM
Senior Surgical Neurophysiologist
Specialty Care Neurological
    Monitoring
Nashville, Tennessee

Arnima Bhasin, BS
Research Assistant
Department of Neurology
St. Francis Medical Center
Peoria, Illinois

Haim D. Blecher, MD
Clinical Assistant Professor
UMDNJ–Robert Wood Johnson
   Medical School
Department of Orthopedic Surgery
New Brunswick, New Jersey

Daniel J. Blizzard, MD, MHS
Resident
Department of Orthopaedic Surgery
Duke University School of Medicine
Durham, North Carolina

Irina G. Bogacheva, PhD
Chief Administrator
The Back Institute
Los Angeles, California

Christopher M. Bono, MD
Associate Professor of Orthopaedic
   Surgery
Harvard Medical School
Chief, Orthopaedic Spine Service
Brigham and Women's Hospital
Co-Director, Combined MGH-BWH
   Spine Surgery Fellowship
Boston, Massachusetts

Brett A. Braly, MD
Resident
Department of Orthopaedic Surgery
University of Pittsburgh Medical
   Center
Pittsburgh, Pennsylvania

Keith H. Bridwell, MD
J. Albert Key Distinguished Professor
   of Orthopaedic Surgery
Professor of Neurological Surgery
Department of Orthopaedic Surgery
Washington University
St. Louis, Missouri

Rocco Richard Calderone, MD
Private Practice
Spine and Orthopedic Surgery
St. John's Regional Medical Center
Oxnard, California
St. John's Pleasant Valley Hospital
Camarillo, California

Kanit Chamroontaneskul, MD
Orthopedic Spine Surgeon
Bangkok Hospital
Bangkok, Thailand

Fernando J. Checo, MD
Clinical Instructor
Spine Surgery Fellow
New England Baptist Hospital
Boston, Massachusetts

Antonia F. Chen, MD, MBA
Resident
Department of Orthopaedics
University of Pittsburgh Medical
   Center
Pittsburgh, Pennsylvania

Norman B. Chutkan, MD, FACS
Professor and Chairman
Department of Orthopaedic Surgery
Georgia Health Sciences University
Augusta, Georgia

Richard Derby, MD, FIPP
Medical Director
Spinal Diagnostics and Treatment
   Center
Daly City, California

Vincent J. Devlin, MD
Orthopaedic Spine Surgeon
Edmond, Oklahoma

Ashvin K. Dewan, MD
Resident
Department of Orthopaedic Surgery
Johns Hopkins Hospital
Baltimore, Maryland

David A. Ditsworth, MD
Chief
Department of Neurosurgery
The Back Institute
Los Angeles, California

Doniel Drazin, MD, MA
Resident
Neurosurgery
Cedars-Sinai Medical Center
Los Angeles, California

Noam Z. Drazin, MD
Hematology/Oncology
Cedars-Sinai Medical Group/
    Cancer Center
Clinical Instructor
UCLA School of Medicine
Beverly Hills, California

Marcel F. Dvorak, MD, FRCSC
Professor of Orthopaedics
Head, Division of Spine
Cordula and Gunther Paetzold Chair
    in Spinal Cord Clinical Research
University of British Columbia
Vancouver, British Columbia, Canada

Matthew R. Eager, MD
Spine Surgeon
SUN Orthopaedic Group
Lewisburg, Pennsylvania

Mostafa H. El Dafrawy, MG, BCh
Research Fellow
Department of Orthopaedic Surgery
Johns Hopkins University School of
    Medicine
Baltimore, Maryland

Steven M. Falowski, MD
St. Luke's University Health Network
Director, Functional Neurosurgery
St. Luke's Neurosurgical Associates
Bethlehem, Pennsylvania

Daniel R. Fassett, MD, MBA
Head of Neurosurgery
Director of Spinal Surgery
Illinois Neurological Institute
University of Illinois College of
    Medicine–Peoria
Peoria, Illinois

Charles G. Fisher, MD, MHSc, FRCSC
Director of Spine Fellowship Program
Combined Neurosurgical and
    Orthopaedic Spine Program
Vancouver General Hospital
Associate Professor
Department of Orthopaedic Surgery
University of British Columia
Vancouver, British Columbia, Canada

Peter G. Gabos, MD
Co-Director
The Spine and Scoliosis Center
Nemours' Alfred I. DuPont Hospital
    for Children
Wilmington, Delaware
Assistant Clinical Professor of
    Orthopaedic Surgery
Jefferson Medical College
Philadelphia, Pennsylvania

Sapan D. Gandhi, BS
Medical Student
Drexel University College of Medicine
Philadelphia, Pennsylvania

Gregory Gebauer, MD, MS
Orthopedic Spine Surgeon
Advanced Orthopedic Center
Port Charlotte, Florida

Peter C. Gerszten, MD, MPH, FACS
Peter E. Sheptak Professor of
    Neurological Surgery and Radiation
    Oncology
Department of Neurological Surgery
University of Pittsburgh Medical
    Center
Pittsburgh, Pennsylvania

George M. Ghobrial, MD
Neurosurgery Resident
Thomas Jefferson University Hospital
Philadelphia, Pennsylvania

Laura E. Gill, MD, MBBS
Resident
Department of Orthopaedics
University of Virginia
Charlottesville, Virginia

Alex Gitelman, MD
Spine Surgeon
White Plains, New York

Maurice Goins, MD
Spine Surgeon
Resurgens Orthopaedics
Fayetteville, Georgia

Matthew J. Goldstein, MD
Chief Resident
Department of Orthopedic Surgery
North Shore–Long Island Jewish
    Health System
New Hyde Park, New York

Jonathan Newman Grauer, MD
Associate Professor
Department of Orthopaedics and
    Rehabilitation
Yale University School of Medicine
New Haven, Connecticut

Qusai Hammouri, MBBS
Pediatric Orthopaedic Fellow
Department of Orthopaedics
Columbia University
New York, New York

James S. Harrop, MD
Associate Professor
Departments of Neurological and
    Orthopedic Surgery
Director
Division of Spine and Peripheral
    Nerve Surgery
Jefferson Medical College
Philadelphia, Pennsylvania

Alan S. Hilibrand, MD
Professor of Orthopaedic Surgery and
    Neurosurgery
Director of Medical Education
Department of Orthopaedic Surgery
The Rothman Institute
Jefferson Medical College
Philadelphia, Pennsylvania

Joshua William Hustedt, BA
Medical Student
Department of Orthopaedics and
    Rehabilitation
Yale University School of Medicine
New Haven, Connecticut

Raymond W. Hwang, MD, MEng, MBA
Orthopaedic Spine Surgeon
Midwest Orthopaedic Institute
Sycamore, Illinois

Ryan R. Janicki, MD, MSc PT, FRCSC
Neurosurgeon
Department of Surgery
Lions Gate Hospital
North Vancouver, British Columbia,
    Canada

Iain H. Kalfas, MD
Staff Neurosurgeon
Department of Neurosurgery
Cleveland Clinic
Cleveland, Ohio

Daniel G. Kang, MD
Orthopaedic Surgery Resident
Department of Orthopaedic Surgery
    and Rehabilitation
Walter Reed National Military
    Medical Center
Bethesda, Maryland

Christopher K. Kepler, MD, MBA
Fellow, Spine Surgery
Department of Orthopaedic Surgery
Thomas Jefferson University
The Rothman Institute
Philadelphia, Pennsylvania

Stewart Kerr, MD
Chief of Orthopaedic Spinal Surgery
Naval Medical Center
San Diego, California

Tagreed M. Khalaf, MD
Staff Physician
Center for Spine Health
Cleveland Clinic
Cleveland, Ohio

Safdar N. Khan, MD
Assistant Professor of Orthopaedic
   Surgery
Chief
Divison of Spine Surgery
Department of Orthopaedic Surgery
The Ohio State University Medical
   Center
Columbus, Ohio

A. Jay Khanna, MD, MBA
Associate Professor of Orthopaedic
   Surgery and Biomedical Engineering
Johns Hopkins University Baltimore,
   Maryland
Johns Hopkins Orthopaedic and
   Spine Surgery–Greater Washington
   Region
Bethesda, Maryland

Loukas Koyonos, MD
Orthopaedic Resident
Department of Orthopedic Surgery
Thomas Jefferson University
   Hospitals
The Rothman Institute
Philadelphia, Pennsylvania

Paul Kraemer, MD
Assistant Professor
Indiana Spine Group
Department of Orthopaedics
Indiana University
Indianapolis, Indiana

Joon Y. Lee, MD
Associate Professor
Department of Orthopaedic Surgery–
   Spine Division
University of Pittsburgh Medical
   Center
Pittsburgh, Pennsylvania

Larry Lee, MD
Resident
Department of Orthopaedics
Tufts Medical Center
Boston, Massachusetts

Ronald A. Lehman Jr., MD
Chief, Pediatric and Adult Spine
Associate Professor
Division of Orthopaedics
Uniformed Services University of the
   Health Sciences
Department of Orthopaedics and
   Rehabilitation
Walter Reed National Military
   Medical Center
Washington, DC

Peter Lewkonia, MD, MSc
Clinical Assistant Professor
Division of Orthopaedics
Department of Surgery
University of Calgary
Calgary, Alberta, Canada

Moe R. Lim, MD
Assistant Professor
Department of Orthopaedics
University of North Carolina
Chapel Hill, North Carolina

Luis A. Lombardi, MD
Spine Surgery
Back Institute
Beverly Hills, California

John P. Lubicky, MD, FAAOS, FAAP
Professor of Orthopaedic Surgery and
  Pediatrics
West Virginia University School of
  Medicine
Morgantown, West Virginia

Steven C. Ludwig, MD
Associate Professor
Chief of Spine Surgery
Director of Spine Fellowship
Department of Orthopaedics
University of Maryland Medical
  System
Baltimore, Maryland

Jeffrey Thomas P. Luna, MD
Orthopaedic Spine, Adult Joint
  Reconstruction and Tumor Surgery
Trinity Orthopaedics
Trinity Regional Medical Center
Fort Dodge, Iowa

Rex A. W. Marco, MD
Associate Professor
Department of Orthopaedic Surgery
University of Texas–Houston
Shriner's Hospital for Children
The Methodist Hospital
Houston, Texas

Daniel Mazanec, MD
Associate Director
Center for Spine Health
Neurological Institute
Cleveland Clinic
Associate Professor
Cleveland Clinic Lerner College of
  Medicine
Cleveland, Ohio

Beck D. McAllister, MD
Orthopaedic Spine Surgery Fellow
Department of Orthopaedic Surgery
UCLA Comprehensive Spine Center
Los Angeles, California

Irina L. Melnik, MD
Spinal Diagnostics and Treatment
  Center
Daly City, California

Amin J. Mirhadi, MD
Faculty Physician
Department of Radiation Oncology
Cedars-Sinai Medical Center
Los Angeles, California

Sergey Mlyavykh, MD
Chief
Deparment of Neurosurgery
Research Institute of Traumatology
  and Orthopedics
Nizhniy Novgorod, Russia

David M. Neils, MD
Resident
Department of Neurosurgery
University of Illinois College of
  Medicine–Peoria
Peoria, Illinois

Douglas G. Orndorff, MD
Board Eligible Orthopedic Surgeon
  Fellowship
Trained Spine Surgeon
Department of Spine Surgery
Spine Colorado
Durango, Colorado

Michael A. Pahl, MD
Orthopedic Surgeon
Memorial Orthopedic Surgical Group
Long Beach, California

Alpesh A. Patel, MD, FACS
Associate Professor
Department of Orthopaedic Surgery
  and Rehabilitation
Loyola University Chicago Medical
  Center
Chicago, Illinois

Katie A. Patty, MS, CCRC
Clinical Research Coordinator
Durango Orthopedic Associates, PC
Spine Colorado
Durango, Colorado

David L. Penn, MS
Medical Student
Department of Neurological Surgery
Thomas Jefferson University
Philadelphia, Pennsylvania

Olga A. Perlmutter, MD
Leading Scientific Fellow
Department of Neurosurgery
Research Institute of Trauma and
    Orthopaedics
Nizhny Novgorod, Russia

Frank M. Phillips, MD
Professor
Co-Director, Spine Fellowship
Head, Section of Minimally Invasive
    Spine Surgery
Department of Orthopaedic Surgery
Rush University Medical Center
Chicago, Illinois

Kornelis A. Poelstra, MD, PhD
President
The Spine Institute
Destin-Fort Walton Beach, Florida

Kris Radcliff, MD
Assistant Professor
Department of Orthopedic Surgery
Rothman Institute
Thomas Jefferson University
Philadelphia, Pennsylvania

Y. Raja Rampersaud, MD, FRCS(C)
Associate Professor
Department of Surgery
University Health Network
University of Toronto
Toronto, Ontario, Canada

Brandon J. Rebholz, MD
Orthopaedic Spine Surgery Fellow
Department of Orthopaedic Surgery
UCLA Comprehensive Spine Center
Los Angeles, California

Conor Regan, MD
Resident
Department of Orthopaedics
University of North Carolina
Chapel Hill, North Carolina

Jeffrey A. Rihn, MD
Associate Professor
Department of Orthopaedic Surgery
Thomas Jefferson University Hospital
The Rothman Institute
Philadelphia, Pennsylvania

Lee H. Riley III, MD
Chief, Orthopaedic Spine Division
Associate Professor
Departments of Orthopaedic Surgery
    and Neurosurgery
The Johns Hopkins University School
    of Medicine
Baltimore, Maryland

Samuel R. Rosenfeld, MD
Associate Clinical Professor
Department of Orthopaedic Surgery,
University of California–Irvine
Director Neuromuscular Clinics
CHOC Children's Hospital
Orange, California

Rick C. Sasso, MD
Professor
Chief of Spine Surgery
Clinical Orthopaedic Surgery
Indiana University School of Medicine
Indiana Spine Group
Indianapolis, Indiana

Amirali Sayadipour, MD
Resident
Department of Psychiatry
Drexel University College of Medicine
Hahnemann University Hospital
Philadelphia, Pennsylvania

Andrew J. Schoenfeld, MD
Assistant Professor
Department of Orthopaedic Surgery
William Beaumont Army Medical
    Center
Texas Tech University Health Sciences
    Center
El Paso, Texas

Daniel M. Schwartz, PhD
Surgical Monitoring Associates, Inc.
Bala Cynwyd, Pennsylvania

Kwan Sik Seo, MD, PhD
Assistant Professor
Department of Physical Medicine and
    Rehabilitation Medicine
Seoul National University
Seoul, South Korea

**Anthony K. Sestokas, PhD, DABNM,
    FASNM**
Chief Clinical Officer
Department of Intraoperative
    Neuromonitoring
Specialty Care
Nashville, Tennessee

Ashwini Sharan, MD
Associate Professor of Neurosurgery
Thomas Jefferson University
Philadelphia, Pennsylvania

Francis H. Shen, MD
Professor of Orthopaedic Surgery
Division Head, Division of Spine
    Surgery
Director, Spine Fellowship
Co-Director, Spine Center
University of Virginia Medical Center
Charlottesville, Virginia

Adam L. Shimer, MD
Assistant Professor
Department of Orthopaedic Surgery
University of Virginia
Charlottesville, Virginia

Jeff S. Silber, MD, DC
Associate Professor
Hofstra Medical School
Associate Chairman
Department of Orthopedics
Chief
Division of Spinal Surgery
Long Island Jewish Medical Center
Great Neck, New York

Andrew K. Simpson, MD, MHS
Resident
Harvard Orthopaedic Surgery
Massachusetts General Hospital
Boston, Massachusetts

Harvey E. Smith, MD
Assistant Clinical Professor
Department of Orthopaedic Surgery
Tufts University School of Medicine
New England Baptist Hospital
Boston, Massachusetts

Jeremy S. Smith, MD
Assistant Professor
Department of Orthopaedic Surgery
Co-Director, USC Center for Spinal
    Surgery
University of Southern California
Los Angeles, California

William Ryan Spiker, MD
Resident Surgeon
Orthopaedic Surgery
University of Utah
Salt Lake City, Utah

Richard M. Spiro, MD, FACS, FICS
Chief, Spinal Surgery
Department of Neurological Surgery
University of Pittsburgh
Pittsburgh, Pennsylvania

Daniel J. Sucato, MD, MS
Chief of Staff
Texas Scottish Rite Hospital
Professor
Department of Orthopaedic Surgery
University of Texas at Southwestern
    Medical School
Dallas, Texas

Ishaq Y. Syed, MD, MS
Assistant Professor
Department of Orthopedic Surgery
Wake Forest University Baptist
    Medical Center
Winston-Salem, North Carolina

Chadi A. Tannoury, MD
Orthopaedic Spine Fellow
Rush University Medical Center
Chicago, Illinois

Tony Tannoury, MD
Department of Orthopedics
Boston University
Director of Spine and Fellowship
    Programs
Founding President
Society for Progress and Innovations
    for the Near East
Boston, Massachusetts

Brett A. Taylor, MD
Private Practice
Adult Spine Surgeon
The Orthopedic Center of St. Louis
St. Louis, Missouri

Louise E. Toutant, MSN
Nurse Practitioner
General Surgery
Anacapa Surgical Associates
Ventura, California

Dominick A. Tuason, MD
Pediatric Orthopaedic Fellow
Texas Scottish Rite Hospital for
    Children
Dallas, Texas

Jonathan A. Tuttle, MD
Assistant Professor
Department of Neurosurgery and
    Orthopaedics
Medical College of Georgia
Augusta, Georgia

Alexander R. Vaccaro, MD, PhD
The Everrett J. and Marion Gordon
    Professor of Orthopaedic Surgery
Professor of Neurosurgery
Co-Director, Delaware Valley Spinal
    Cord Injury Center
Co-Chief, Spine Surgery
Co-Director, Spine Fellowship
    Program
Thomas Jefferson University
The Rothman Institute
Philadelphia, Pennsylvania

Jeffrey C. Wang, MD
Vice Chairman
UCLA Department of Orthopaedic
    Surgery
Chief, Orthopaedic Spine Service
Professor of Orthopaedic Surgery and
    Neurosurgery
UCLA Comprehensive Spine Center
Santa Monica, California

William C. Welch, MD, FACS, FICS
Professor of Neurosurgery
Chair, Department of Neurosurgery
Pennsylvania Hospital
Vice-Chair, Department of
    Neurosurgery
Perelman School of Medicine
University of Pennsylvania
Philadelphia, Pennsylvania

Brian C. Werner, MD
Resident
Department of Orthopaedic Surgery
University Virginia
Charlottesville, Virginia

Andrew P. White, MD
Assistant Professor
Harvard Medical School
Department of Orthpaedic Surgery
Beth Israel Deaconess Medical Center
Boston, Massachusetts

Chengyuan Wu, MD, MSBmE
Resident
Department of Neurological Surgery
Thomas Jefferson University
  Hospitals
Philadelphia, Pennsylvania

Moshe Yanko, MD
Hillel Yaffe Medical Center
Hadera, Israel and Meir Medical
  Center
Kfar Saba, Israel

Jim A. Youssef, MD
Board certified Orthopedic Surgeon
Fellowship Trained Spine Surgeon
Durango Orthopedic Associates, PC/
  Spine Colorado
Durango, Colorado

Lukas P. Zebala, MD
Assistant Professor of Orthopaedic
  Surgery
Washington University in St. Louis,
Department of Orthopaedic Surgery
St. Louis, Missouri

Matthew G. Zmurko, MD
Orthopaedic Spine Surgeon
Vermont Orthopaedic Clinic
Rutland Regional Medical Center
Rutland, Vermont

I Cervical Trauma

Suspected Occipito-Atlantal Injury

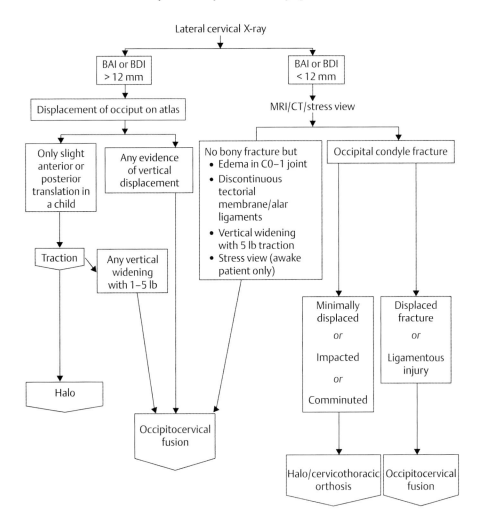

BAI, basion-axial interval; BDI, basion–dental interval; CCI, occipital condyle–cervical 1 interval; CT, computed tomography; MRI, magnetic resonance imaging

1

Occipito-Atlantal Injuries

Andrew J. Schoenfeld and Christopher M. Bono

Injuries at the occipito-atlantal (OA) junction exist on a spectrum, from simple posterior ligamentous strain to fracture of the occipital condyles and true OA dissociation, which represents the complete disruption of the osseo-ligamentous complex of the OA joint. OA dislocations manifest as varying degrees of subluxation, or disarticulation, of the occipital condyle(s) from the articular surface of the first cervical vertebra (atlas). These injuries are often precipitated by massive forces applied across the OA junction and usually result from high-speed motor vehicle accidents, falls from substantial heights, or accidents in which a pedestrian is struck by a motor vehicle. OA dislocation/dissociation in particular is feared because of high associated rates of neurologic injury and mortality. Until recently, OA dislocations were considered uniformly fatal, but, thanks to advances in emergency medical response and scientific understanding regarding these injuries, successful interventions and cases of OA dissociation without neurological deficit have recently been reported.

Classification

Occipital condyle fractures were classified in the system described by Anderson and Montesano (**Fig. 1.1**). In this classification, type I and II fractures are considered stable, while type III fractures may be unstable because of compromised ligamentous structures. Tuli and colleagues attempted to derive a classification of occipital condylar injuries that is more capable of informing outcome. In this system, type 1 fractures are nondisplaced, type 2a fractures are displaced but stable because ligamentous structures are competent, and type 2b fractures are displaced and unstable secondary to compromised ligaments. OA dislocations were initially classified by Traynelis et al. in a purely descriptive system based on the direction of displacement (**Fig. 1.2**). This classification has been

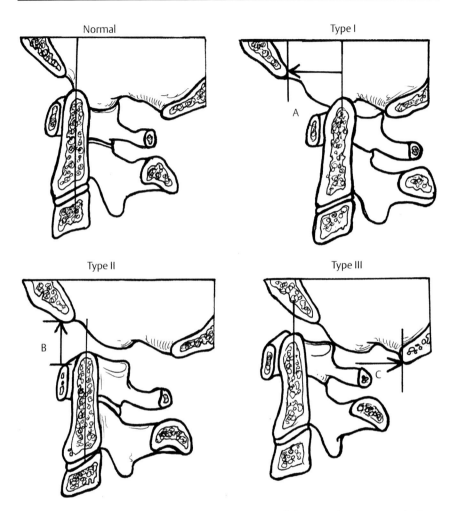

Fig. 1.1 Classification system for OA dislocations. Type I dislocations have anterior displacement. Type II dislocations have vertical (upward) displacement of the occiput from the atlas (OA dissociation). (Note: Some authors have divided these into type IIa and IIb, in which the latter has vertical separation of the atlas from the axis; however, this is more accurately categorized as atlanto-axial instability and is discussed in Chapter 3.) Type III dislocations are posteriorly displaced.

criticized on the grounds that it does not inform treatment or outcome and that in severe OA dissociations, hypermobility may enable a single patient to be classified in all three categories depending on the location of the occiput at the time various imaging studies are obtained. Recently, Bellabarba et al. and Horn et al. have both derived newer schemes intended to inform treatment of OA dislocations. Both classifications employ computed tomography (CT) and magnetic resonance (MR) imaging (MRI), and the system of Bellabarba et al.

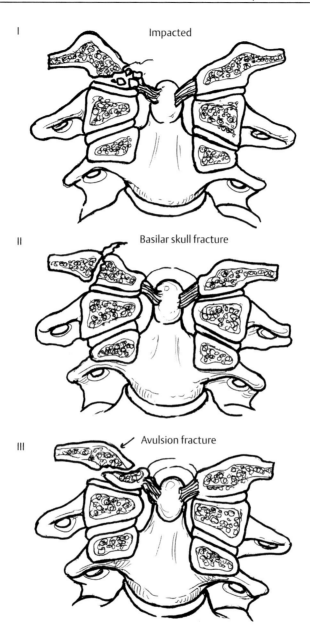

Fig. 1.2 Classification system for occipital condyle fractures as described by Anderson and Montesano. Type I fractures are considered impaction fractures and are stable. Type II fractures are basilar skull fractures that extend through the condyle and communicate with the foramen magnum. These are also usually stable. Type III fractures are unstable, as they are avulsion fractures that primarily represent ligamentous incompetence.

also employs provocative traction. In Bellabarba et al.'s classification, type I injuries are aligned within 2 mm of normal by CT and distract <2 mm with provocative traction, type II dislocations distract more than 2 mm, and type III injuries are grossly misaligned on CT imaging alone. Horn et al. employ a more simple system in which type I injuries are considered stable and type II injuries are unstable. To be considered stable in the system of Horn et al., a patient's CT must be essentially normal at the OA junction, and any evidence of ligamentous injury in the posterior structures, or OA joints, solely detectable by MRI.

Workup

History

OA injuries must be suspected in individuals who have suffered high-energy accidents and in those with cranial or cervical injuries and associated respiratory distress, neurological deficits, obvious cranial nerve injury, and/or sympathetic disruption. Because of the substantial force required to precipitate an OA dislocation, patients with these injuries often present intubated, with multisystem trauma. The initial detection of an OA injury may be delayed in patients in extremis from other injuries, patients who are already intubated and require mechanical ventilation, and patients for whom a full neurological examination is not possible. Patients with isolated occipital condyle fractures usually present without neurological injury. The main complaint in these situations is pain localized to the occipital region.

Physical Examination

All patients should receive a complete neurological evaluation, including rectal exam and evaluation of the bulbocavernosus reflex. Those patients suspected of having an OA dislocation should also undergo a rigorous examination of the cranial nerves, as deficits of these nerves may be present in as many as 40% of patients (cranial nerves IX, X, and XII are commonly involved in the event of condylar fractures, whereas VI, X, and XII are often reported in the setting of OA dislocations). Patients who are awake and cooperative may complain of pain in the occipitocervical region and have reproducible symptoms with palpation. If an OA dislocation is suspected, sandbags should be used for head immobilization during the initial evaluation. A cervical collar should be avoided, as it can distract the damaged OA joint. Once an OA dislocation has been confirmed by imaging, halo immobilization can be applied as a temporary means of stabilization. Axial traction should be avoided because it recreates the mechanism of injury and may lead to further neurological injury.

Spinal Imaging

Initial plain-film images and/or CT scans performed as part of the standard trauma evaluation should be obtained in all patients suspected of OA injuries. Condylar fractures are most commonly identified by CT examination but may be evident on plain radiographic imaging, particularly the open-mouth odontoid view. Lateral plain-film radiographs and sagittal CT reconstructions of the OA junction should be scrutinized using the basion–dental interval (BDI) and basion–axial interval (BAI) described by Harris and colleagues (**Fig. 1.3**). Neither of these parameters should exceed 12 mm on lateral plain film or sagittal CT of the OA junction. A recent study has correlated poor prognosis for survival with BDI > 16 mm. Recently, Pang et al. advocated the use of occipital condyle–C1 interval (CCI) as the diagnostic gold standard for OA dislocation. These authors maintained that a CCI > 4 mm has the highest diagnostic sensitivity and specificity for dislocations and is the only radiographic parameter interrogating the actual joint compromised in OA injuries. Additionally, widening of the CCI is not influenced by patient positioning or the location of the occiput during imaging studies. MR imaging is often used as an adjunct to CT or as a means to detect ligamentous injury at the occipitocervical (OC) junction when CT scan

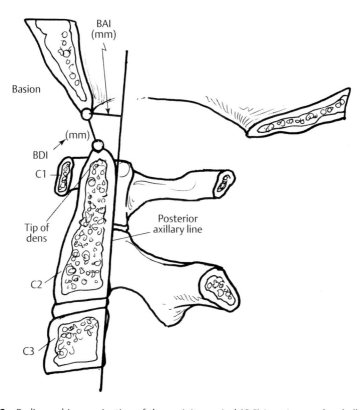

Fig. 1.3   Radiographic examination of the occipitocervical (OC) junction can be challenging. Harris et al. described the basion–axial interval (BAI) and the basion–dental interval (BDI). The BDI is measured from the tip of the odontoid process (dens) to the basion (anterior portion of the foramen magnum). The BAI is measured from the basion to a line drawn perpendicular to the body of the axis (C2). If these intervals are greater than 12 mm, an OA dislocation should be highly suspected.

is normal and "autoreduction" of an OC dislocation is suspected. Edema within the OA joint on MRI is a hallmark of capsular injury, as is disruption of the tectorial membrane or alar ligaments.

Special Diagnostic Tests

If a vertebral artery injury is considered possible by history or physical examination findings, a CT angiogram or MR angiogram (MRA) may be performed to assess the patency of the vertebral arteries. Unilateral vertebral artery injury is often well tolerated, but bilateral occlusion may result in catastrophic stroke, and consideration for intervention is necessary.

Treatment

Stable occipital condylar fractures can be treated in a cervical orthosis or a cervicothoracic brace. Fractures associated with ligamentous compromise (Anderson and Montesano type III, Tuli type 2b) may necessitate occipitocervical fusion. Patients with no radiographic abnormalities at the OC junction but with MR evidence of posterior ligamentous or OA joint edema (Horn type I or Bellabarba type I injuries) may be treated in a halo–thoracic vest for 3 months. Any individual with associated neurological compromise, or radiographic evidence of gross OA incompetence, should be considered for posterior OC fusion (**Fig. 1.4**) with or without decompression. In most cases fusion is performed from the occiput to C2, allowing for better screw purchase and a more rigid construct. C1-C2 transarticular screws have been used frequently in the past (**Fig. 1.4**), although C1 lateral mass and C2 pars interarticularis screws are becoming increasingly popular.

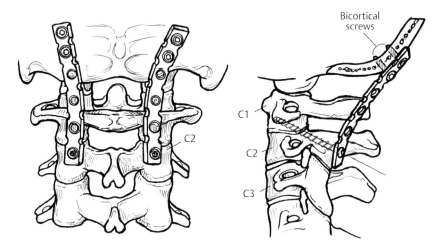

Fig. 1.4 Rigid forms of internal fixation include plates and screws that are used to stabilize the OC junction.

Outcome

Most occipital condylar fractures heal uneventfully with nonoperative management. Posterior occipitocervical fusion reliably achieves solid arthrodesis, but loss of craniocervical motion should be anticipated. Slightly more than 100 individuals are reported in the literature as having survived an OC dislocation. Regardless of the type of treatment, long-term survival for patients with OC dislocations is estimated at only 33%. The most important prognostic factors for patients is the degree of neurological deficit at the time of initial presentation, especially to the phrenic nerve controlling the diaphragm, and the rapidity of effective treatment for the OC dislocation. Individuals without neurological deficit have the best long-term prognosis.

Complications

The most significant complication of injuries to the OC junction is neurological injury. This can occur from the initial traumatic event or from inappropriate immobilization in the case of unrecognized injury. Significant neurological deterioration has been reported in patients with unstable OC dislocations that were not diagnosed at the time of initial presentation. A high level of suspicion based on mechanism and patient presentation, as well as effective immobilization and treatment, are paramount to prevent the development or progression of neurological deficits. Complications commonly associated with OC fusion procedures include infection, vertebral artery or cervical nerve root injury, dural tear, nonunion, and/or failure of instrumentation.

Suggested Readings

Anderson PA, Montesano PX. Morphology and treatment of occipital condyle fractures. Spine (Phila Pa 1976) 1988;13(7):731–736

> *This paper describes the most commonly utilized classification system for occipital condyle fractures.*

Bellabarba C, Mirza SK, West GA, et al. Diagnosis and treatment of craniocervical dislocation in a series of 17 consecutive survivors during an 8-year period. J Neurosurg Spine 2006;4(6): 429–440

> *A retrospective review of 17 patients who survived OA dislocations. This study emphasizes the importance of early detection and also proposes a new classification system capable of informing treatment.*

Chaput CD, Torres E, Davis M, Song J, Rahm M. Survival of atlanto-occipital dissociation correlates with atlanto-occipital distraction, injury severity score, and neurological status. J Trauma 2011;71(2):393–395

> *A retrospective review of 14 patients with OA dissociation. All patients with BDI >16 mm died. Complete neurological injury and higher ISS scores were also associated with mortality.*

Dickman CA, Papadopoulos SM, Sonntag VK, Spetzler RF, Rekate HL, Drabier J. Traumatic occipitoatlantal dislocations. J Spinal Disord 1993;6(4):300–313

This work highlights the importance of utilizing CT and MRI in the evaluation of patients with suspected OA dislocation. In several patients presented in this series, cervical traction led to neurological deterioration.

Fisher CG, Sun JC, Dvorak M. Recognition and management of atlanto-occipital dislocation: improving survival from an often fatal condition. Can J Surg 2001;44(6):412–420

The authors identify at-risk patients for OA injuries, including individuals struck by motor vehicles or those involved in high-speed accidents.

Garrett M, Consiglieri G, Kakarla UK, Chang SW, Dickman CA. Occipitoatlantal dislocation. Neurosurgery 2010;66(3, Suppl):48–55

This excellent review article summarizes the current literature on OA dislocations. Treatment options and fusion techniques for this injury are discussed in detail.

Harris JH Jr, Carson GC, Wagner LK, Kerr N. Radiologic diagnosis of traumatic occipitovertebral dissociation: 2. Comparison of three methods of detecting occipitovertebral relationships on lateral radiographs of supine subjects. AJR Am J Roentgenol 1994;162(4):887–892

This paper describes the use of the BAI and BDI in the diagnosis of OA dislocations.

Horn EM, Feiz-Erfan I, Lekovic GP, Dickman CA, Sonntag VKH, Theodore N. Survivors of occipitoatlantal dislocation injuries: imaging and clinical correlates. J Neurosurg Spine 2007;6(2):113–120

This important work represents the largest series of survivors of OA dislocations to be published in the literature. The article describes the natural history and grim prognosis for most patients who survive the initial injury. A novel classification and treatment protocol are also proposed.

Pang D, Nemzek WR, Zovickian J. Atlanto-occipital dislocation—part 2: The clinical use of (occipital) condyle-C1 interval, comparison with other diagnostic methods, and the manifestation, management, and outcome of atlanto-occipital dislocation in children. Neurosurgery 2007;61(5):995–1015, discussion 1015

This paper reviews the various radiographic parameters used in the diagnosis of OA dislocation. The authors highlight the importance of the occipital condyle–C1 interval (CCI) in radiographic assessment of this injury.

Su TM, Lui CC, Cheng MH, Tsai SC. Occipital condyle fracture with hypoglossal nerve palsy: case report. J Trauma 2000;49(6):1144–1146

This case report focuses on the association of occipital condyle fractures with cranial nerve injuries.

Traynelis VC, Marano GD, Dunker RO, Kaufman HH. Traumatic atlanto-occipital dislocation. Case report. J Neurosurg 1986;65(6):863–870

In this article, the authors propose a classification system for OA dislocations based on the direction of displacement.

Tuli S, Tator CH, Fehlings MG, Mackay M. Occipital condyle fractures. Neurosurgery 1997;41(2):368–376, discussion 376–377

This article proposes a classification system for occipital condyle fractures based on the degree of fracture displacement as well as ligamentous integrity.

Ring Atlas (C1) Fracture

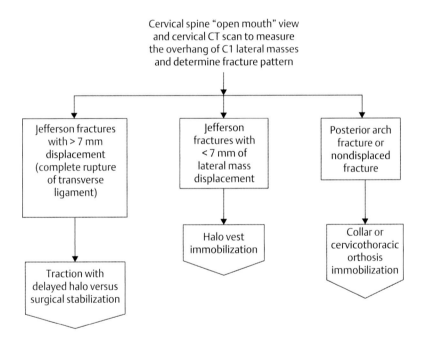

2

C1 Ring Fractures

Gregory Gebauer, Michael A. Pahl, Chadi A. Tannoury, and
D. Greg Anderson

Fractures of the C1 vertebra, or atlas, make up 2–13% of all spine fractures and 1–2% of skeletal fractures. C1 ring fractures were first described by Cooper in 1822 but are better known from the descriptions of Jefferson in 1920, whose name is often associated with the four-part C1 ring fracture. Historically, these fractures were thought to be universally fatal, although in reality most fractures were missed until the advent of modern imaging modalities, with many isolated C1 ring fractures recovering without complications. In current practice, over half of C1 ring fractures are associated with other musculoskeletal injuries.

The anatomy of the C1 ring is unique and contributes to the typical fracture patterns that are seen. Two arches of bone, one anterior and one posterior, are joined together by two lateral masses to form a ring. Superiorly, the lateral masses support the occipital condyles, and inferiorly they articulate with the upper surface of the axis. The atlas ring surrounds both the odontoid process and the spinal cord. The odontoid process is held firmly to the posterior aspect of the anterior arch of the atlas by the transverse ligament. This complex enables the unique mobility of the head in relation to the spine. The vertebral arteries pass laterally through the foramen transversarium, then curve medially across the posterior/inferior portion of the ring before entering the cranium.

Neurologic injuries are rare with isolated C1 ring fractures, because of the ample size of the spinal canal in relation to the spinal cord.

Classification

There are four basic types of C1 fractures. The most common type is an isolated fracture of the posterior arch (**Fig. 2.1A**), which accounts for almost two-thirds of all atlas fractures. This injury occurs after forced hyperextension of the skull and cervical spine. The relatively weak posterior arch is compressed between the occiput and the neural arch of the axis. The injury is best seen on a lateral radiograph or sagittal and axial computed tomography (CT) images.

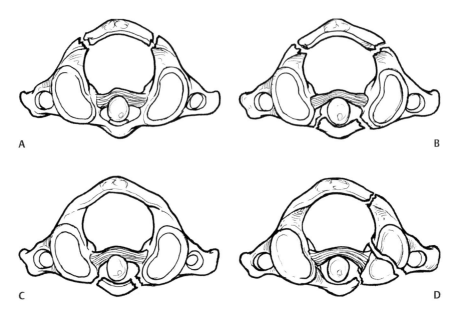

Fig. 2.1 **(A)** A posterior arch fracture; **(B)** burst (Jefferson) fracture; **(C)** anterior arch fracture; **(D)** lateral mass fracture.

Burst fractures (Jefferson fractures) (**Fig. 2.1B**) make up about a third of atlas fractures and result from an axial load applied to the skull. The force is transmitted through the lateral condyles, which fracture and are then forced laterally outward. Classically, there are four breaks in the ring; in front of and behind each of the lateral masses; however, other variations are seen. Severe variants of this injury are associated with a rupture of the transverse ligament, which allows the lateral masses to spread widely.

Less common fracture patterns involve anterior arch fractures (**Fig. 2.1C**) or comminuted fractures of the lateral masses (**Fig. 2.1D**).

 Workup

Patients with neck pain following trauma should be treated with a high index of suspicion regarding a possible cervical fracture. Initial radiological evaluation includes odontoid (open-mouth), anteroposterior (AP), and lateral views of the cervical spine, which will pick up 80–95% of atlas fractures. CT scans are useful to evaluate the fracture pattern further. A magnetic resonance imaging (MRI) scan is useful for those with associated neurological injuries or suspected ligamentous instability.

Fractures of the atlas are considered unstable when the transverse ligament is ruptured. This can be evaluated on plain radiographs by measuring the distance from the lateral edge of C1 to the lateral edge of C2 on both sides on the AP open-mouth radiograph or coronal CT scan. If the sum of these two distances (lateral mass displacement, or LMD) is greater than 7 mm, complete rupture of the transverse ligament is presumed to be present. Approximately 53% of atlas fractures are associated with other spinal fractures. The most common associated fractures involve the odontoid process.

Treatment

Stable, minimally displaced (< 7 mm LMD) atlas fractures are treated by immobilization in a semi-rigid cervical collar or halo vest for 8–12 weeks. Unstable C1 ring fractures can generally be reduced by the application of cranial traction. After 3–6 weeks in traction, when the fracture begins to heal, a halo vest orthosis can be applied for an additional 6–10 weeks.

Surgical treatment may be useful for unstable fractures or for polytrauma patients with associated injuries that require early mobilization. Various surgical approaches have been described, including C1–C2 transarticular fixation and occipitocervical (OC) fusion.

Outcomes

The treatment of atlas fractures depends on the nature of the fracture and the severity of associated injuries. Patients with isolated, stable fractures generally do well. Those with severe disruption of the joint surfaces of the occiput, C1, and/or C2 may have significant neck pain and stiffness due to post-traumatic arthritis.

Complications

Most C1 fractures heal with a low associated complication rate. Potential complications include malunion, nonunion, post-traumatic arthritis, greater occipital nerve neuralgia, and injuries to the vertebrobasilar vascular system.

Suggested Readings

Dvorak MF, Johnson MG, Boyd M, Johnson G, Kwon BK, Fisher CG. Long-term health-related quality of life outcomes following Jefferson-type burst fractures of the atlas. J Neurosurg Spine 2005;2(4):411–417

> Long-term follow-up (average 75 months) on 34 patients with Jefferson burst fractures is presented. Patients' perceived health status had not returned to preinjury levels and was less than that of a comparative normal population. Concomitant injuries and significant bony displacement were associated with poorer outcomes.

Kakarla UK, Chang SW, Theodore N, Sonntag VK. Atlas fractures. Neurosurgery 2010;66(3, Suppl):60–67

> A detailed review of atlas fractures, including their incidence, diagnosis, and treatment.

Landells CD, Van Peteghem PK. Fractures of the atlas: classification, treatment and morbidity. Spine (Phila Pa 1976) 1988;13(5):450–452

A review of 35 patients with C1 fractures showed that long-term morbidity is not as low as previously thought, with 13 of 23 patients (56%) followed up a minimum of 1 year posttrauma having significant symptoms of scalp dysesthesia, neck pain, and/or neck stiffness.

Levine AM, Edwards CC. Fractures of the atlas. J Bone Joint Surg Am 1991;73(5):680–691

Thirty-four patients who had fractures of the atlas were reviewed at an average follow-up of 4.5 years. Seventeen patients had bilateral fracture of the posterior arch, six patients had a fracture in the area of the lateral mass, and eleven patients sustained a Jefferson, or burst, fracture. Initial patient management varied depending upon their fracture patterns and confounding injuries. No atlanto-axial instability was evident in any patient at follow-up.

Longo UG, Denaro L, Campi S, Maffulli N, Denaro V. Upper cervical spine injuries: indications and limits of the conservative management in halo vest. A systematic review of efficacy and safety. Injury 2010;41(11):1127–1135

Forty-seven studies including 1078 patients treated in halo vests for C1–C2 fractures were reviewed. A discussion of the safety and efficacy of halo vest is presented.

Scher AT. The value of retropharyngeal swelling in the diagnosis of fractures of the atlas. S Afr Med J 1980;58(11):451–452

A case report discussing the diagnostic value of seeing increased retropharyngeal swelling on plain radiographs and distinguishing a Jefferson fracture from a posterior arch fracture of the atlas.

Schlicke LH, Callahan RA. A rational approach to burst fractures of the atlas. Clin Orthop Relat Res 1981;(154):18–21

Discusses the decision-making process in treating Jefferson fractures, including indications for atlanto-axial arthrodesis.

Segal LS, Grimm JO, Stauffer ES. Non-union of fractures of the atlas. J Bone Joint Surg Am 1987;69(9):1423–1434

Eighteen patients with fractures of the atlas were evaluated clinically by CT at an average of 46 months follow-up to determine the effect of fracture pattern, bony healing, and method of initial immobilization on long-term follow-up.

Sherk HH, Nicholson JT. Fractures of the atlas. J Bone Joint Surg Am 1970;52(5):1017–1024

A review of C1 fracture patterns and classifications.

Teo EC, Ng HW. First cervical vertebra (atlas) fracture mechanism studies using finite element method. J Biomech 2001;34(1):13–21

The authors constructed a detailed three-dimensional finite element model of the human atlas with geometrical data obtained using a three-dimensional digitizer. Then, using material properties from literature, the finite element model was exercised under simulated axial compressive loading stresses to investigate the sites of failure reported in vivo and in vitro.

Injury to C1–2 Complex

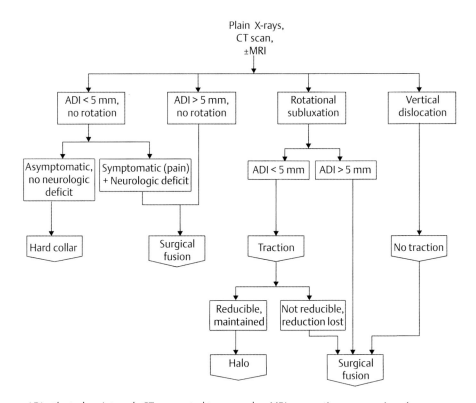

ADI, atlantodens interval; CT, computed tomography; MRI, magnetic resonance imaging

3

Atlanto-Axial Instability

Andrew J. Schoenfeld and Christopher M. Bono

The atlanto-axial (AA) junction is one of the most mobile joints in the entire spine, accounting for ~50% of the head's rotational ability about the torso. Motion at the AA junction occurs through the articulation of the atlas on the dens, with the C1 ring rotating around the fixed post of the C2 odontoid process. The stability of this articulation is ensured by several strong ligamentous structures: the transverse ligament, which spans the interval posterior to the odontoid and connects the lateral masses of C1; the apical ligament; and the alar ligaments, which stabilize both the occipitocervical (OC) and AA junctions. AA instability may result from injuries to the osseo-ligamentous structures, such as in conjunction with a C1 ring Jefferson fracture or odontoid fracture, or the ligaments alone can be disrupted.

AA injuries exist on a continuum, from disruption of a single ligament to true AA instability, which represents the complete disruption of all ligamentous stabilizers of the articulation. Traumatic AA injuries are rare and are usually precipitated by significant forces applied across the articulation, as may occur from high-speed motor vehicle accidents or falls from a height. These injuries, although somewhat similar in terms of the structures involved, are different from the more common nontraumatic AA instability encountered in patients with rheumatoid arthritis, and treatment for these injuries cannot reliably be informed by studies describing management in the rheumatoid population.

Classification

The two most commonly encountered injuries involving the AA junction are traumatic disruption of the transverse ligament and rotational instability. Based on their experience with 39 patients, Dickman and colleagues graded transverse ligament injuries in a four-part classification system (**Fig. 3.1**). The classification is largely descriptive in nature, based on the location of the ligamentous injury and the presence of associated fracture, but the system does provide a means of informing treatment. Rotational instability at the AA junction was classified by Fielding and Hawkins (**Fig. 3.2**). This classification consists of four grades and accounts for the amount of displacement of C1 on C2, the degree of lateral mass subluxation, and widening of the atlanto–dens interval (ADI). This grading scheme, derived from the authors' experience with 17 patients, has not been validated. Yet it remains a descriptive classification, although its reliability, reproducibility, and ability to direct treatment are yet to be substantiated.

Workup

History

Traumatic AA injuries usually occur as a result of significant high-impact trauma, such as motor vehicle accidents, falls from a height, or accidents in which a pedestrian is struck by a motor vehicle. Frontal-impact motor vehicle accidents

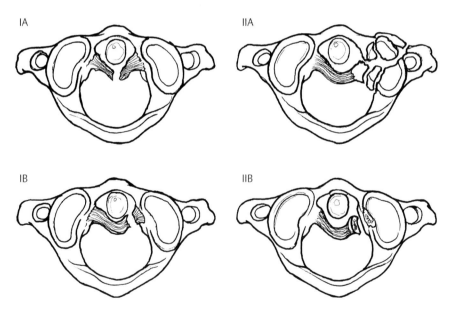

Fig. 3.1 Classification of transverse ligament injuries described by Dickman et al. Type IA: midsubstance tear; Type IB: tear at the periosteal attachment; Type IIA: comminuted fracture of the lateral mass at the ligament insertion (which technically is not a ligament injury but results in ligament incompetence); Type IIB: small osseous avulsion of the ligament from C1.

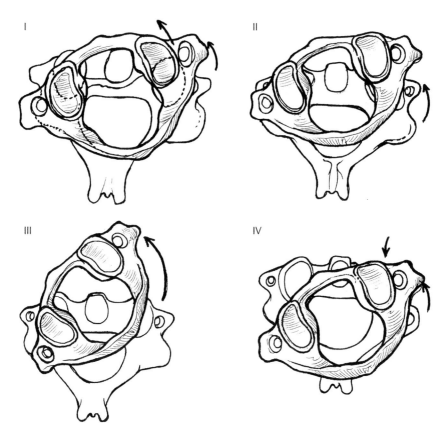

Fig. 3.2 The Fielding and Hawkins classification of traumatic rotatory AA instability. Type I is a pure, fixed rotation with no widening of the atlanto–dens interval (ADI); Type II is a rotation injury with an ADI less than 5 mm (transverse ligament alone disrupted) and one lateral mass joint intact; Type III is rotation with more than 5 mm of widening of the ADI and asymmetric lateral mass subluxation; Type IV consists of posterior subluxation and rotation. The rare Type IV manifestation presumably results from an extension mechanism.

have frequently been cited as precipitating trauma at the AA junction. All patients with an appropriate injury mechanism and complaints of substantial upper cervical or OC pain should be considered as potentially having an AA injury until proven otherwise. Those who present with a fixed torticollis should be suspected of having AA rotatory instability. Patients with a longstanding history of rheumatoid arthritis and children with Grisel's syndrome (retropharyngeal infection) may be prone to developing AA injuries following minimal or no trauma. The similarity between these nontraumatic etiologies and traumatic AA instability remains unclear.

Physical Examination

All patients with suspected, or confirmed, AA instability should undergo a complete neurological evaluation. Those who are alert, cooperative, and lack other distracting injuries may complain of pain at the occipitocervical (OC) junction or upper cervical spine and can have reproducible pain on palpation. A cervical collar should be placed, immobilizing the cervical spine until definitive imaging can be performed. Patients with vertical dislocation of the AA joint should be immobilized with sandbags placed on either side of the head. The application of a collar, or halo traction, can worsen injury in these situations. If rotatory AA instability has been confirmed by imaging, a halo ring can be placed as a temporary means of stabilization and gentle traction may be applied. In children, this intervention alone can be capable of reducing the rotatory subluxation.

Spinal Imaging

Plain-film radiographs and computed tomography (CT) imaging of the cervical spine, performed as part of the standard trauma workup, should be reviewed in those individuals suspected of having an injury at the AA junction. The plain-film lateral should be scrutinized for evidence of retropharyngeal soft-tissue swelling in the upper cervical region. Soft-tissue swelling greater than 6 mm anterior to the C2 body may be considered highly suggestive of injury. The ADI should also be examined on plain-film or sagittal CT reconstruction images (**Fig. 3.3**). Widening of this space more than 3 mm in an adult or 5 mm in a child indicates potential injury or rupture of the transverse ligament. The posterior cervical line, or spinolaminar line, should also be evaluated between C1 and C2 (**Fig. 3.3**). Normally, this line is a smooth concave arc running from the occiput through the posterior processes of C2. Any disruption in the contour of this curve should be considered indicative of an abnormal articular relationship between C1 and C2. Rotatory abnormalities between C1 and C2 are difficult to assess on plain radiographs, although some indication may be evident on the open-mouth odontoid view. A more robust examination of this articulation may be made using axial CT images, and the definitive diagnosis of rotational AA subluxation can occur with this study alone. If the patient's medical condition and cognitive status will allow, dynamic axial CT examination can be performed with the patient attempting to rotate the head to the left and then to the right. The degree of rotational instability can best be assessed using this technique. MR imaging may be employed as an adjunct, to evaluate for the presence of edema within the AA joints, or to visualize the transverse ligament directly.

Treatment

Injuries at the AA junction may be amenable to conservative management or may necessitate surgical intervention, depending on the type of injury and degree of instability. Transverse ligament injuries that involve an avulsion fracture of the C1 ring and that are not associated with neurological injury can be

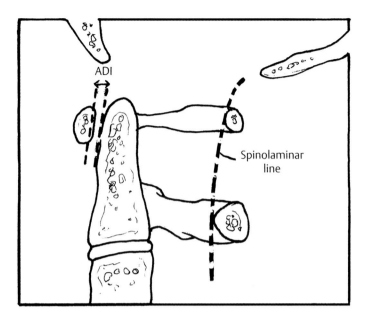

Fig. 3.3 The ADI should be evaluated in all cases of suspected AA instability. The spinolaminar line, drawn by connecting points along the anterior portion of the posterior rings of each vertebra, should consist of a confluent arc.

treated with rigid immobilization in a cervicothoracic orthosis, or halo–thoracic vest. Purely ligamentous disruptions of the transverse ligament that result in instability should be treated with AA arthrodesis. Traditionally, such fusion constructs have consisted of transarticular screws with posterior sublaminar wiring and interposition bone grafting (**Fig. 3.4**). More recently, C1 lateral mass screws and C2 isthmus screws, along with C2 laminar screws and unilateral fixation techniques, have gained popularity. Studies have shown the C1 lateral mass, C2 isthmus screw constructs to be biomechanically comparable to transarticular screws. Unilateral instrumentation is biomechanically inferior to bilateral constructs, but clinical studies have shown no difference in outcome between these two fusion methods.

AA rotatory instability can be reduced with the application of a halo ring and gentle traction. Manipulative reduction through a halo ring can also be employed based on the treating surgeon's discretion and experience. Once the rotatory subluxation is reduced, patients can be maintained in a cervicothoracic orthosis or halo–thoracic vest for 3 months if the injury is considered stable. If the reduction cannot be satisfactorily maintained through external means, an AA arthrodesis is required. AA fusion is also indicated in the event of complete ligamentous disruption of the stabilizers of the AA joint (vertical dislocation of the AA joint, or ADI >5 mm), and if neurological injury is present. In the case of vertical dislocation of the AA joint, provisional traction is contraindicated.

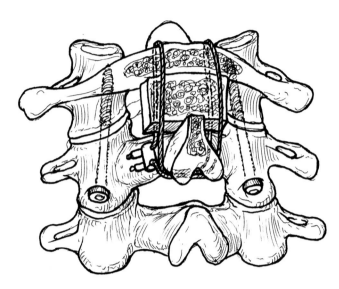

Fig. 3.4 Transarticular screws combined with posterior sublaminar wiring and interposition bone grafting results in one of the most biomechanically stable constructs for fixing AA injuries.

Outcome

There are no studies available in the literature describing outcomes of AA injuries among a large series of adult patients. Most investigations are limited to cohorts with less than 20 patients collected over several years. Early reduction of rotatory subluxation and fusion in cases of instability seem to result in satisfactory outcomes for patients. Posterior AA arthrodesis for rotational instability, or transverse ligament injury, predictably leads to healing in most instances, although a significant loss of cervical rotation must be expected. Rotational injuries that have been missed, or those that have been fixed for a long period of time, are not likely to be reducible using closed traction techniques.

Complications

Those patients with AA injuries treated with nonoperative interventions commonly have sequelae of cervical pain and stiffness. A loss of some cervical rotation can be expected following healing, although the degree and significance of limitations in range of motion vary on a case-by-case basis. Residual instability and late neurologic deterioration may also occur, but these consequences are exceedingly rare. Immediate complications associated with surgical intervention include wound infection, nonunion, hardware failure, iatrogenic spinal cord injury, and vertebral artery injury from the placement of lateral mass screws at

C1, isthmus screws at C2, or transarticular screws across the C1–C2 junction. If vertebral artery injury occurs during screw tract preparation, screws may be still be placed on the ipsilateral side. Contralateral screw placement is contraindicated, however. A significant loss of cervical rotation should be anticipated in the setting of AA arthrodesis.

Suggested Readings

Hue YH, Chun HJ, Yi HJ, Oh SH, Oh SJ, Ko Y. Unilateral posterior atlantoaxial transarticular screw fixation in patients with atlantoaxial instability: comparison with bilateral method. J Korean Neurosurg Soc 2009;45(3):164–168

This study compared outcomes and fusion rates among patients with AA instability treated with unilateral and bilateral transarticular screw fusion techniques. There was no statistically significant difference in fusion between the two treatment groups, and outcomes were similar.

Claybrooks R, Kayanja M, Milks R, Benzel E. Atlantoaxial fusion: a biomechanical analysis of two C1-C2 fusion techniques. Spine J 2007;7(6):682–688

This biomechanical investigation compared C1 lateral mass and C2 pedicle screw constructs to C1 lateral mass and C2 laminar screws. The two constructs were comparable biomechanically, but lateral mass and pedicle screw instrumentation provided superior restraint in flexion/extension and anteroposterior translation.

Dickman CA, Greene KA, Sonntag VK. Injuries involving the transverse atlantal ligament: classification and treatment guidelines based upon experience with 39 injuries. Neurosurgery 1996;38(1):44–50

This paper described a classification system for transverse ligament injuries. Type I injuries involve the ligament alone, while type II injuries are associated with C1 fractures. Type II injuries were felt to be amenable to conservative management, but type I injuries required surgical intervention.

Fielding JW, Hawkins RJ. Atlanto-axial rotatory fixation. (Fixed rotatory subluxation of the atlanto-axial joint.) J Bone Joint Surg Am 1977;59(1):37–44

A review of 17 patients with AA rotatory subluxation. The authors proposed surgical intervention as the most effective treatment for these injuries and described a classification scheme that is still in use today.

Mihara H, Onari K, Hachiya M, Toguchi A, Yamada K. Follow-up study of conservative treatment for atlantoaxial rotatory displacement. J Spinal Disord 2001;14(6):494–499

A retrospective review of 35 children treated for AA rotatory instability. Treatment included halter traction for 2–3 weeks and a soft collar. The authors found that conservative treatment for these injuries generally resulted in satisfactory outcome.

Rocha R, Sawa AG, Baek S, et al. Atlantoaxial rotatory subluxation with ligamentous disruption: a biomechanical comparison of current fusion methods. Neurosurgery 2009;64(3, Suppl):137–143, discussion 143–144

In this biomechanical study, the authors found that C1 lateral mass and C2 pedicle screws provided comparable stability for AA rotatory injuries relative to transarticular constructs. Unilateral variants of both techniques were found to be biomechanically inferior.

Weiner BK, Brower RS. Traumatic vertical atlantoaxial instability in a case of atlanto-occipital coalition. Spine (Phila Pa 1976) 1997;22(9):1033–1035

This case report describes a patient with congenital occipito-atlantal coalition who sustained a vertical dislocation at the AA joint. The patient was treated with a posterior cervical fusion.

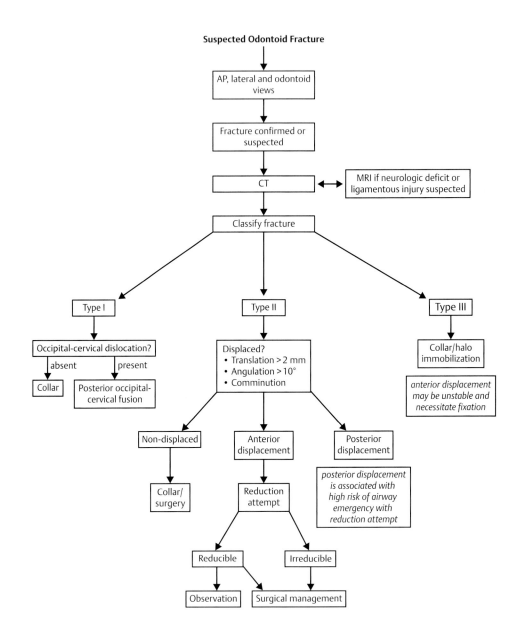

Suspected Odontoid Fracture

AP, lateral and odontoid views

Fracture confirmed or suspected

CT ↔ MRI if neurologic deficit or ligamentous injury suspected

Classify fracture

Type I

Type II

Type III

Occipital-cervical dislocation?

absent present

Collar

Posterior occipital-cervical fusion

Displaced?
• Translation > 2 mm
• Angulation > 10°
• Comminution

Collar/halo immobilization

anterior displacement may be unstable and necessitate fixation

Non-displaced

Anterior displacement

Posterior displacement

Collar/surgery

Reduction attempt

posterior displacement is associated with high risk of airway emergency with reduction attempt

Reducible

Irreducible

Observation

Surgical management

4

Odontoid Fractures

Harvey E. Smith, Raymond W. Hwang, Jeremy S. Smith, and Alexander R. Vaccaro

Odontoid fractures are the most common cervical spine fracture in the elderly, and their incidence is increasing.[1] The odontoid process of C2 serves as a peg on which the C1 ring rotates: sixty degrees of axial rotation occurs at the C1–C2 articulation.[2] Anterior translation of C1 relative to C2 is prevented primarily by the transverse ligament and secondarily by the alar and apical ligaments. Posterior translation is prevented by the odontoid articulation against the anterior arch of C1. Fractures of the odontoid may result in instability because the C1–odontoid complex can translate relative to the body of C2. Because of the capacious nature of the spinal canal in the upper cervical spine, odontoid fractures are rarely associated with an acute neurological deficit. However, in the setting of chronic instability due to an odontoid nonunion, late-onset myelopathy has been observed.[3]

Classification

Anderson and D'Alonzo[4] described the most commonly used classification system for odontoid fractures (**Fig. 4.1**).Type I fractures represent a fracture of the tip of the odontoid, cephalad to the transverse ligament. Type II fractures denote a fracture through the base of the dens but not involving the body of C2, while Type III fractures extend into the body of C2. It has been noted that there is relatively poor inter-observer agreement in differentiating Type II and Type III fractures.[5] Grauer et al.[6] suggested modifying the Anderson classification to consider fracture displacement, obliquity, and comminution. This modification also further distinguishes between Type II and III fractures, with Type III fractures defined as those involving the C2 superior articular facet.

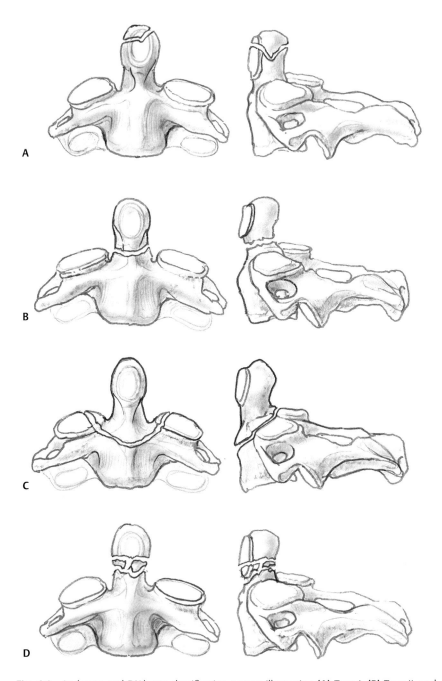

Fig. 4.1 Anderson and D'Alonzo classification system illustrating **(A)** Type I, **(B)** Type II, and **(C)** Type III odontoid fractures. Note the subset **(D)** IIA added by Haley, which denotes comminution. (From Stannard et al., Surgical Treatment of Orthopaedic Trauma. Thieme, NY. 2006. Reprinted with permission.)

Workup

History

The incidence of odontoid fractures has a bimodal age distribution: younger patients have predominantly high-energy mechanisms, whereas older patients generally present with low-energy mechanisms, such as falls from standing. When evaluating an elderly patient with a history of repeated falls, one must consider the possibility of a chronic fracture.

Imaging

Anteroposterior (AP), lateral, and open-mouth odontoid views should be routinely obtained in the setting of a suspected fracture. If a fracture is identified or cannot be excluded, a computed tomography (CT) scan with sagittal and coronal reconstructions should be obtained to aid with fracture classification and treatment planning. Odontoid fractures are associated with other cervical fractures, such as C1 arch fractures, and the clinician must carefully evaluate the entire cervical spine on CT scan. If the fracture involves the foramen transversarium, magnetic resonance (MR) angiography should be considered to assess the vertebral artery. The presence of a neurological deficit is an absolute indication to obtain MR imaging (MRI). An MRI should also be considered if a ligamentous injury is suspected.

Treatment

The management of Type I and Type III odontoid fractures has little controversy. In the setting of a Type I fracture, upper cervical instability and occipitocervical (OC) dislocation must be excluded. In the absence of dislocation or instability, these injuries can be managed with a collar until symptoms subside. Type III fractures occur through the C2 body, which has a relatively robust blood supply and healing potential; following closed reduction, these injuries will usually heal with immobilization in a hard cervical orthosis or halo vest. However, Type III fractures with anterior displacement may be biomechanically unstable and are at risk for repeat displacement with closed management. In the setting of anterior displacement, management with internal fixation should be considered.[7]

Type II odontoid fractures present a management challenge because of the confluence of several factors. The blood supply of C2 is sparse at the base of the dens because of the presence of a true synovial joint. Coupled with a relative thinning of the trabeculae,[8] the biological environment is not conducive to bony union. Fracture displacement and age > 50 years are the predominant risk factors for nonunion with closed management. Union rates for C2 fractures with closed management (cervical orthosis) have been reported to be as low as 15% in the elderly.[9] With surgical intervention, union rates with direct osteosynthesis (anterior odontoid screw) range from 80 to 100%,[7,10–13] and posterior fusion rates with modern instrumentation techniques exceed 90%.[14] The outcome of a nonunion in the elderly is controversial. If there is minimal fracture displacement, some consider a stable fibrous nonunion to be an acceptable outcome.[15] In the setting of an unstable nonunion, there is significant concern both for the risk of catastrophic neurological injury with a subsequent fall and for the potential development of late-onset myelopathy.

Nonoperative Management

Nonoperative management consists of immobilization in either a cervical orthosis or a halo vest. The success of immobilization is predicated, in large part, on the degree of fracture displacement. Studies that have documented high nonunion rates for Type II odontoid fractures have had fracture displacements that exceeded 2 mm. Therefore, particularly in the elderly, it is unlikely that a displaced fracture will achieve a stable union with immobilization. In the setting of a minimally displaced odontoid fracture, successful outcomes with nonoperative management have been demonstrated to range from 74 to 90%,[15,16] if one accepts a stable fibrous nonunion. Bony union with closed management, even in the setting of minimal displacement, is unlikely to exceed 50%.[15]

Nonoperative management necessitates close surveillance and consideration of C1–C2 stability. Particularly given the fall risk inherent to a subset of the elderly population, the relative merits of a fibrous nonunion and the relative risk of C1–C2 instability in the setting of a nonunion, compared with the risk of operative intervention, are patient-specific.

Operative Management

The goal of operative intervention is to achieve either direct osteosynthesis of C2 (anterior procedure) or C1–C2 stability via a posterior C1–C2 fusion.

Anterior Odontoid Screw Fixation

Anterior screw fixation and direct osteosynthesis were first described by Bohler et al.[11] Union rates have been reported to be between 70 and 96%,[10,12,17–19] with higher rates of nonunion in the elderly.[18] Fracture reduction prior to fixation is crucial, and an irreducible fracture is an absolute contraindication to anterior fixation. Similarly, an incompetent transverse ligament is also a contraindication, as there will be continued C1–C2 translational instability after fixation. A significant advantage of anterior direct osteosynthesis is the maintenance of axial rotation due to the avoidance of a posterior C1–C2 fusion.[20,21] The fixation, achieved via a lag-screw technique and cortical screw purchase, is integral to achieving compression at the fracture site. Increased rates of instrumentation failure have been reported in the elderly population, and it is hypothesized that this is due to osteoporosis.[17] A chronic fracture is a relative contraindication to anterior fixation because of the increased incidence of nonunion.[10]

Posterior Fusion

Posterior management aims to fuse the posterior elements of C1 and C2. Historically, this was accomplished with Brooks fusion technique. With modern instrumentation the technique has evolved to C1–C2 transarticular instrumentation and fusion (Magerl) and C1 lateral mass/C2 pars instrumentation (popularized by Harms). Fusion rates generally exceed 90% with either technique. Harms technique is increasingly supplanting transarticular fixation,[1] largely because of the perceived lower risk of injury to the vertebral artery. In addition to the higher rate of fusion, with the use of modern instrumentation, surgeons are increasingly opting for a cervical orthosis postoperatively in lieu of halo vest immobilization.

 ## Complications

Multiple studies indicate that Type II odontoid fractures are associated with significant morbidity in the elderly, with either surgical or nonsurgical management.[22–25] There is increased recognition of the morbidity of halo vest immobilization in the elderly, with some observing acute mortality rates as high as 42% in patients managed with halo vest immobilization.[26] Conversely, others have reported relatively few significant problems with the use of halo vests.[15,27,28] As these studies are retrospective and of single-center cohorts, the divergence in results likely reflects that halo vest management necessitates specialized care, and the role of halo vest use is likely institution-specific. Postoperatively, the clinical team must be prepared for potential airway and swallowing complications, which, although observed with both anterior and posterior approaches, are more prevalent in the former.[1]

References

1. Smith HE, Vaccaro AR, Maltenfort M, et al. Trends in surgical management for type II odontoid fracture: 20 years of experience at a regional spinal cord injury center. Orthopedics 2008;31(7):650
2. Panjabi MM, Crisco JJ, Vasavada A, et al. Mechanical properties of the human cervical spine as shown by three-dimensional load-displacement curves. Spine (Phila Pa 1976) 2001;26(24):2692–2700
3. Crockard HA, Heilman AE, Stevens JM. Progressive myelopathy secondary to odontoid fractures: clinical, radiological, and surgical features. J Neurosurg 1993;78(4):579–586
4. Anderson LD, D'Alonzo RT. Fractures of the odontoid process of the axis. J Bone Joint Surg Am 1974;56(8):1663–1674
5. Barker L, Anderson J, Chesnut R, Nesbit G, Tjauw T, Hart R. Reliability and reproducibility of dens fracture classification with use of plain radiography and reformatted computer-aided tomography. J Bone Joint Surg Am 2006;88(1):106–112
6. Grauer JN, Shafi B, Hilibrand AS, et al. Proposal of a modified, treatment-oriented classification of odontoid fractures. Spine J 2005;5(2):123–129
7. Maak TG, Grauer JN. The contemporary treatment of odontoid injuries. Spine (Phila Pa 1976) 2006;31(11, Suppl):S53–S60, discussion S61
8. Heggeness MH, Doherty BJ. The trabecular anatomy of the axis. Spine (Phila Pa 1976) 1993;18(14):1945–1949
9. Ryan MD, Taylor TK. Odontoid fractures in the elderly. J Spinal Disord 1993;6(5):397–401

10. Apfelbaum RI, Lonser RR, Veres R, Casey A. Direct anterior screw fixation for recent and remote odontoid fractures. J Neurosurg 2000;93(2, Suppl):227–236
11. Böhler J. Anterior stabilization for acute fractures and non-unions of the dens. J Bone Joint Surg Am 1982;64(1):18–27
12. Börm W, Kast E, Richter HP, Mohr K. Anterior screw fixation in type II odontoid fractures: is there a difference in outcome between age groups? Neurosurgery 2003;52(5):1089–1092, discussion 1092–1094
13. ElSaghir H, Böhm H. Anderson type II fracture of the odontoid process: results of anterior screw fixation. J Spinal Disord 2000;13(6):527–530, discussion 531
14. Jeanneret B, Magerl F. Primary posterior fusion C1/2 in odontoid fractures: indications, technique, and results of transarticular screw fixation. J Spinal Disord 1992;5(4):464–475
15. Koech F, Ackland HM, Varma DK, Williamson OD, Malham GM. Nonoperative management of type II odontoid fractures in the elderly. Spine (Phila Pa 1976) 2008;33(26):2881–2886
16. Müller EJ, Schwinnen I, Fischer K, Wick M, Muhr G. Non-rigid immobilisation of odontoid fractures. Eur Spine J 2003;12(5):522–525
17. Harrop JS, Przybylski GJ, Vaccaro AR, Yalamanchili K. Efficacy of anterior odontoid screw fixation in elderly patients with Type II odontoid fractures. Neurosurg Focus 2000;8(6):e6
18. Platzer P, Thalhammer G, Ostermann R, Wieland T, Vécsei V, Gaebler C. Anterior screw fixation of odontoid fractures comparing younger and elderly patients. Spine (Phila Pa 1976) 2007;32(16):1714–1720
19. Subach BR, Morone MA, Haid RW Jr, McLaughlin MR, Rodts GR, Comey CH. Management of acute odontoid fractures with single-screw anterior fixation. Neurosurgery 1999;45(4):812–819, discussion 819–820
20. Platzer P, Thalhammer G, Oberleitner G, Schuster R, Vécsei V, Gaebler C. Surgical treatment of dens fractures in elderly patients. J Bone Joint Surg Am 2007;89(8):1716–1722
21. Jeanneret B, Vernet O, Frei S, Magerl F. Atlantoaxial mobility after screw fixation of the odontoid: a computed tomographic study. J Spinal Disord 1991;4(2):203–211
22. Smith HE, Kerr SM, Maltenfort M, et al. Early complications of surgical versus conservative treatment of isolated type II odontoid fractures in octogenarians: a retrospective cohort study. J Spinal Disord Tech 2008;21(8):535–539
23. Bednar DA, Parikh J, Hummel J. Management of type II odontoid process fractures in geriatric patients; a prospective study of sequential cohorts with attention to survivorship. J Spinal Disord 1995;8(2):166–169
24. Hanigan WC, Powell FC, Elwood PW, Henderson JP. Odontoid fractures in elderly patients. J Neurosurg 1993;78(1):32–35
25. Müller EJ, Wick M, Russe O, Muhr G. Management of odontoid fractures in the elderly. Eur Spine J 1999;8(5):360–365
26. Tashjian RZ, Majercik S, Biffl WL, Palumbo MA, Cioffi WG. Halo-vest immobilization increases early morbidity and mortality in elderly odontoid fractures. J Trauma 2006;60(1):199–203
27. Bransford RJ, Stevens DW, Uyeji S, Bellabarba C, Chapman JR. Halo vest treatment of cervical spine injuries: a success and survivorship analysis. Spine (Phila Pa 1976) 2009;34(15):1561–1566
28. Platzer P, Thalhammer G, Sarahrudi K, et al. Nonoperative management of odontoid fractures using a halothoracic vest. Neurosurgery 2007;61(3):522–529, discussion 529–530

Suggested Readings

Crockard HA, Heilman AE, Stevens JM. Progressive myelopathy secondary to odontoid fractures: clinical, radiological, and surgical features. J Neurosurg 1993;78(4):579–586

Description of late-onset progressive myelopathy in a cohort of ondontoid fracture nonunions. Crockard et al. found that the transverse ligament was frequently interposed in the fracture.

Grauer JN, Shafi B, Hilibrand AS, et al. Proposal of a modified, treatment-oriented classification of odontoid fractures. Spine J 2005;5(2):123–129

> *Vaccaro et al. proposed a modified classification of odontoid fractures incorporating fracture obliquity, displacement, and comminution. These factors are important considerations for type of treatment and surgical technique (if operative treatment is utilized).*

Maak TG, Grauer JN. The contemporary treatment of odontoid injuries. Spine (Phila Pa 1976) 2006;31(11, Suppl):S53–S60, discussion S61

> *A thorough literature review of the treatment of odontoid fractures.*

Smith HE, Kerr SM, Fehlings MG, et al. Trends in epidemiology and management of type II odontoid fractures: 20-year experience at a Model System Spine Injury tertiary referral center. J Spinal Disord Tech 2010;23(8):501–505

> *A review of the historical trends in the epidemiology and management of odontoid fractures. There is a marked epidemiological trend of increased incidence of this injury in an aging population and an increasing probability of operative management.*

Tashjian RZ, Majercik S, Biffl WL, Palumbo MA, Cioffi WG. Halo-vest immobilization increases early morbidity and mortality in elderly odontoid fractures. J Trauma 2006;60(1):199–203

> *Tashjian et al. identify a significant incidence of complications and a high relative risk of mortality in elderly patients with the use of halo vest immobilization.*

Suspected Injury to C2

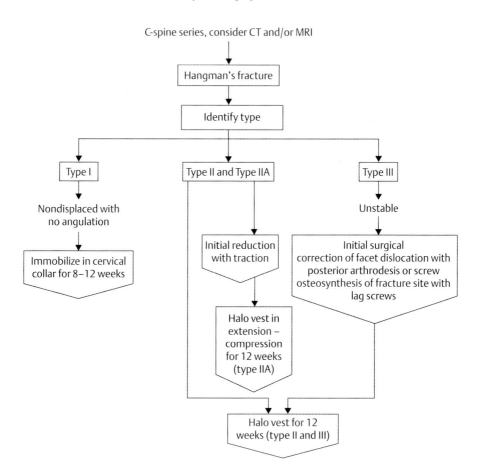

CT, computed tomography; MRI, magnetic resonance imaging

5

Traumatic Spondylolisthesis of the Axis (Hangman's Fracture)

D. Greg Anderson and Gregory Gebauer

Traumatic spondylolisthesis of the axis, or hangman's fracture, refers to a fracture through the neural arch of the axis (pars interarticularis) with or without disruption of the C2–C3 articulation. The pars interarticularis is the narrow isthmus of bone connecting the superior and inferior articular facets. Despite the colloquial name, the typical mechanism is quite different from that observed with judicial hangings. Judicial hangings produce a forceful distraction and hyperextension of the spine, while most hangman's fractures occur with a blunt impact to the head causing forced hyperflexion or hyperextension.

Classification

The classification system of Effendi and Levine is most commonly used and is based on angulation and/or subluxation of the fracture fragments (**Fig. 5.1**). A Type I fracture has a fracture line traversing the C2 pars with minimal displacement (less than 3 mm) and with no angulation. The Type II fracture pattern is similar but demonstrates significant angulation and displacement of greater than 3 mm. Type IIA fractures show significant angulation without much displacement. This injury pattern results from flexion and distraction of the C2–C3 segment with disruption of the posterior longitudinal ligament, leaving the anterior longitudinal ligament intact. Traction should be avoided with the Type IIA injuries, as it may lead to increased angulation.

Type III injuries are the most severe and involve displacement and angulation of the fracture line in combination with a unilateral or bilateral facet dislocation of the C2–C3 facet joint. Type III injuries result in a high rate of spinal cord injury and are most commonly treated with open reduction. The atypical hangman's fracture, or Type IA, involves a fracture line that traverses the C2 body obliquely, leaving bony fragments anterior to the spinal cord. This injury is more likely to be associated with a spinal cord injury than are other Type I and Type II injuries.

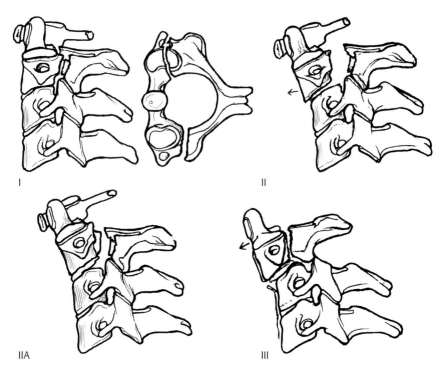

Fig. 5.1 The four types of fracture of the neural arch of the axis, known as hangman's fractures. Type I: minimally displaced with no angulation. Type II: angulated and displaced. Type IIA: minimal displacement with angulation. Type III: severely angulated and displaced with uni/bilateral facet dislocation.

Workup

Any patient sustaining a significant injury to the head/neck region should be immobilized until radiological studies can be completed. The most common causes of hangman's fractures are significant falls or motor vehicle collisions. Patients with hangman's fractures present with neck pain and tenderness over the upper cervical region, especially at the C2 spinous process. A thorough neurological examination is required to rule out a spinal cord injury. Closed head injuries are frequently seen in patients with hangman's fractures and may significantly affect outcome.

Radiographic studies, including anteroposterior (AP), lateral, and open-mouth views, are routinely done when a cervical injury is suspected. When a cervical fracture is noted (or the region of the cervical spine is poorly visualized), a cervical computed tomography (CT) scan should be obtained. Magnetic resonance imaging (MRI) is useful for patients with spinal cord injuries or when a ligamentous disruption is suspected.

Treatment

Type I and Type IA fractures are stable and are treated with a semi-rigid cervical collar for 8 to 12 weeks. Type II fractures are less stable; some advocate initial reduction with skeletal traction (placing the neck in slight hyperextention and applying 10–15 lbs of cranial traction). Fractures with less than 4 or 5 mm of displacement and 15 degrees of angulation may be considered for early mobilization in a halo vest, which is worn for ~8–12 weeks. Patients with less stable injuries may first be treated with initial traction for several weeks until fracture callus begins to form, followed by placement of halo vest orthosis.

With Type IIA fractures, traction should be avoided. These injuries are best treated with early application of a cervical orthosis (halo vest) in slight extension and compression for 8–12 weeks.

Type III injuries are generally not amenable to closed reduction and require open reduction of the facets, followed by arthrodesis using internal fixation. Neurologically intact patients should be studied with MRI prior to the reduction to ensure that a traumatic disk herniation is not present that would preclude a safe reduction of the fracture.

As an alternative, unstable fractures (Types II and III) have been successfully treated by direct screw osteosynthesis of the fracture site, placing lag screws across the fractured pars interarticularis.

Outcome

Outcomes depend on the fracture type. Types I and IA fractures do well, with union rates approaching 98%. The most frequent long-term complication involves post-traumatic degeneration of the C2–C3 facet joint, which is seen in 10%. Type II fractures with uncorrectable displacement of 5 mm or greater have a high incidence of nonunion, but commonly undergo fusion of the C2–C3 disk space, providing stability to the segment in 70% of patients. Type III fractures have high rates of union following surgical arthrodesis. Patients sustaining a spinal cord injury in the setting of a hangman's fracture have outcomes similar to other neurologically injured patients, with the long-term outcome dependent on the severity of the spinal cord injury.

Complications

Nonunion, post-traumatic arthritis, and neurological deficits may occur. Complications of fracture treatment, such as halo pin loosening, infection, and skull perforation, must be watched for. Associated injuries, particularly closed head injuries, often complicate the treatment of hangman's fractures.

Recommended Reading

Bucholz RW, ed. Orthopaedic Decision Making. 2nd ed. St Louis, MO: Mosby; 1996:420–423

This chapter provides useful descriptions of radiographic evaluation of trauma patients with suspected cervical spine injuries. An overview of the treatment of hangman's fractures based on the Levine and Edwards classification is also discussed.

Pepin JW, Hawkins RJ. Traumatic spondylolisthesis of the axis: Hangman's fracture. Clin Orthop Relat Res 1981;(157):133–138

The authors give an overview of the etiology of hangman's fractures. They also describe a classification system based on fractures being either displaced or non-displaced, to be used in determining treatment options. However, this did not completely address the issue of instability.

DeLee JC, Drez D Jr, Miller MM, eds. DeLee and Drez's Orthopaedic Sports Medicine. 2nd ed. Philadelphia, PA: Saunders; 2003:834

The author gives an introduction to hangman's fractures, including mechanism of injury, patient presentation, evaluation and treatment.

Levine AM, Edwards CC. The management of traumatic spondylolisthesis of the axis. J Bone Joint Surg Am 1985;67(2):217–226

This article introduces the Levine and Edwards classification system of hangman's fractures, most widely used today for treatment. The classification was based on their study of 52 patients and takes stability into account.

Longo UG, Denaro L, Campi S, Maffulli N, Denaro V. Upper cervical spine injuries: Indications and limits of the conservative management in halo vest. A systematic review of efficacy and safety. Injury 2010;41(11):1127–1135

Forty-seven studies including 1078 patients treated in halo vests for C1–C2 fractures were reviewed. A discussion of the safety and efficacy of halo vest is presented.

Ma W, Xu R, Liu J, et al. Posterior short-segment fixation and fusion in unstable hangman's fractures. Spine (Phila Pa 1976) 2011;36(7):529–533

The authors present a series of 35 patients treated with posterior C2–C3 fusion using C2 pedicle screws and either C3 pedicle screws or lateral mass screws. Fusion was noted in 29 patients, and few surgery-related complications were noted.

Schneider RC, Livingston KE, Cave AJE, Hamilton G. "Hangman's fracture" of the cervical spine. J Neurosurg 1965;22:141–154

This article gives a historical introduction of the etiology, presentation, and treatment of hangman's fractures. The author first coined the term "hangman's fractures" for C2 fractures resulting from vehicular accidents, after noting the similarity with those sustained in judicial hangings.

Sherk HH, Howard T. Clinical and pathologic correlations in traumatic spondylolisthesis of the axis. Clin Orthop Relat Res 1983;(174):122–126

This article correlates the clinical treatment and prognosis of hangman's fractures with the anatomic lesion. The authors report that fractures that occur through the superior articular facet have a high potential for union because of the well-vascularized cancellous bone of the area, versus those that occur through the thin cortical bone of the pars interarticularis.

Vaccaro AR, Madigan L, Bauerle WB, Blescia A, Cotler JM. Early halo immobilization of displaced traumatic spondylolisthesis of the axis. Spine (Phila Pa 1976) 2002;27(20):2229–2233

In this retrospective study of early halo immobilization in Type II and IIa fractures in 31 patients, the authors found that patients with initial angulation of greater than 12 degrees on lateral radiographic films required an extended period of traction.

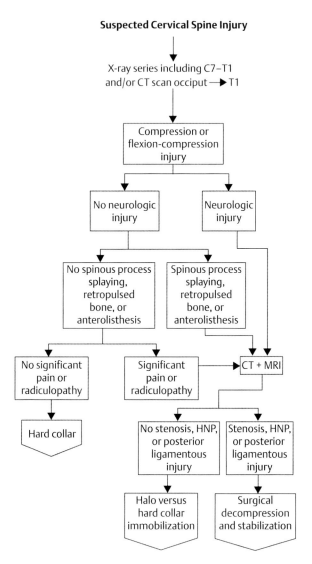

Suspected Cervical Spine Injury

X-ray series including C7–T1
and/or CT scan occiput ⟶ T1

Compression or
flexion-compression
injury

No neurologic
injury

Neurologic
injury

No spinous process
splaying,
retropulsed
bone, or
anterolisthesis

Spinous process
splaying,
retropulsed
bone, or
anterolisthesis

No significant
pain or
radiculopathy

Significant
pain or
radiculopathy

CT + MRI

Hard collar

No stenosis, HNP,
or posterior
ligamentous
injury

Stenosis, HNP,
or posterior
ligamentous
injury

Halo versus
hard collar
immobilization

Surgical
decompression
and stabilization

CT, computed tomography; HNP, herniated nucleus pulposus;
MRI, magnetic resonance imaging

6

Flexion-Compression Injuries of the Cervical Spine

John M. Beiner

Classification

The classification of cervical spine injuries has evolved considerably in the last decade. Previous classification schemes have relied on assumptions based on imaging, injury mechanisms, and force vectors, with no one method being universally accepted. The most popular classification system used for compression injuries of the cervical spine was described by Allen et al. in 1982.[1] This system is based on the interpretation of plain-film radiographs and clinical history and includes a comprehensive biomechanical classification system for each subtype of compression injury of the cervical spine. Compression-flexion injuries were most commonly due to motor vehicle or diving accidents. Adopting the terminology used for thoracolumbar fractures,[2] the anterior column, consisting of the vertebral bodies and intervertebral disks, fails in compression, with variable failure of the middle column (posterior vertebral body) and posterior column (the facet joints and posterior ligamentous complex) in distraction. According to Allen and Ferguson, there are five stages of flexion-compression injuries (**Fig. 6.1**). Stage 1 involves rounding over of the superior endplate. Stage 2 involves further collapse of the endplate, with beaking, or anterior fracture, of the vertebral body. The middle and posterior columns are spared in these early stages. With progression to Stage 3, the well-known "teardrop" fracture is observed, with splaying of the posterior spinous processes and more significant coronal or sagittal fractures of the vertebral body. In Stage 4, there is mild (<3 mm) retrolisthesis of the vertebral body into the spinal canal. The final stage, Stage 5, involves complete rupture of the posterior column in distraction, and retropulsion of bone into the spinal canal of 3 mm or more. These latter stages can also be termed cervical "burst" fractures.

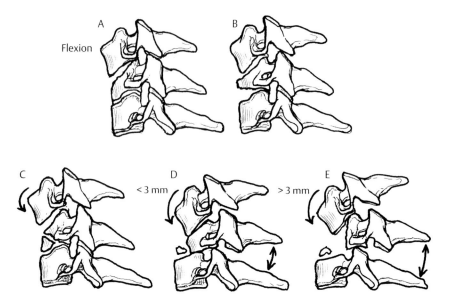

Fig. 6.1 Five stages of flexion-compression injuries.

Vertical compression injuries are commonly caused by a direct blow to the head, such as occurs during a diving accident or from the largely abandoned technique of "spear-tackling" in football. In these injuries, divided into three stages by Allen et al.,[1] failure occurs with progressive loading of a rigid segmental column (**Fig. 6.2**). Stage 1 involves a central depression fracture of the endplate. In Stage 2 injuries, both endplates are commonly involved, with fracture through the body. Injuries that involve displacement of the vertebral body into the spinal canal are classified as Stage 3, and are similar to the higher-stage flexion compression injuries. Lamina or facet fractures can occur in the higher stages.

In 2007 the Spine Trauma Study Group developed a new classification system: the Subaxial Injury Classification (SLIC),[3] which has since been validated as teachable and reproducible, with intra-observer reliability comparable to the Allen and Ferguson classification.[4,5] This system offers a simple, reproducible way of incorporating information about the injury that is considered the most clinically relevant (**Table 6.1**). This classification system uses three main descriptors: injury morphology, integrity of the discoligamentous complex (DLC), and neurological status of the patient.[3] The first category of injury morphology is compression, including loss of height and vertebral body fractures, and comprises injuries traditionally known as compression fractures, burst fractures, and "teardrop" fractures. Posterior or lateral element fractures can also occur if the spine experiences load in extension or lateral flexion. As the severity of the injury increases, the SLIC score increases as well. Translational injuries, including facet dislocations, are covered under a separate category. This system offers a more comprehensive and simpler method of classification than the Allen and Ferguson system.

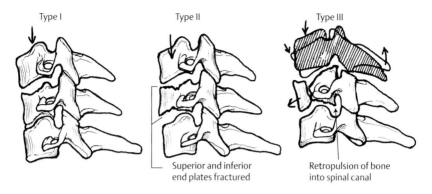

Fig. 6.2   Vertical compression fractures as staged by Allen and Ferguson.

Table 6.1   SLIC Scale

	Points
Morphology	
No abnormality	0
Compression	1
Burst	+1 = 2
Distraction (e.g., facet perch, hyperextension)	3
Rotation/translation (e.g., facet dislocation, unstable teardrop or advanced stage flexion-compression injury)	4
Discoligamentous complex (DLC)	
Intact	0
Indeterminate (e.g., isolated interspinous widening, MRI signal change only)	1
Disrupted (e.g., widening of disk space, facet perch, or dislocation)	2
Neurological status	
Intact	0
Root Injury	1
Complete cord injury	2
Incomplete cord injury	3
Continuous cord compression in setting of neuro deficit (neuro modifier)	+1

Source: Vaccaro AR, Hulbert RJ, Patel AA, et al.: The Subaxial Cervical Spine Injury Classification System. A novel approach to recognize the importance of morphology, neurology, and integrity of the disko-ligamentous complex. Spine 2007;32:2367. Reprinted with permission.

Workup

Spinal Imaging

Workup of these patients involves a careful neurological examination and appropriate imaging. While a thorough discussion of imaging requirements is outside the scope of this chapter, many trauma centers have adopted the use of computed tomography (CT) and magnetic resonance imaging (MRI) for all cervical spine injuries. When a fracture is identified, radiographs and possibly MRI of the entire spine should be obtained to rule out noncontiguous injuries. With more sensitive imaging, noncontiguous injuries have been found in up to 28% of patients.[6]

Treatment

Treatment is based on the neurological status as well as the amount of instability that results from the injury. The SLIC scale assigns points for each of the three components to give an overall stability assessment. In compression injuries, one point is given for a simple compression injury and two points for a burst component. In contrast to distraction and translational injuries, many compression fractures do not include injury to the DLC. In injuries without disruption of the DLC, no neurological injury is present, and according the SLIC scale, there is no significant instability present. These patients may be treated with a rigid orthosis or, infrequently, halo immobilization. Injuries with focal collapse and kyphosis due to disruption of facet capsules and the interspinous ligament result in higher SLIC scores. Although halo immobilization is an option for these patients, the alignment must be neutral or lordotic to avoid subsequent deformity.[7] Higher-energy burst fractures, which under the Allen and Ferguson classification involve distraction of the posterior elements, include interspinous widening and segmental kyphosis (> 11 degrees); higher instability is reflected in a higher SLIC score due to DLC disruption (**Fig. 6.3**).

Neurological status is also used in stratifying instability, with the highest score going to incomplete spinal cord injury. The sum total of the three components of the SLIC scale is used to direct treatment, with surgery recommended for scores with total points > 5. This method resulted in agreement for surgery in 92% of cases.[3] Confounding variables, such as ankylosing spondylitis, are also considered.

When angulation exceeds 11 degrees, or a neurological deficit is present, the SLIC score will be higher, and surgical treatment is generally recommended. Surgery may include an anterior corpectomy and instrumented fusion, or a combined anterior/posterior procedure.[8] A technique for reduction of the fracture using a posterior-alone method has also been described.[9] There is no widespread agreement on when supplemental posterior instrumentation and fusion are necessary, but we recommend this approach in cases where endplate integrity is compromised and/or posterior structures are completely disrupted.[5,10]

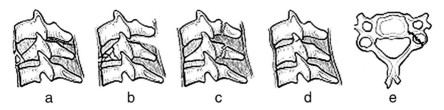

Fig. 6.3 SLIC classification for compression injuries: Simple compression morphology is identified by a visible loss of height in the anterior column **(a)**. Compression may be accompanied by definite DLC disruption **(b)** or laminar fractures **(c)**. Nondisplaced lateral mass and/or facet fractures are also compression injuries **(d)**. Axial view of lateral mass fracture with vertical fracture line **(e)**. (Reproduced with permission from Vaccaro AR, Hulbert RJ, Patel AA, et al. The Subaxial Cervical Spine Injury Classification System. A novel approach to recognize the importance of morphology, neurology, and integrity of the disko-ligamentous complex. Spine 2007;32:2367.)

Outcome

Outcome for these patients is most closely linked to their neurological status after injury. As is the case with most spinal cord injuries regardless of mechanism, complete injuries (American Spinal Injury Association [ASIA] Grade A) generally show poor potential for recovery. Incomplete lesions (ASIA B/C/D) generally improve a variable amount and may include recovery of a cephalad root function (80%) or recovery of an ASIA grade or more in function. Patients' functional outcome can also be related to the need for, and duration of, immobilization (more surgery may mean less immobilization) or easier treatment of other musculoskeletal injuries, but no consensus exists on the duration of immobilization necessary to stabilize the spine. Inadequately stabilized injuries can go on to progressive kyphosis or deformity and can be a major source of long-term morbidity.

References

1. Allen BL Jr, Ferguson RL, Lehmann TR, O'Brien RP. A mechanistic classification of closed, indirect fractures and dislocations of the lower cervical spine. Spine (Phila Pa 1976) 1982; 7(1):1–27
2. Denis F. Spinal instability as defined by the three-column spine concept in acute spinal trauma. Clin Orthop Relat Res 1984;189(189):65–76
3. Vaccaro AR, Hulbert RJ, Patel AA, et al.; Spine Trauma Study Group. The Subaxial Cervical Spine Injury Classification System: a novel approach to recognize the importance of morphology, neurology, and integrity of the disco-ligamentous complex. Spine (Phila Pa 1976) 2007;32(21):2365–2374
4. Zehnder SW, Lenarz CJ, Place HM. Teachability and reliability of a new classification system for lower cervical spinal injuries. Spine (Phila Pa 1976) 2009;34(19):2039–2043
5. Dvorak MF, Fisher CG, Fehlings MG, et al. The surgical approach to subaxial cervical spine injuries: an evidence-based algorithm based on the SLIC classification system. Spine (Phila Pa 1976) 2007;32(23):2620–2629

6. Choi SJ, Shin MJ, Kim SM, Bae SJ. Non-contiguous spinal injury in cervical spinal trauma: evaluation with cervical spine MRI. Korean J Radiol 2004;5(4):219–224
7. Fisher CG, Dvorak MFS, Leith J, Wing PC. Comparison of outcomes for unstable lower cervical flexion teardrop fractures managed with halo thoracic vest versus anterior corpectomy and plating. Spine (Phila Pa 1976) 2002;27(2):160–166
8. Vaccaro AR, Cook CM, McCullen G, Garfin SR. Cervical trauma: rationale for selecting the appropriate fusion technique. Orthop Clin North Am 1998;29(4):745–754
9. Signoret F, Jacquot FP, Feron JM. Reducing the cervical flexion tear-drop fracture with a posterior approach and plating technique: an original method. Eur Spine J 1999;8(2):110–116
10. Kim HJ, Lee KY, Kim WC. Treatment outcome of cervical tear drop fracture. Asian Spine J 2009;3(2):73–79

Suggested Reading

Vaccaro AR, Hulbert RJ, Patel AA, et al.; Spine Trauma Study Group. The Subaxial Cervical Spine Injury Classification System: a novel approach to recognize the importance of morphology, neurology and integrity of the disco-ligamentous complex. Spine (Phila Pa 1976) 2007;32(21): 2365–2374

> *The authors devise a new, comprehensive classification system for subaxial cervical trauma based on literature review and expert opinion, and they validate it with a multicenter trial involving cervical trauma.*

Dvorak MF, Fisher CG, Fehlings MG, et al. The surgical approach to subaxial cervical spine injuries: an evidence-based algorithm based on the SLIC classification system. Spine (Phila Pa 1976) 2007;32(23):2620–2629

> *The members of the Spine Trauma Study Group refine the algorithm of treatment of spinal trauma and attempt to guide the answers to "Should I operate?" and "Which surgical approach should I select?"*

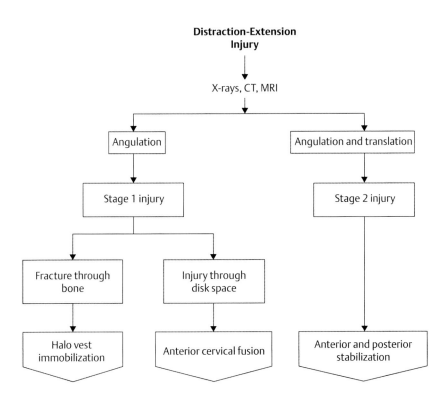

CT, computed tomography; MRI, magnetic resonance imaging

7

Cervical Distraction-Extension Injuries

Amirali Sayadipour and D. Greg Anderson

Cervical distraction-extension injuries (CDEIs) are responsible for 5–22% of all structurally significant traumas to the subaxial cervical spine. Surprisingly, there are relatively few published studies regarding the CDEI pattern.

The majority of CDEIs occur in elderly patients with spondylosis or in patients with ankylosing spondylitis or diffuse idiopathic skeletal hyperostosis (DISH). The common factor for all these diseases is that the flexibility of the cervical spine is dramatically decreased. A CDEI is generally caused by hyperextension of the stiff cervical spine, especially following motor vehicle accidents or falls. The hyperextension forces disrupt the anterior longitudinal ligament (ALL) and disk and may, in severe cases, result in disruption of posterior ligamentous structures. In severe cases, where the posterior longitudinal ligament and facet joint capsules are involved, posterior translation of the superior vertebral body with respect to the subjacent vertebrae will be noted on the lateral radiograph. Such translation markedly compromises the stability of the cervical spine.

Neurologic and vascular complications may occur in cases with significant displacement or angulation. Mild cases of CDEI require a high index of suspicion, as the spine may show minimal or no displacement because of a spontaneous postural reduction of the injury. Elderly patients with a history of a significant traumatic mechanism and spondylosis should be examined for this type of trauma. In such cases, magnetic resonance imaging (MRI) scanning can be a valuable tool; high T2-weighted signal within the disk space is consistent with the traumatic disruption.

Classification

CDEI as classified by Allen and Ferguson has been divided into two stages. In stage 1 CDEI, the disruption involves the ALL and disk (with or without an adjacent vertebral fracture) and one may observe widening of the anterior disk space (**Fig. 7.1A,B**). In a stage 2 CDEI, the disruption additionally involves the posterior ligamentous structures and leads to retrolisthesis of the superior vertebral body (**Fig. 7.2A,B**). These more severe injuries are severely unstable, with a higher risk of neurological injury.

Samartzis et al.[1] studied a cadaver model with serial disruption of the ligamentous structures and expanded the CDEI classification into four categories (DES-1, DES-2A, DES-2B, and DES-3), based on the degree of posterior translation and angulation noted on the lateral radiograph (**Table 7.1**).

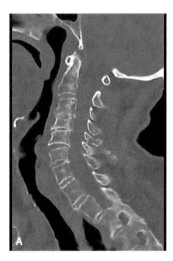 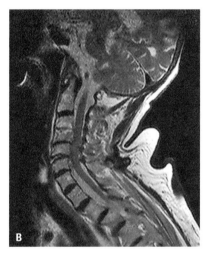

Fig. 7.1 85-year-old woman with cervical spine trauma following a ground-level fall. **(A)** Sagittal CT reconstruction. Notice the preexisting spondylosis resulting in a stiff cervical spine. A subtle widening of the anterior disk space is seen at the C5–C6 level. **(B)** MRI showing increased T2-weighted signal within the C5–C6 disk space (*arrow*), which is indicative of the disruption. Using the Allen–Ferguson classification, this would be a Type 1 injury.

Table 7.1 Classification of Subaxial CDEI Stages Based on Soft-tissue Injury

Staging	Soft-Tissue Injuries	Radiographic View
CDEI-1	ALL	Angulation
CDEI-2A	ALL and disk	Angulation and posterior translation
CDEI-2B	ALL, disk, and PLL	Angulation and posterior translation with instability
CDEI-3	ALL, disk, PLL, and facet capsule ± remaining PLL	Angulation and posterior translation with gross instability

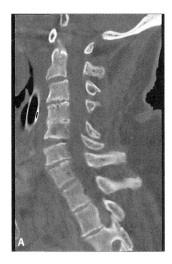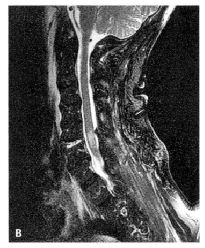

Fig. 7.2 73-year-old man with cervical spine injury after rolling down an embankment on his lawn tractor. **(A)** Reconstructed sagittal CT scan. Notice the subtle posterior translation of the upper vertebral body in addition to severe angulation on the **(B)** MRI study. Notice that the posterior translation is not seen because some spontaneous postural reduction at the injury site has occurred. However, there is evidence of bright signal within the substance of the spinal cord (*arrow*), consistent with an acute spinal cord injury.

Workup

Physical Examination

Advanced trauma life support (ATLS) protocol should be initially instituted, including immobilization of the cervical spine and support of the patient's airway, breathing, and circulation. Steroid protocols can be considered for patients with an incomplete spinal cord injury presenting in the first 8 hours following the blunt trauma. Medical comorbidities should be assessed and included in the treatment plan, particularly when dealing with these often elderly or medically frail patients.

Spinal Imaging

Spinal column radiography and computed tomography (CT) scanning are standard imaging modalities following acute cervical spine trauma, and they may demonstrate either angulation or posterior translation of the vertebral body at the side of the injury. However, it is important to remember that these studies may not identify all cases of CDEI because of spontaneous reduction of the spinal column. Therefore, when the index of suspicion for a CDEI is high, MRI should be performed. MRI is more sensitive to the presence of soft-tissue disruptions, including rupture of the disk and ligaments. T2-weighted MRI images will generally exhibit bright signal within the disrupted disk space, leading to the correct diagnosis.

Treatment

Early and continuous immobilization of the spinal column should be instituted following this type of injury using most commonly a semi-rigid cervical collar. Some patients, such as those with ankylosing spondylitis, are particularly prone to displacement at the site of the disruption and thus may be considered for halo immobilization during transportation for imaging studies and medical tests leading up to a definitive stabilization procedure. For patients exhibiting *only* angulation at the site of the disruption, simple anterior discectomy with structural grafting and anterior plating is able to restore stability. In more severe cases, with significant posterior translation of the vertebral body or in the setting of severe osteoporosis, circumferential stabilization should be considered. Patients with significant preexisting stenosis with an incomplete spinal cord injury may benefit as well from decompression of the cord at the time of surgery.

Complications

Few studies have addressed outcome following the CDEI pattern. However, Vaccaro et al.[2] in one study reported 100% successful bony stabilization following aggressive surgical treatment, leading to improvements in neurological condition in 94% of patients. Patients with CDEI may experience a wide variety of complications depending on the form of treatment employed and the presence of pre-injury medical comorbidities. Complications, including dysphagia, halo pin loosening or calvarium penetration, infection, and neurological deterioration, have been described. Vaccaro et al. reported a 42% mortality rate in their study.

References

1. Samartzis D, Wein SM, Shen FH, Beazell J, Francke EI, Anderson DG. A revisitation of distractive-extension injuries of the subaxial cervical spine: a cadaveric and radiographic soft tissue analysis. Spine (Phila Pa 1976) 2010;35(4):395–402
2. Vaccaro AR, Klein GR, Thaller JB, Rushton SA, Cotler JM, Albert TJ. Distraction extension injuries of the cervical spine. J Spinal Disord 2001;14(3):193–200

Suggested Readings

Samartzis D, Wein SM, Shen FH, Beazell J, Francke EI, Anderson DG. A revisitation of distractive-extension injuries of the subaxial cervical spine: a cadaveric and radiographic soft tissue analysis. Spine (Phila Pa 1976) 2010;35(4):395–402

>*CDEI injuries were evaluated in a cadaveric model using a serial ligament sectioning study. It was found that the anterior facet capsule and posterior longitudinal ligament were primary stabilizers, and disruption of these structures led to posterior subluxation as seen clinically with the Stage II injury. Treatment considerations based on this study are discussed in the manuscript.*

Vaccaro AR, Klein GR, Thaller JB, Rushton SA, Cotler JM, Albert TJ. Distraction extension injuries of the cervical spine. J Spinal Disord 2001;14(3):193–200

>*Cervical distraction extension injuries (CDEI) are responsible for 8–22% of subaxial cervical spine injuries. CDEI carries a high mortality rate, particularly in elderly patients. Surgical and nonsurgical management of CDEI are addressed in this article.*

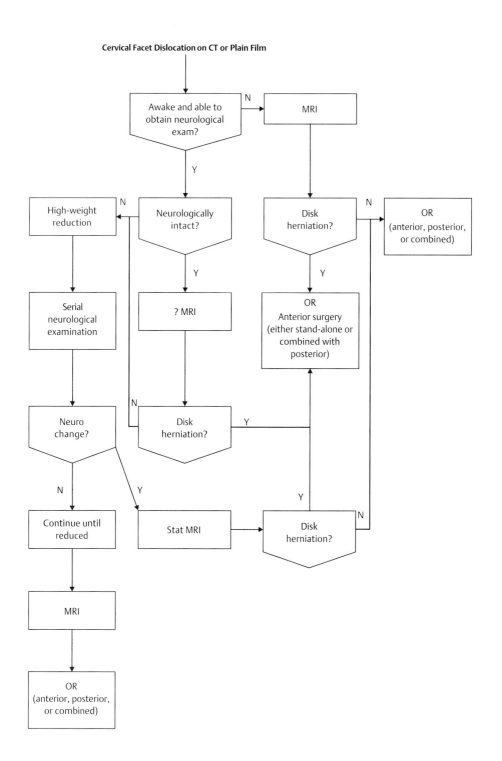

Cervical Facet Dislocation on CT or Plain Film

Awake and able to obtain neurological exam?

N → MRI

Y ↓

Neurologically intact?

N → High-weight reduction → Serial neurological examination → Neuro change?

N → Continue until reduced → MRI → OR (anterior, posterior, or combined)

Y → Stat MRI → Disk herniation?

Y ↓

? MRI

Disk herniation?

N

Y →

Disk herniation?

N → OR (anterior, posterior, or combined)

Y → OR Anterior surgery (either stand-alone or combined with posterior)

8

Cervical Facet Dislocations

Gregory Gebauer and Brett A. Taylor

Facet dislocations are flexion-distraction injuries to the cervical spine that result from high-energy trauma. Motor vehicle crashes and falls are common modes of injury, and many patients may present with multiple other injuries in addition to their facet dislocation. Depending on the nature of the dislocation, the presence of associated fractures, and the amount of concomitant soft-tissue injury, the spine may be highly unstable. This instability may in turn lead to neurologic injury. Prompt recognition and treatment are essential for these injuries.

Classification

Facet dislocations represent a spectrum of injury. Allen and Ferguson described four levels of severity: (1) facet subluxation, (2) unilateral facet dislocation, (3) bilateral facet dislocation, and (4) complete dislocation or spondyloptosis. These injuries are often also associated with facet fractures, endplate or vertebral body fractures, and discoligamentous injury. Radiographically, facet subluxation may appear with widening of the facet joint or with the facets "perched," with the inferior artciular process from the superior level sitting atop the superior articular process from the subjacent level. Unilateral facet dislocations involve frank dislocation of one set of facet joints and subluxation of the contralateral joint. Generally, anterolisthesis of the superior body is less than 25% of anterior-posterior diameter of the vertebral body. Bilateral dislocations may have 50% anterolisthesis or more.

Workup

Physical Exam

Any patient suspected of having a facet dislocation should undergo a complete physical exam. As these injuries are associated with high-energy trauma, all patients should have a thorough examination of the head, body, and extremities to exclude any other injuries. A complete neurologic examination is essential and should include evaluation of sensation, motor function, reflexes, and rectal tone and sensation.

Imaging

Historically, all patients suspected of having a cervical spine injury or involved in a high-energy trauma were initially screened with plain-film radiographs. Recently, the increased availability and accuracy of computed tomography (CT) have led to plain films' being bypassed and patients' being sent directly for CT scans. The CT scan should include the entire cervical spine, including the occipitocervical and cervicothoracic junctions. The images should be reviewed to identify any associated fractures of the facets or vertebral bodies. Imaging of the thoracic and lumbar spine (either by plain-film radiographs or CT) should be obtained to exclude noncontiguous fracture.

While magnetic resonance imaging (MRI) should be obtained on all patients with a facet dislocation, the timing of the study is a matter of debate (this is discussed further in the Treatment section of this chapter). Regardless of the time, the MRI should be used to evaluate for compression of the spinal cord or exiting nerve roots, herniations and injuries to the intervertebral disk, and ligamentous injury.

Treatment

The treatment of facet dislocation depends on the nature and severity of the injury, the presence or absence of any concomitant fractures, the neurologic status of the patient, and whether or not a reliable neurologic exam can be obtained from the patient. Facet subluxations can represent a spectrum of injury, ranging from relatively minor "sprains," or injuries only to the facet capsule, to full dislocations that have spontaneously reduced prior to radiographs' being obtained. An MRI may help to demonstrate the extent of ligamentous injury. Minor injuries may be treated in a hard collar, with frequent radiographs taken to ensure that no late-onset instability has occurred. Injuries that become unstable or that demonstrate extensive soft-tissue injury should be stabilized with surgery.

Patients with either unilateral or bilateral facet dislocations will require reduction of the joint. Early reduction may help to reduce any tension on the spinal cord and neural elements, minimize swelling, and theoretically help to reduce the risk of or treat any existing neurologic injury. The timing of the reduction depends on the neurologic status of the patient and the ability to obtain a thorough neurologic exam on the patient. The need for MRI prior to reduction is a matter of great debate.

Patients who are awake and who have complete neurologic injuries should be treated with immediate high-weight reduction. There is no need for MRI prior to reduction. Expedient reduction relieves pressure on the spinal cord as quickly as possible and gives the patient the best chance for recovery. An MRI should be obtained after reduction to identify any sites of continued spinal cord compression and to evaluate for any epidural hematoma. Surgical stabilization is then undertaken.

Controversy exists regarding whether or not to obtain MRI prior to reduction in both patients who are awake with intact neurologic exams and patients with only radicular-type symptoms. This concern is driven by a case report describing a patient who was initially neurologically intact but then underwent anesthesia while a posterior open reduction and fusion was performed. She awoke quadriplegic. Subsequent radiographic evaluation revealed an anterior disk herniation, which was believed to have extruded into the canal during the reduction maneuver. This has led some to suggest that MRI should be obtained prior to any attempt at reduction to identify disks that may be at risk for possible posterior extrusion. These patients could then be treated with anterior discectomy prior to reduction to minimize the risk of further spinal cord injury. However, there is no clear definition as to what constitutes a disk that is at risk for herniation. If no disk herniation is present, the patient can be treated with high-weight reduction, with careful observation to make sure that there is no change in the neurologic exam.

For patients whose neurologic status cannot be assessed, either because the patient is unconscious, uncooperative, or intoxicated or because there are communication barriers or distracting injuries, an MRI should be performed to assess the patient's injury fully and to exclude the presence of a large disk herniation. Treatment can then be based on the MRI findings.

High-Weight Reduction

Traction can be used to perform a closed reduction of facet dislocations. This can be used in patients with complete neurologic deficits or in patients who are neurologically intact and from whom a reliable neurologic exam can be obtained. To perform a high-weight reduction, the patient is first positioned onto a bed with the traction apparatus attached at the head. Gardner-Wells tongs, made of stainless steel to prevent pin bending during reduction, are then applied to the skull with the pins 1 cm superior to the pinnae of the ears. Local anesthetic agents as well as narcotics should be used to help with the pain. The bed can be tipped into a reverse Trendelenburg position to help counter the force of the traction. The pulleys should be arrayed such that they enable both axial traction and slight flexion of the head. Flexing the head allows the facet joints to disengage and will permit reduction. Traction is started at 5 or 10 lb and then increased in 5 or 10 lb increments. In between the placements of additional weight, the patient's neurologic status should be assessed and a lateral radiograph taken. Weight is added until the cephalad facets appear to have cleared the caudal facets. At this point, the neck can be extended and the traction shifted to a more axial vector. A lateral cervical spine film is again obtained, and if it shows reduction of the dislocation, the weight is gradually reduced.

During the course of the reduction procedure, the process should be aborted if the lateral radiograph demonstrates excessive disk space widening, roughly defined at a disk space 1.5 times as great as that of adjacent levels. Likewise, if there is any change in the neurologic status, the weight should be removed and the patient taken for an emergent MRI scan. In addition to a disk herniation, other causes of neurologic injury, such as an epidural hematoma, should be excluded. The patient should then be taken emergently to the operating room for surgical decompression, reduction, and fusion.

Surgery

Surgery is indicated if a reduction cannot be obtained by closed reduction, if there is evidence of neural compression resulting in a neurologic deficit, or if the injury is felt to be unstable even after reduction. The approach selected depends on the goals of the surgery. Most dislocations without significant disk herniations can be treated with posterior instrumentation, reduction, and fusion. A large herniation may necessitate an anterior approach to remove the disk material, followed by reduction, grafting, and plate fixation. Some authors have asserted that anterior fixation alone may provide enough mechanical stability; however, many feel that anterior surgery alone is not sufficiently stable and should be backed up by posterior instrumentation. Injuries that are highly unstable or that are in patients with complete paralysis may be treated with both anterior and posterior fixation to provide maximal stability.

Outcomes

Children with minor subluxations generally heal well when treated with collar immobilization. Soft-tissue healing in the adult patient is less predictable, and surgical intervention is often considered. Some patients may develop persistent neck or radicular pain when treated nonoperatively. These patients may be candidates for elective decompression and fusion. The outcome of patients with unilateral and bilateral facet dislocations depends on the severity of their injuries at the time of presentation and, particularly, their neurologic status. Typically these injuries will require surgical stabilization to prevent redislocation, late instability, and persistent pain.

Suggested Reading

Dvorak MF, Fisher CG, Aarabi B, et al. Clinical outcomes of 90 isolated unilateral facet fractures, subluxations, and dislocations treated surgically and nonoperatively. Spine (Phila Pa 1976) 2007; 32(26):3007–3013

> *The authors retrospectively reviewed 90 patients with isolated unilateral facet dislocations or fractures. They concluded that these injuries resulted in long-term pain and disability and that patients treated operatively had better outcomes, despite more serious injury patterns, than patients treated without surgery.*

Grauer JN, Vaccaro AR, Lee JY, et al. The timing and influence of MRI on the management of patients with cervical facet dislocations remains highly variable: a survey of members of the Spine Trauma Study Group. J Spinal Disord Tech 2009;22(2):96–99

> *The authors surveyed 25 fellowship-trained spine surgeons regarding the need for MRI and its role in determining whether or not to proceed with open or closed reduction of a dislocated facet type injury. No consensus could be reached on the role of MRI or the type of reduction to be performed.*

Newton D, England M, Doll H, Gardner BP. The case for early treatment of dislocations of the cervical spine with cord involvement sustained playing rugby. J Bone Joint Surg Br 2011;93(12): 1646–1652

> *The authors report a series of 57 patients who sustained a facet dislocation while playing rugby. Thirty-two of these patients were completely paralyzed at presentation. Eight patients had their dislocations reduced within 4 hours. Of these, 5 had a complete recovery. Of the 24 patients who were paralyzed and whose dislocations were reduced after 4 hours, none had a complete recovery, and only 1 had meaningful improvement.*

Fracture of Cervicothoracic Junction

Minor fracture, stable
(lamina, spinous process, etc.)

Unstable
fracture

Brace
(CTO)

Surgery

Stable
anterior
column

Unstable
anterior
column

Posterior fusion
instrumentation

Anterior-posterior
fusion instrumentation

CTO, cervicothoracic orthosis

9

Cervicothoracic Fractures and Dislocations

Norman B. Chutkan and Jonathan A. Tuttle

Fractures of the cervicothoracic junction account for 9% of all cervical fractures. These injuries can frequently be missed on initial radiographic evaluation because of the difficulty imaging this area with plain-film radiographs. The problem is more often found in muscular or obese individuals. The cervicothoracic junction, like the occipitocervical and thoracolumbar junctions, is at particular risk for injury. This is because the cervicothoracic junction is a transition zone between the flexible and mobile cervical spine and the rigid thoracic spine. The complex biomechanical forces acting on this region make immobilization with external orthosis challenging. For unstable injuries and in patients with neurologic deficits in particular, surgical stabilization is preferred.

Classification

Very little has been written on cervicothoracic injuries, and there is no specific classification system. They have often been classified using systems devised for the subaxial cervical spine. The system most frequently used was developed by Allen and Ferguson et al. A newer classification system, called the Subaxial Injury Classification system (SLIC), was recently proposed by the Spine Trauma Study Group (**Table 9.1**). This scoring system is helpful in guiding treatment. Scores of 5 or higher usually require surgical management, and scores of 3 or lower can usually be treated nonoperatively. A score of 4 may be considered for either operative or nonoperative management. The biomechanical differences between the subaxial cervical spine and the cervicothoracic junction may make using a subaxial classification scheme less ideal, but to date it is the best option to help guide treatment. Common fracture patterns seen in this region include unilateral or bilateral facet dislocations, burst fractures, and fracture dislocations.

Table 9.1 Subaxial Injury Classification Scoring System

	Points
Morphology	
No abnormality	0
Compression	1
Burst	+1 = 2
Distraction (e.g., facet perch, hyperextension)	3
Rotation/translation (e.g., facet dislocation, unstable teardrop or advanced-stage flexion-compression injury)	4
Discoligamentous complex (DLC)	
Intact	0
Indeterminate (e.g., isolated interspinous widening, MRI signal change only)	1
Disrupted (e.g., widening of disk space, facet perch, or dislocation)	2
Neurological status	
Intact	0
Root injury	1
Complete cord injury	2
Incomplete cord injury	3
Continuous cord compression in setting of neuro deficit (neuro modifier)	+1

Workup

Physical Examination

Initial management of patients with cervicothoracic injuries should follow the same principles as for any trauma patient. Cervical spine immobilization should be maintained during the resuscitation and evaluation phase. The multiply injured patient is at increased risk for missed fractures as attention is focused on other, more obvious injuries.

Spinal Imaging

A thorough radiographic evaluation is mandated in these patients. The lateral cervical spine view should include the top of T1 and allow visualization of the C7–T1 disk space and the C7–T1 facet joints posteriorly. If the lateral cervical spine view is inadequate, a swimmer's view should be obtained. This can sometimes be difficult to interpret because of overlying structures, particularly in patients who are muscular or obese or who have short necks. If there is any question with the swimmer's view, a computed tomography (CT) scan with thin cuts and sagittal reconstructions should be performed (**Fig. 9.1**). Most trauma centers now routinely obtain cervical CT scans in trauma patients. When a disk herniation, epidural hematoma, or ligamentous injury is suspected, a magnetic resonance imaging (MRI) scan can be helpful. Widening of the interspinous distance or subtle facet subluxation needs to be carefully evaluated to rule out a ligamentous injury.

Treatment

Management of cervicothoracic injuries depends on the stability of the specific fracture. Stable fractures, such as spinous process fractures, lamina fractures, stable burst fractures, and facet fractures without subluxation, can be treated with an external orthosis, such as a rigid cervical collar, a cervicothoracic orthosis (CTO), or a halo vest. Patients with unstable injuries (such as facet dislocations, fracture dislocations, or unstable burst fractures) and patients with a neurologic injury are best treated with surgical management. This allows for restoration of normal spinal alignment, immediate stabilization, and rapid rehabilitation. In patients with fracture dislocations or subluxations, immediate closed reduction with traction may be attempted. These injuries are sometimes difficult to reduce closed; however, there are reports of high rates of successful closed reductions using weights up to 60% of body weight or greater.

Options for surgical intervention include anterior procedures, posterior procedures, or combined anterior and posterior procedures. Anterior procedures are primarily indicated for anterior vertebral column injuries, such as burst fractures with canal compromise in patients with a neurologic deficit. The complex anatomy in this region can make this approach quite challenging. In patients with long, thin necks, a low anterior cervical approach may be adequate; however, for many individuals some form of sternotomy is required,

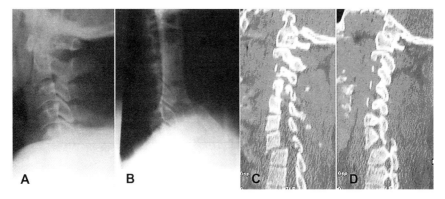

Fig. 9.1   A 36-year-old man fell 70 feet from a scaffold. **(A)** Inadequate initial lateral. **(B)** Inadequate swimmer's view. **(C,D)** Sagittal reconstruction CT showing C7–T1 fracture dislocation.

particularly at the T2 and T3 levels. Modifications of the classic sternal splitting approach involving osteotomies of the clavicle and medial portion of the manubrium have also been described with less morbidity. The posterior approach is the most widely used approach for the management of cervicothoracic injuries. Most fractures and fracture dislocations can be treated via this approach. Clinical results using thoracic pedicle screws and cervical lateral mass screws have shown a high rate of success and are biomechanically superior to wiring or hook instrumentation.

 ## Outcome

There are very few data on the outcome of treatment of cervicothoracic injuries in the literature. Patients with a complete spinal cord syndrome have a poor prognosis for recovery.

Complications

There is also a paucity of data on complication rates. There are specific complications related to the type of treatment selected. In appropriate fractures, closed management with an external orthosis has a low complication rate, although pin-site infections can be seen with the use of a halo. The posterior approach also has relatively low complication rate. Wound healing can be a problem at the cervicothoracic junction, particularly in thin patients with prominent bony anatomy. Neurovascular structures are also at risk from malposition of thoracic pedicle screws or cervical lateral mass screws. The anterior approach to the cervicothoracic junction is more difficult because of the presence of the sternum, clavicle, and great vessels and the transition from cervical lordosis to thoracic kyphosis. These approaches have the potential for significant morbidity.

Suggested Readings

Allen BL, Ferguson RL, Lehman TR, O'Brien RP. A mechanistic classification of closed, indirect fractures and dislocations of the lower cervical spine. Spine 1982;7:1–27

> *After studying 165 cases to demonstrate the various spectra of injury, the authors create a classification scheme to formulate a rational treatment plan for injuries to the cervical spine.*

An HS, Vaccaro A, Cotler JM, Lin S. Spinal disorders at the cervicothoracic junction. Spine 1994;19:2557–2564

> *In this retrospective study of 36 patients undergoing surgeries for rare cervicothoracic junctional problems, the authors discuss diagnostic methods, surgical approaches, surgical outcomes, and associated complications.*

Birch R, Bonney G, Marshall RW. A surgical approach to the cervico-thoracic spine. J Bone Joint Surg Br 1990;72:904–907

> *The authors describe a method for approaching the lower cervical and upper thoracic spine, the brachial plexus, and related vessels. They report this practice in 17 cases with few complications and good results.*

Chapman JR, Anderson PA, Pepin C, Toomey S, Newell DW, Grady SM. Posterior instrumentation of the unstable cervicothoracic spine. J Neurosurg 1996;84:552–558

In this case report on 23 patients with instability of the cervicothoracic region, the authors analyze neurologic status, spine anatomy and reconstruction, and complications during the pre- and postoperative treatment period. They conclude that posterior plate fixation is a satisfactory method of treatment.

Dvorak MF, Fisher CG, Fehlings MG, et al. The surgical approach to subaxial cervical spine injuries: an evidence-based algorithm based on the SLIC classification system. Spine 2007;32: 2620–2629

This article applies the SLIC system to multiple subaxial injury models and suggests possible treatment options, including surgical approach (anterior versus posterior).

Evans DK. Dislocations at the cervicothoracic junction. J Bone Joint Surg Br 1983;65:124–127

The author concludes that on theoretical grounds it is justified to embark on operative reduction of displacements at the C7–T1 level only if the cord lesion is incomplete (and nerve root recovery therefore possible) and if the operation can be performed soon after the injury.

Jelly LM, Evans DR, Easty MJ, Coats TJ, Chan O. Radiography versus spiral CT in the evaluation of cervicothoracic injuries in polytrauma patients who have undergone intubation. Radiographics 2000;20:S251–S259

The authors suggest that routine CT of the cervicothoracic junction in a highly select group of severely injured patients helped detect occult fracture in seven of 73 patients (10%); however, most of these fractures were not clinically significant.

Nichols CG, Young DH, Schiller WR. Evaluation of cervicothoracic junction injury. Ann Emerg Med 1987;16:640–642

The authors recommend that adequate visualization of the cervical spine through the cervicothoracic junction must be the standard for trauma care.

O'Brien JR, Dmitriev AE, Yu W, Gelb D, Ludwig S. Posterior-only stabilization of 2–column and 3-column injuries at the cervicothoracic junction. A biomechanical study. J Spinal Disord Tech 2009;22(5):340–346

The authors performed in-vitro biomechanical studies of posterior-only instrumentation at two levels above and two levels below cervicothoracic junction two- or three-column injury. The authors concluded that C6 lateral mass screws and C7–T2 pedicle screws with a cross-link between the T1 and T2 screws provided sufficient stabilization of either two- or three-column injuries.

Vaccaro AR, An HS, Lin S, Sun S, Balderston RA, Cotler JM. Noncontiguous injuries of the spine. J Spinal Disord 1992;5:320–329

In this case report evaluating 372 patients, the authors recommend complete spinal roentgenographic evaluation in the workup of suspected spinal column injury patients. Additional imaging modalities may be necessary in those areas of the spine difficult to visualize.

Vaccaro AR, Hurlbert RJ, Fisher CG, et al. The sub-axial cervical spine injury classification system (SLIC): a novel approach to recognize the importance of morphology, neurology and integrity of the disco-ligamentous complex. Spine 2007;32:2365–2374

The authors propose a new classification system, similar to the thoracolumbar classifications system (TLICS), that can be applied to subaxial cervical spine trauma. The system was a result of a literature review and expert opinion among surgeons in the Spine Trauma Study Group.

Isolated Subaxial Cervical Spine Facet Injury

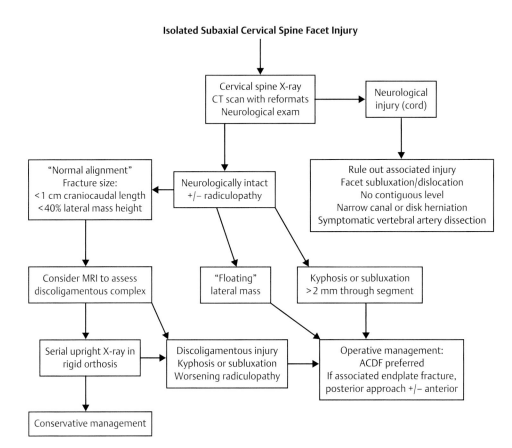

10

Facet Fractures

Ryan R. Janicki, Marcel F. Dvorak, and James S. Harrop

Facet fractures account for ~7% of all cervical spine fractures. Ninety percent of injuries occur at the C5–C7 levels. Isolated facet/lateral mass fractures of the cervical spine are rarely distinguished from subluxed, perched, locked, or dislocated facets in the literature. Subluxations and dislocations are commonly produced by a flexion moment, axial compression, and anterior shear, and may frequently be associated with neurological injury. The management of perched, locked, and dislocated facet injuries is addressed in Chapter 8.

In contrast, isolated facet fractures are thought to be due to extension, side bending and rotation forces, or rotational forces on a flexed neck. The most common injury pattern is that of an undisplaced or minimally displaced superior facet fracture, followed by a more obviously displaced superior facet fracture. Facet fractures are often missed on initial presentation and may lead to axial neck pain, radiculopathy, or focal kyphosis if they displace. Acute instability may occur if associated with discoligamentous injury. Fractures of both the facet and pedicle/lamina result in fracture-separation/"floating" lateral mass, which is considered an unstable injury (**Fig. 10.1**). This presents a challenge because two motion segments are involved, although subluxation occurs most frequently at the more caudal of the two disrupted motion segments. Neurological injury may occur as a result of foraminal injury to a single nerve root. Patients with congenitally small or spondylotic spinal canals may exhibit signs of cord injury secondary to cervical hyperextension or associated traumatic disk herniation.

Classification

There is no universally accepted classification for facet fractures of the subaxial cervical spine. Isolated facet fractures have been classified by Allen and Ferguson's mechanistic system as stage I compression-extension injuries. This includes unilateral fractures with or without antero-rotary vertebral displacement. Fracture patterns may consist of linear, nondisplaced, compressive, or pedicle

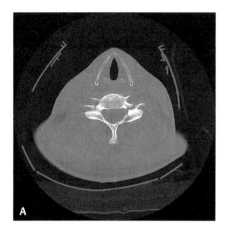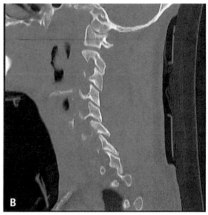

Fig. 10.1 Unilateral fracture involving both pedicle and lamina. **(A,B)** Axial CT scan demonstrating "floating lateral mass." **(B)** Sagittal reformats demonstrating the "horizontalized" C6 facet/lateral mass complex.

and laminar fractures producing a floating lateral mass. White and Panjabi did not specifically address facet fractures but defined clinical instability based on patterns of displacement (sagittal plane translation > 3.5 mm or kyphosis > 11 degrees), anterior/posterior column destruction, and clinical findings. The AO classification, based on mechanism of injury, was developed for the thoracolumbar spine but is often applied to the cervical spine. The AO classification is not really relevant to, nor has it been validated in, the subaxial cervical spine. Vaccaro described the Subaxial Injury Classification (SLIC) severity scoring system, which gives gradated points for injury morphology, discoligamentous injury, and neurological status. The SLIC system uses the aggregate score to direct management to either surgical or nonoperative paradigms. Kotani proposed a unique classification system for lateral mass fractures based on morphology (separation, comminution, split types and traumatic spondylolysis) based on a series of 31 patients. Dvorak classified unilateral facet injuries based on the presence of facet fracture, the degree and pattern of subluxation or dislocation, or the combined presence of fracture and subluxation or dislocation (**Fig. 10.2**).

Workup

History

Facet fractures are most commonly the result of motor vehicle accidents, falls, or sports injury. Acutely, patients describe axial neck pain aggravated by neck movement. Transient or persistent radiculopathy due to impingement on the root in the intervertebral foramen may cause significant arm symptoms of pain, numbness, and weakness and may be the patient's sole complaint. New radicular symptoms may develop in a delayed fashion due to progressive slip.

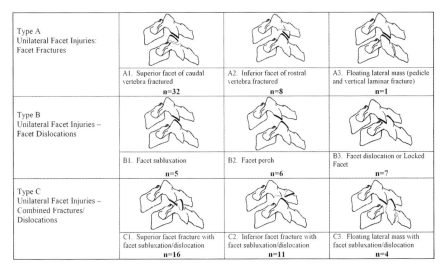

Type A Unilateral Facet Injuries: Facet Fractures			
	A1. Superior facet of caudal vertebra fractured **n=32**	A2. Inferior facet of rostral vertebra fractured **n=8**	A3. Floating lateral mass (pedicle and vertical laminar fracture) **n=1**
Type B Unilateral Facet Injuries – Facet Dislocations			
	B1. Facet subluxation **n=5**	B2. Facet perch **n=6**	B3. Facet dislocation or Locked Facet **n=7**
Type C Unilateral Facet Injuries – Combined Fractures/ Dislocations			
	C1. Superior facet fracture with facet subluxation/dislocation **n=16**	C2. Inferior facet fracture with facet subluxation/dislocation **n=11**	C3. Floating lateral mass with facet subluxation/dislocation **n=4**

Fig. 10.2 Classification system for unilateral subaxial facet injuries based on 90 unilateral facet injuries. Type A fractures may be treated nonoperatively with external orthosis and close follow-up if there is no kyphosis or displacement on upright radiographs. Type B and C injuries that are subluxed are generally treated operatively. Type C injuries associated with dislocation or locked facets are addressed in Chapter 8 of this volume. (From Dvorak MF, Fisher CG, Aarabi B, et al. Clinical outcomes of 90 isolated unilateral facet fractures, subluxations, and dislocations treated surgically and nonoperatively. Spine 2007;32:3007–3013. Reprinted with permission.)

Physical Examination

Simple isolated facet fractures rarely present with spinal cord injury (SCI), although SCI may occur as a result of either a concomitant disk herniation at the level of the fracture, a congenitally narrow spinal canal, or the possibility that a nearly dislocated facet may have reduced and may masquerade as a less severe injury. Neck pain on palpation may localize the injury. Radiculopathy resulting in motor, sensory, and reflex loss should be elicited. Unexplained neurological deficits may be secondary to other noncontiguous injuries or possibly even a traumatic vertebral artery dissection. A careful examination of the visual fields and cerebellar and lower cranial nerve function may suggest a more central neurological etiology, which may have resulted from an embolic event.

Spinal Imaging

Facet fractures can easily be missed on screening radiographs. Understanding fracture morphology, associated vertebral body fracture, and involvement of the upper or lower facet complex can be achieved by reviewing both the axial and reformatted computed tomography (CT) scanning images. Evidence of disco-ligamentous injury (segmental kyphosis and vertebral translation) should be measured on sagittal reformatted CT images or on plain radiographs. Vaccarro predicted failure of nonoperative management if the craniocaudal height of the fracture fragment was > 1 cm or the ratio to the intact lateral mass was < 40% based on sagittal CT images (**Fig. 10.3A,B**). Magnetic resonance imaging (MRI) is the most reliable modality for identifying diskoligmentous injury, disk herniation, and neurovascular injury.

Special Diagnostic Tests

CT or MR angiogram should be ordered if vertebral artery injury is suspected. The head and brain should be included in the imaging when there is suspicion of embolic events or a more central neurological deficit. Patients treated nonoperatively should be mobilized in an external orthosis. Upright radiographs and an assessment of the patient's pain and clinical neurological status are an important component of clinical management. When there is an increase in the patient's local neck pain, new or progressive nerve root deficit, radiographic evidence of vertebral translation of greater than > 2 mm, or significant segmental kyphosis, then the treating physician should consider the possibility of surgical management (**Fig. 10.4A,B**). MR imaging is useful to document discoligamentous injury.

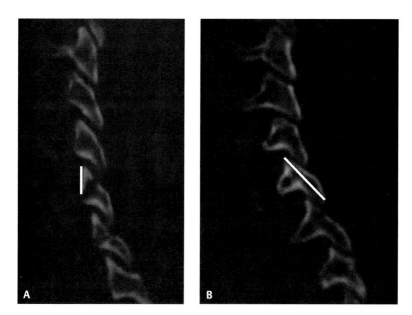

Fig. 10.3 **(A,B)** CT sagittal reformats. **(A)** Measurement of height of facet fracture. **(B)** Height of intact lateral mass. In this study, no patient with facet fracture height to intact lateral mass height ratio <40% or absolute facet fracture height >1 cm failed nonoperative management. (From Spector LR, Kim DH, Affonso J, Albert TJ, Hilibrand AS, Vaccaro AR. Use of computed tomography to predict failure of nonoperative treatment of unilateral facet fractures of the cervical spine. Spine 2006;31:2827–2835. Reprinted with permission.)

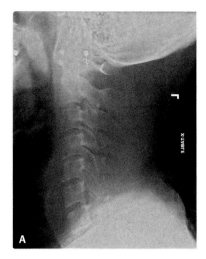 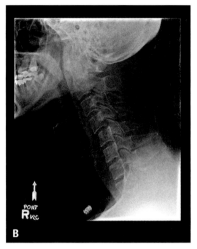

Fig. 10.4   40-year-old man involved a rollover motor vehicle accident presenting with axial neck pain. **(A)** Initial cross-table lateral demonstrates subtle opening of the C4–C5 facet and a laminar fracture. Based on initial imaging, nonoperative management was contemplated. **(B)** Upright radiograph demonstrates segmental kyphosis and the anterior translation through the C4–C5 disk space. CT demonstrated an undisplaced fracture through the inferior facet and lamina; the pedicle was intact. The patient went on to have a C4–C5 ACDF and plating.

Treatment

Nonoperative management in a cervical orthosis is appropriate for simple un-displaced or minimally displaced fractures without a neurological root deficit and without profound discoligamentous injury as seen on MRI. An early 1- to 2-week upright anteroposterior (AP) and lateral radiograph will identify those who develop increased subluxation, angular kyphosis, or lateral tilt and thus would be deemed to have failed nonoperative management. The anterolateral rotary instability associated with these injuries is not addressed effectively by rigid halo immobilization. If present, operative management is appropriate. Anterior, posterior, and combined approaches have been advocated. Anterior cervical discectomy and fusion (ACDF) is a familiar and efficient procedure that limits the arthrodesis to one motion segment. Associated anterior compression from disk material can be addressed. Indirect decompression of the interver-tebral foramen will usually address any radiculopathy. When there is even a minimal endplate compression fracture or extensive comminution and disrup-tion of the posterior facets, then anterior fusion alone is not recommended.

Posterior approaches directly address the pathology but have inherent drawbacks, including a higher risk of infection and the need to position the pa-tient prone. Fractures of the lateral mass may preclude segmental fixation and mandate incorporation of additional motion segments. Posterior fixation alone may lead to focal segmental kyphosis, since the disk is often disrupted and loses height as the posterior fusion progresses toward union.

Combined approaches are indicated in specific cases of higher-energy injuries, such as those with significant anterior disk disruption and herniation, when either the reduction cannot be fully achieved through an anterior-only approach or when there is a concomitant endplate compression or substantial posterior comminution.

Outcome

Isolated facet fractures do well relative to other cervical spine fractures associated with spinal cord injury. The goal should be a return to their preinjury health status. Delayed diagnosis or failure of nonoperative treatment may lead to neck pain, persistent radiculopathy, and kyphotic deformity. In the only randomized controlled study on unilateral facet injuries, Kwon demonstrated that there is a trend favoring anterior surgery based on postoperative pain, segmental kyphosis, and infection rate. Dvorak looked at operative versus nonoperative management of isolated unilateral facet injuries (fractures, subluxations, dislocations). Although the operative group had more severe injuries, their outcomes were significantly better.

Complications

Misdiagnosis of an isolated facet fracture (missing a profound ligamentous injury where the facets have autoreduced, or associated cord-compromising disk herniation) may result in avoidable neurological injury. Delayed diagnosis or failure of nonoperative management may lead to kyphotic deformity and pain. Anterior surgical approaches are preferred when feasible due to their low inherent risk and their familiarity to the surgeon, high technical success rate, and low risk of pseudarthrosis. Posterior approaches have been employed successfully; however, they carry with them a heightened risk of infection and kyphotic deformity. For more complex or higher-energy injuries, combined anterior and posterior approaches are recommended.

Suggested Readings

Dvorak MF, Fisher CG, Aarabi B, et al. Clinical outcomes of 90 isolated unilateral facet fractures, subluxations, and dislocations treated surgically and nonoperatively. Spine (Phila Pa 1976) 2007; 32(26):3007–3013

> A cross-sectional outcome study compared operative versus nonoperative management of unilateral facet injuries (fractures, subluxations, dislocations). Although nonoperatively managed patients had less severe initial injuries, they had poorer 18-month pain outcomes. This study provides a classification system for unilateral facet injuries based on fracture morphology and degree of subluxation or dislocation.

Johnson MG, Fisher CG, Boyd M, Pitzen T, Oxland TR, Dvorak MF. The radiographic failure of single segment anterior cervical plate fixation in traumatic cervical flexion distraction injuries. Spine (Phila Pa 1976) 2004;29(24):2815–2820

> *This is a retrospective review of 87 patients with unilateral or bilateral facet injuries who had undergone ACDF and plating within 1 week of injury. Seventy-five percent of patients had bilateral injuries. Radiographic failure was strongly correlated with endplate fractures. Many fractures were identified only on sagittal CT reconstructions.*

Kotani Y, Abumi K, Ito M, Minami A. Cervical spine injuries associated with lateral mass and facet joint fractures: new classification and surgical treatment with pedicle screw fixation. Eur Spine J 2005;14(1):69–77

> *This article describes a series of patients with lateral-mass/facet fractures and proposes a unique classification system for lateral mass fractures. All patients were imaged with MRI. Seventy-six percent had MRI imaging suggestive of anterior longitudinal ligament and/or disk injury. Surgical management included pedicle screw fixation in all patients, with osteosynthesis of the lateral mass fragment alone in one patient.*

Kwon BK, Fisher CG, Boyd MC, et al. A prospective randomized controlled trial of anterior compared with posterior stabilization for unilateral facet injuries of the cervical spine. J Neurosurg Spine 2007;7(1):1–12

> *Forty-two patients with unilateral cervical facet injuries (fractures, subluxations, dislocations) without spinal cord injury were randomized into ACDF versus posterior fusion. Primary outcome measure failed to reach statistical significance, but secondary outcome measures (pseudarthrosis and infection) favored an anterior approach.*

Spector LR, Kim DH, Affonso J, Albert TJ, Hilibrand AS, Vaccaro AR. Use of computed tomography to predict failure of nonoperative treatment of unilateral facet fractures of the cervical spine. Spine (Phila Pa 1976) 2006;31(24):2827–2835

> *This is a retrospective chart review of patients with isolated unilateral facet fractures at one or more cervical spine levels. Patients with isolated unilateral facet fractures with >3.5 mm displacement or 11 degrees of angulation were treated operatively and not included. Failure of operative management did not occur in any patients with fracture height <40% of the height of the intact facet or absolute fracture height <1 cm. No other radiographic variables were predictors of failure in this group.*

II Thoracolumbar Trauma

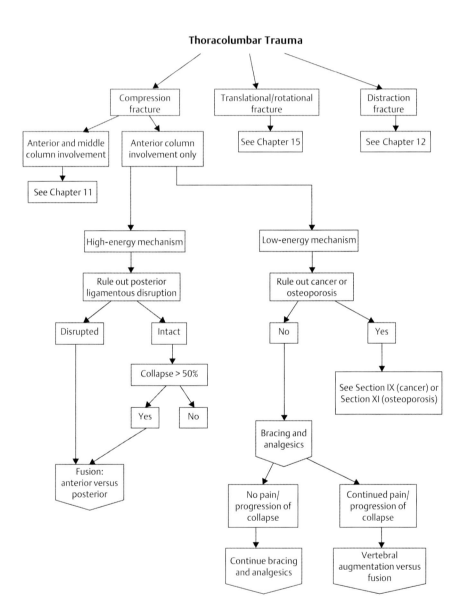

11

Thoracic and Lumbar Vertebral Compression Fractures

Stewart Kerr, Andrew K. Simpson, and Andrew P. White

Thoracic and lumbar compression fractures are of a bimodal etiology. Most osteoporotic compression fractures result from low-energy injuries, but high-energy trauma sustained in falls from height and vehicular collision contributes a significant quantity of these injuries annually in younger and middle-aged patients. The decrease in bone mineral density seen in osteoporosis is a predisposition to many fractures. These insufficiency fractures occur commonly at the distal radius, hip, and spine, with the majority of vertebral compression fractures occurring in the mid-thoracic to upper lumbar region. With the aging of the baby boomers, with a median age of 65 in 2010, there has been an increased prevalence of vertebral compression fractures in the United States.[1] The National Osteoporosis Foundation has estimated that more than 100 million people worldwide are at risk for fragility fractures.[2] Many of the fractures that occur within the axial skeleton can be effectively managed with activity modification, bracing, and analgesics. Only a small percentage of patients who cannot be mobilized with these conservative efforts require surgical treatment. Of those with insufficiency fractures treated operatively, most are managed with vertebral augmentation procedures, such as kyphoplasty or vertebroplasty, rather than fusion.

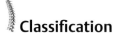

Classification

In North America, a common classification for thoracolumbar fracture is the Denis system, which divides the axial skeleton into anterior, middle, and posterior columns (**Fig. 11.1**).[3] Utilizing this system, Denis described four injury types: compression fractures, burst fractures, flexion-distraction fractures (e.g., seat belt injuries), and fracture dislocations. Another effective method described by Vaccaro for evaluation of thoracolumbar injury is the Thoracolumbar Injury Classification System (TLICS).[4] This system provides treatment recommendations after evaluating fracture morphology, neurologic findings, and the integ-

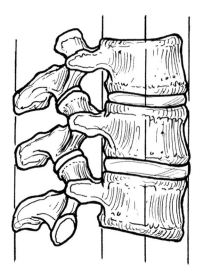

Fig. 11.1 Vertebral body outlining the Denis three-column support structure of the spinal column. The anterior column consists of the anterior half of both the vertebral body and the disks, along with the anterior longitudinal ligament (ALL). The middle column consists of the posterior longitudinal ligament (PLL) and the posterior half of the disk and vertebral body. The posterior column consists of the bony neural arch, posterior spinous ligaments, and ligamentum flavum as well as the facet joints.

rity of the posterior osseoligamentous complex. Several studies have validated this system's usefulness.[5]

All vertebral compression fractures involve loading to the anterior spine. They are distinguished from burst fractures, which additionally have posterior vertebral wall involvement and commonly have bone retropulsion into the spinal canal. Vertebral compression fractures are rarely unstable and do not tend to present with spine-related neurologic deficits. Evaluation of the posterior tension band, which is composed of the dorsal osseous and ligamentous structures, is necessary, as high-energy injuries may be unstable despite presenting only as simple anterior vertebral compression fracture injuries on initial radiographs.

 Workup

High-energy, compression-type spinal injuries require an evaluation that determines the stability of the dorsal spinal column. Along with a purposeful physical examination, this may include computed tomography (CT) and magnetic resonance imaging (MRI) studies to evaluate the posterior spinal tension band fully. Patients with low-energy, pathologic fracture etiology should be worked up for neoplasm and osteoporosis and treated accordingly. This may entail additional imaging studies in addition to a CT-guided or other method of spinal biopsy.

Spinal Imaging

Initial imaging studies include anteroposterior (AP) and lateral radiographs (**Fig. 11.2A**). Plain radiographs in the acute trauma setting are often difficult to obtain and interpret because of other injuries and artifact from immobilization backboards, surrounding soft tissues, and bony overlap. CT imaging is a relatively quick and reliable study to determine whether an unstable pattern exists

(**Fig. 11.2B**). Additional information regarding available space in the spinal canal for neural elements can be discerned in those patients with burst fractures that could not be fully appreciated on plain radiography.

MRI is perhaps the most clinically useful study in patients with vertebral compression fractures (**Fig. 11.2C**). Fracture maturity and healing can often be inferred from the amount of bony edema on T2-weighted sequences when vertebral augmentation is considered. Additionally, MRI is useful in determining the extent of both osseous and soft-tissue involvement in both primary and metastatic neoplastic processes if reconstruction is being considered. For patients with high-energy trauma mechanisms, MRI is useful if there is concern for a posterior ligamentous complex disruption. In the atypical case of compression fracture with neurologic deficit, MRI can be useful in determining extent and localization of neural insult along with etiology (for example, fracture-related epidural hematoma versus direct compression of neural elements from retropulsed bone and tissue). In patients who are unable to have MRI scans, a bone scan can be used to determine whether fractures are acute or chronic.

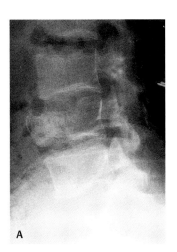

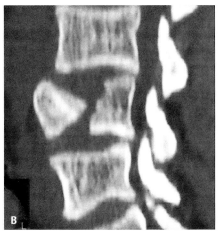

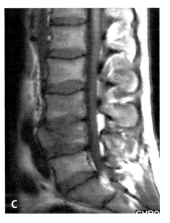

Fig. 11.2   (A) Lateral plain radiograph, (B) CT scan with sagittal reconstruction, and (C) T1-weighted sagittal MRI of the lumbar spine demonstrating an L4 vertebral compression fracture. It is a stable fracture as defined by the Denis classification system. Note that there is not posterior extension of the fracture into the spinal canal and no distal spinal cord compression.

Treatment

Fortunately, the majority of patients with osteoporotic vertebral compression fractures can be treated nonsurgically with bracing, analgesics, and temporary activity modifications. In select injuries, however, operative treatment with vertebral augmentation may be indicated. These indications include painful, progressive collapse in the setting of pathologic fracture and continued pain despite compliance with nonsurgical measures.[6] Vertebroplasty or kyphoplasty may be the most appropriate treatment of osteoporotic fractures in patients who cannot be mobilized from bed or discharged from the hospital through conservative care means.[7] In these cases, vertebral augmentation procedures may be considered useful in restoring mobility and reducing the risk of otherwise life-threatening complications, including thromboembolism, skin decubiti, and pulmonary infections. Patients who can be mobilized are at low risk for these serious complications and typically do not require vertebral augmentation. These patients are likely to heal their fractures uneventfully and may not benefit from vertebral augmentation more than from placebo surgery, as demonstrated in recently published studies.[8]

Patients with flexion-distraction injuries require instrumented stabilization and arthrodesis of the posterior tension band with or without anterior column reconstruction. Requirements for anteroposterior reconstruction are loosely defined and are dependent on several factors, including co-morbid injuries, focal kyphotic angle and extent of anterior spinal bony loss, fracture morphology, bone quality, non-union risks, body habitus, and patient compliance.[9]

Vertebral augmentation is a procedure that injects polymethylmethacrylate (PMMA) into weakened vertebral bodies via cannulas that are advanced fluoroscopically through the pedicle.[10] Following vertebral augmentation in osteoporosis, patients should be periodically evaluated for adjacent-level fracture; one study showed a 4.6-fold increased risk, which fortunately can be decreased with teriparatide and raloxifine administration.[11,12]

Outcomes

The majority of patients with vertebral compression fractures respond well with nonsurgical care; pain resolution is gradual, allowing return to activity as tolerated in 6 to 8 weeks. Nonetheless, these fractures do represent an overall decline in health and are associated with increased age-adjusted mortality rates, in women in particular.[13] Patients with pathologic fractures failing to respond favorably with conservative measures or those with progressive collapse generally experience good pain relief with vertebral augmentation.[14,15] Vertebral compression fractures with posterior ligament complex disruption have variable results reported in the literature. Many of these patients also sustain concomitant musculoskeletal extremity injury. Also, treatment for vertebral compression injury is variable with respect to extent of reconstruction. Several studies show favored results following anteroposterior surgery for patients with spinal instability due to anterior spinal fracture combined with posterior column injury (ligament disruption or combined soft-tissue and osseous injury). However, to date there is no established "gold standard" for treating these injuries despite many reports and multicenter studies. For those patients with high-energy injury mechanisms, validated outcomes do not result in complete recovery despite satisfactory restoration of sagittal and coronal alignment through contemporary arthrodesis techniques.

Complications

Vertebral compression fractures treated operatively have the usual risks of surgical intervention, including hemorrhage, infection, pseudarthrosis, inadvertent durotomy, neurological injury, pneumonia, and instrumentation-related complications. Cement extravasation into the spinal canal or venous system has been reported; patients with multiple-level (>3 levels) vertebral PMMA augmentation performed in the same procedure have succumbed, presumably due to monomer toxicity. Meta-analysis results comparing vertebroplasty to kyphoplasty have shown that although both procedures are effective and safe, vertebroplasty is associated with a statistically significant increased rate of procedure-related complications.[16]

Patients treated nonsurgically also experience complications. These are often related to mobilization difficulty and can include a variety of complications in the elderly population, including deep venous thrombosis, pulmonary embolus, decubitus ulcers, deconditioning, and worsened osteoporosis. Some vertebral compression fractures demonstrate progressive collapse, which can develop into a burst component with neural compromise or may lead to a progressive kyphotic deformity with associated worsened back pain and, at times, neurologic compromise.

References

1. Consensus Statement NIH. Osteoporosis prevention, diagnosis, and therapy. NIH Consens Statement 2000;17(1):1–45
2. National Osteoporosis Foundation. America's Bone Health: The State of Osteoporosis and Low Bone Mass in Our Nation. Washington, DC: National Osteoporosis Foundation; 2002
3. Denis F. The three column spine and its significance in the classification of acute thoracolumbar spinal injuries. Spine (Phila Pa 1976) 1983;8(8):817–831
4. Patel AA, Vaccaro AR. Thoracolumbar spine trauma classification. J Am Acad Orthop Surg 2010;18(2):63–71
5. Joaquim AF, Fernandes YB, Cavalcante RA, Fragoso RM, Honorato DC, Patel AA. Evaluation of the thoracolumbar injury classification system in thoracic and lumbar spinal trauma. Spine (Phila Pa 1976) 2011;36(1):33–36
6. Barr JD, Barr MS, Lemley TJ, McCann RM. Percutaneous vertebroplasty for pain relief and spinal stabilization. Spine (Phila Pa 1976) 2000;25(8):923–928
7. Trout AT, Kallmes DF, Gray LA, et al. Evaluation of vertebroplasty with a validated outcome measure: the Roland-Morris Disability Questionnaire. AJNR Am J Neuroradiol 2005; 26(10):2652–2657
8. Buchbinder R, Osborne RH, Ebeling PR, et al. A randomized trial of vertebroplasty for painful osteoporotic vertebral fractures. N Engl J Med 2009;361(6):557–568

9. Knop C, Kranabetter T, Reinhold M, Blauth M. Combined posterior-anterior stabilisation of thoracolumbar injuries utilising a vertebral body replacing implant. Eur Spine J 2009;18(7):949–963
10. Manson NA, Phillips FM. Minimally invasive techniques for the treatment of osteoporotic vertebral fractures. Instr Course Lect 2007;56:273–285
11. Trout AT, Kallmes DF, Kaufmann TJ. New fractures after vertebroplasty: adjacent fractures occur significantly sooner. AJNR Am J Neuroradiol 2006;27(1):217–223
12. Bouxsein ML, Chen P, Glass EV, Kallmes DF, Delmas PD, Mitlak BH. Teriparatide and raloxifene reduce the risk of new adjacent vertebral fractures in postmenopausal women with osteoporosis. Results from two randomized controlled trials. J Bone Joint Surg Am 2009;91(6):1329–1338
13. Kado DM, Browner WS, Palermo L, Nevitt MC, Genant HK, Cummings SR. Study of Osteoporotic Fractures Research Group. Vertebral fractures and mortality in older women: a prospective study. Arch Intern Med 1999;159(11):1215–1220
14. Glassman SD, Alegre GM. Adult spinal deformity in the osteoporotic spine: options and pitfalls. Instr Course Lect 2003;52:579–588
15. Lieberman IH, Dudeney S, Reinhardt MK, Bell G. Initial outcome and efficacy of "kyphoplasty" in the treatment of painful osteoporotic vertebral compression fractures. Spine (Phila Pa 1976) 2001;26(14):1631–1638
16. Lee MJ, Dumonski M, Cahill P, Stanley T, Park D, Singh K. Percutaneous treatment of vertebral compression fractures: a meta-analysis of complications. Spine (Phila Pa 1976) 2009;34(11):1228–1232

Suggested Readings

Buchbinder R, Osborne RH, Ebeling PR, et al. A randomized trial of vertebroplasty for painful osteoporotic vertebral fractures. N Engl J Med 2009;361(6):557–568

This multicenter, randomized, double-blind, placebo-controlled trial of patients with painful osteoporotic compression fractures, treated with vertebroplasty or sham procedure, demonstrates no benefit at 1 week through 6 month interval follow up.

Muijs SP, van Erkel AR, Dijkstra PD. Treatment of painful osteoporotic vertebral compression fractures: a brief review of the evidence for percutaneous vertebroplasty. J Bone Joint Surg Br 2011;93(9):1149–1153

This is a review of the published evidence for percutaneous vertebroplasty.

Patel AA, Vaccaro AR. Thoracolumbar spine trauma classification. J Am Acad Orthop Surg 2010;18(2):63–71

This is the summary paper on the TLICS injury classification system and initial reliability and validation studies.

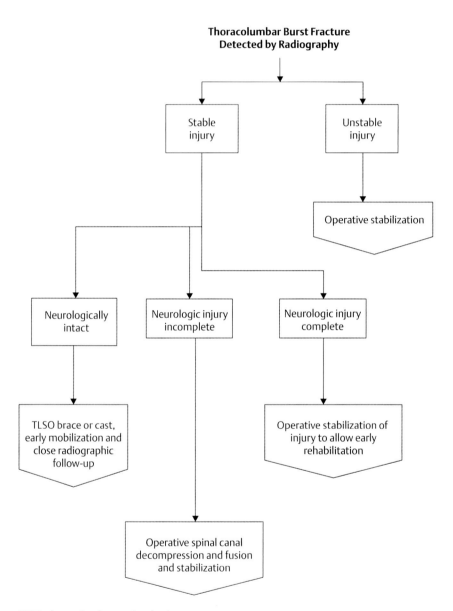

Thoracolumbar Burst Fracture Detected by Radiography

Stable injury

Unstable injury

Operative stabilization

Neurologically intact

Neurologic injury incomplete

Neurologic injury complete

TLSO brace or cast, early mobilization and close radiographic follow-up

Operative stabilization of injury to allow early rehabilitation

Operative spinal canal decompression and fusion and stabilization

TLSO, thoracolumbosacral orthosis

12

Thoracolumbar Burst Fractures

George M. Ghobrial, Alexander R. Vaccaro, and James S. Harrop

Thoracolumbar junctional burst fractures include spinal injuries between the T11 and L2 vertebral levels that result in posterior vertebral wall failure and retropulsion into the spinal canal due to greater than physiologic axial loading forces. The hallmark of these fractures is some degree of bony retropulsion into the spinal canal or violation of the posterior spinal canal cortical margin. Occasionally there will be a herniation of the nucleus pulposus of the intervertebral disk through the respective upper endplate into the vertebral body.

Anatomically, the rigid thoracic spine transitions to a more mobile lumbar spine, which predisposes this junction to increased dispersal of energy and the potential for a fracture. Almost 90% of all burst fractures occur at the thoracolumbar junction, representing a fifth of all spine fractures, occurring most commonly in young males and following high-speed motor vehicle collisions.[1,2]

Classification

No universal classification system for thoracolumbar trauma presently exists. Historically, the most commonly used scheme in North America is the Denis classification system. In this system, the spine is divided into three columns. The anterior column consists of the anterior longitudinal ligament (ALL), annulus fibrosus, and anterior half of the vertebral body. The middle column consists of the posterior longitudinal ligament (PLL), the posterior portion of the annulus fibrosus, and the posterior half of the vertebral body. The posterior column consists of the bony neural arch, the posterior spinous processes, the ligamentum flavum, and the facet joints. A recent and presently more popular thoracolumbar fracture classification system is the TLICS (Thoracolumbar Injury Classification and Severity Score) system, which describes the morphology of the fracture, the status of the posterior ligamentous complex, and the neurologic status of the patient.

Utilizing the Denis system, a burst fracture is then defined as a violation or fracture of the anterior and middle columns, typically as a result of increased axial loading, that results in the retropulsion of bony fragments, including the posterior vertebral body wall, into the spinal canal, potentially resulting in a neurologic injury. Injury to the posterior column is variably present as well. A determination of stability depends on an assessment of the bony fracture in addition to the status of the posterior ligament complex or tension band. A recent focus on the stability of an injury is the neurologic status of a patient. The TLICS emphasizes neurologic status in addition to injury morphology and stability of the posterior ligamentous complex.

Workup

Physical Examination

There should be a high suspicion for a thoracolumbar fracture in all trauma patients. This is particularly true in individuals who fall from heights and land on their feet, since this creates high-energy axial compression at the thoracolumbar junction. Patients who have calcaneal fractures due to falls should be evaluated for a thoracolumbar fracture. Patients with a suspected thoracolumbar fracture should be immobilized and placed on flat bed rest. The patient should be kept immobilized until a trauma evaluation has been completed, including a thorough neurologic exam and review of imaging of the entire spinal axis.

Spinal Imaging

Plain-film radiographs may help as a screening tool; however, all patients suspected of having a burst fracture should be evaluated by computed tomography (CT). There is a high incidence of concurrent noncontiguous fractures for patients with thoracolumbar fractures; therefore, the entire spinal axis should be imaged (**Fig. 12.1A**). Additionally, it is common practice to perform a baseline CT scan of the head to survey for intracranial hemorrhage or contusions. Spinal CT with reconstructed images is excellent at demonstrating spinal alignment, osseous architecture, and canal encroachment from retropulsed bone fragments of the vertebral body or laminae (**Fig. 12.1B, C**). Magnetic resonance imaging (MRI) is particularly valuable for demonstrating injury to the soft tissues. This modality can reveal the extent of damage to the spinal cord and the presence of ligamentous disruption as well as disk protrusions; however, it may be oversensitive in detecting nonspecific soft-tissue injuries (**Fig. 12.1D**).

Treatment

The treatment of thoracolumbar burst fractures is controversial, and there are no uniformly accepted algorithms or protocols. Operative management is often directed by the patient's neurologic examination. Surgery in patients with complete neurologic deficits (ASIA A) rarely results in improvements in neuro-

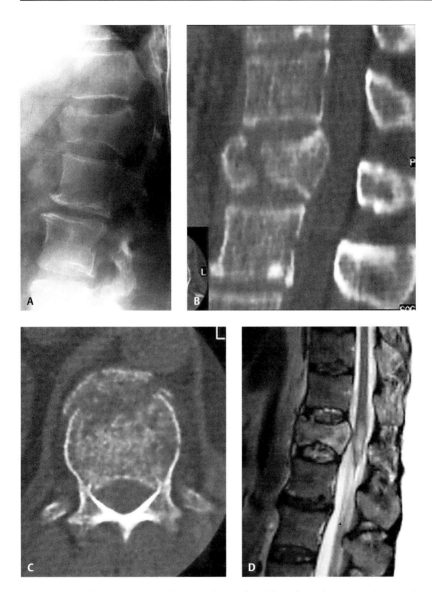

Fig. 12.1   L1 burst fracture with retropulsion of middle column bone into the spinal canal causing canal narrowing. **(A)** Lateral plain radiograph. **(B)** CT scan with sagittal reconstruction. **(C)** Axial CT. **(D)** T2-weighted sagittal MRI of the thoracolumbar spine.

logic function, but it may be indicated to correct a spinal deformity or to confer stability to allow for accelerated rehabilitation. Therefore, the goal of surgery for complete deficits, American Spinal Injury Association (ASIA) A, is to achieve bony healing and stability, and to allow the patient to be mobilized for early rehabilitation. The patient population deriving the greatest benefit from spinal decompression is the neurologically incomplete patient (ASIA B–D). However, operative treatment has yet to be proven in randomized controlled trials to have outcomes superior to those of conservative management in regard to functional outcome and pain scores.[2] Surgical treatment has been correlated with improved correction of kyphotic deformity, earlier return to work, and decreased requirements for external immobilization. The optimal surgical approach and technique for treatment of thoracolumbar burst fractures are still of much debate today.

Nonoperative

The majority of fractures encountered in the thoracolumbar region can be treated with immobilization and do not require surgical intervention. Burst fractures in the absence of a neurologic deficit or disruption of the posterior ligamentous complex are often managed adequately with conservative treatment. The absence of significant kyphosis implies that the posterior ligament complex is not significantly disrupted and the stability of the posterior tension band is preserved.

Some authors recommend prolonged immobilization with bedrest for definitive treatment of these fractures. In the absence of a neurologic deficit or significant disruption of the posterior ligamentous complex, bracing has been shown to be as effective as operative management with regard to postoperative ambulation and pain.[3]

In patients treated with immobilization, serial radiographs and close clinical follow-up are necessary to detect early failure of treatment. Patients typically fail treatment because of a progressive focal increase in kyphosis at the fracture site. The major risk of nonoperative treatment is the acute or chronic development of a neurologic deterioration. Fortunately, this is infrequent. Mechanical pain is often the greatest symptom of potential chronic or glacial instability.

Operative Treatment

There are three general surgical approaches that are commonly employed in the treatment of thoracolumbar burst fractures. The anterior approach is technically a more demanding operative procedure and requires manipulation of the great vessels and retroperitoneal structures. Typically this entails removal of bony fracture fragments from the spinal canal, decompressing the neural elements, and reestablishing spinal alignment, followed by stabilization of the spine with a structural bone graft, cage, and possibly adjunctive spinal instrumentation. This approach is preferred in cases with incomplete neurologic injury with residual anterior thecal sac compression. The anterior approach may provide for a shorter surgical construct (fewer levels fused) than a posterior approach. The posterior approach is less technically demanding and avoids key vascular and visceral structures. The posterior approach allows for a easier reduction and realignment of a fracture dislocation. Long-segment pedicle screw fixation, consisting of immobilizing at least two levels above and below the fracture level, often allows for adequate spinal stability at the expense of loss of range of motion. When the fracture occurs distal to the conus medullaris, a posterior approach can be used to manipulate the neural elements safely to remove offending diskal and bony fragments out of the spinal canal. Finally, a combined approach (anterior and posterior) can be used. This provides for improved stability at the expense of longer surgical times and the potential for a greater number of complications.[2]

 # Complications

Unstable thoracolumbar fractures are at risk for progressive deformity, non-union, or neurologic decline. In the absence of a neurologic deficit, patients with stable burst fractures can be managed with close serial observation and immobilization in a thoracolumbosacral orthosis (TLSO) brace or cast. Patients with an incomplete neurologic injury are typically treated with early operative reduction, decompression, and stabilization. In the patient who has a sustained and complete (ASIA A) neurologic injury, operative treatment is utilized to preserve and maintain sagittal balance and posture and to assist in early patient mobilization.

References

1. Dai LY, Jiang LS, Jiang SD. Conservative treatment of thoracolumbar burst fractures: long-term follow-up results with special reference to the load sharing classification. Spine (Phila Pa 1976) 2008;33(23):2536–2544
2. Dai LY, Jiang SD, Wang XY, Jiang LS. A review of the management of thoracolumbar burst fractures. Surg Neurol 2007;67(3):221–231, discussion 231
3. Wood K, Buttermann G, Mehbod A, Garvey T, Jhanjee R, Sechriest V. Operative compared with nonoperative treatment of a thoracolumbar burst fracture without neurological deficit. A prospective, randomized study. J Bone Joint Surg Am 2003;85-A(5):773–781

Suggested Readings

Dai LY, Jiang LS, Jiang SD. Conservative treatment of thoracolumbar burst fractures: long-term follow-up results with special reference to the load sharing classification. Spine (Phila Pa 1976) 2008;33(23):2536–2544

> *Dai et al. retrospectively review 127 patients with thoracolumbar burst fractures (Denis Type B) conservatively managed. Eighty-seven percent of patients reported improvement to acceptable levels of pain.*

Dai LY, Jiang SD, Wang XY, Jiang LS. A review of the management of thoracolumbar burst fractures. Surg Neurol 2007;67(3):221–231, discussion 231

> *Dai et al. describe their experience with the management of thoracolumbar burst fractures.*

Denis F. The three column spine and its significance in the classification of acute thoracolumbar spinal injuries. Spine (Phila Pa 1976) 1983;8(8):817–831

> *This article summarizes the Denis classification of thoracolumbar spine injuries.*

Vaccaro AR, Lehman RA Jr, Hurlbert RJ, et al. A new classification of thoracolumbar injuries: the importance of injury morphology, the integrity of the posterior ligamentous complex, and neurologic status. Spine (Phila Pa 1976) 2005;30(20):2325–2333

The TLICS emphasizes neurological status in addition to injury morphology and stability of the posterior ligamentous complex. This article further describes the system.

Wood K, Buttermann G, Mehbod A, Garvey T, Jhanjee R, Sechriest V. Operative compared with nonoperative treatment of a thoracolumbar burst fracture without neurological deficit. A prospective, randomized study. J Bone Joint Surg Am 2003;85-A(5):773–781

A randomized, prospective trial of 47 patients, comparing posterior stabilization versus bracing, found no difference in primary and secondary endpoints. There were no significant differences between those that returned to work and the average pain score on follow-up.

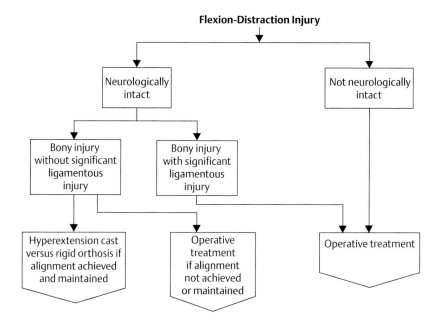

Flexion-Distraction Injury

Neurologically intact

Not neurologically intact

Bony injury without significant ligamentous injury

Bony injury with significant ligamentous injury

Hyperextension cast versus rigid orthosis if alignment achieved and maintained

Operative treatment if alignment not achieved or maintained

Operative treatment

13

Thoracolumbar Flexion-Distraction Injuries

Loukas Koyonos and Jeffrey A. Rihn

Flexion-distraction injuries in the thoracolumbar spine are classically referred to as "seat belt injuries" or Chance fractures. They comprise 5–15% of thoracolumbar fractures. The most common mechanism is a motor vehicle accident in which a lap belt acts as an axis of rotation anterior to the spinal column, causing failure of the spinal column in tension. If the center of rotation involves the anterior portion of the spinal column, it may fail either in compression or in tension. Upwards of 50–60% of patients will suffer concomitant abdominal visceral injuries, which require a high level of suspicion and judicious management by trauma personnel.

Fractures with the aforementioned mechanism involving the bony spinal elements with the axis of rotation anterior to the spine have been given the eponym "Chance fractures" after G. Q. Chance, the first physician to report on this particular pattern of injury.[1] Specifically, Chance noted that in several cases the vertebral body was relatively incompressible and, as he stated, "something has to give way," referring to the posterior bony structures. A traditional Chance fracture involves a horizontal splitting of the vertebra that begins with the spinous process or lamina and extends anteriorly through the pedicles and vertebral body.

Classification

Several classification schemes have been proposed. However, inter- and intra-observer reliability, as well as prognostic value, have been lacking in most cases. In 2005, the Spine Trauma Study Group introduced the Thoracolumbar Injury Classification and Severity Score (TLICS) in an attempt to address the shortcomings of previous methods of classification.[2] Injury morphology, neurologic status, and posterior ligamentous complex integrity were all taken into account, and operative versus nonoperative management was proposed based on the severity of injury.

93

Of relevance to flexion-distraction injuries, in this system, distraction injuries receive the maximal amount of points (4/4) in the morphology category and disruption of the posterior ligamentous complex receives 3/3, again, the maximal amount of points, in its category. Surgical treatment is recommended for a point total greater than 4. Recent evidence suggests that this system can reliably be used to predict surgical management.[3]

Other classification systems that are more specific to flexion-distraction injuries have been described. Denis divided these injuries into four types: (A) one-level injury, primarily bony; (B) one-level injury, primarily soft tissue (i.e., ligamentous and disk); (C) two-level injury, primarily bony, through the posterior vertebral body; and (D) two-level injury, primarily soft tissue, through the posterior vertebral body.

A classification system based on the posterior starting point and symmetry of the fracture was described by Gumley et al.[4] There were three types. Type I fractures start in the spinous process and are symmetrical. Type II fractures start at the base of the spinous process and are symmetrical. Type III fractures are asymmetrical, and the fracture plane is not parallel to the endplates.

Gertzbien and Court-Brown expanded upon Gumley's classification to incorporate the exit point of the fracture and the degree to which the vertebral body was involved.[4] In this scheme, fractures were first classified as I, II, or III based on Gumley's system, and then further classified into subgroups A through E: (A) fracture exits through disk, (B) fracture exits through anterior vertebral body wall, (C1) superior endplate involved, (C2) inferior endplate involved, (D) anterior vertebral body compression, (E) burst component.

 # Workup

History

Flexion-distraction injuries most commonly occur during motor vehicle accidents or falls. It is important to elucidate whether the patient was wearing a seat belt and whether it was a simple lap belt or a belt including a shoulder harness. These injuries are classically associated with lap belt use, though today many injuries occur as a result of other mechanisms, including fall from height.

Physical Examination

Evaluation by a trauma team is paramount when flexion-distraction injury is suspected to rule out concomitant intraabdominal injury. Classically, with enough force, abdominal wall contusions, known as the "seatbelt sign," will be noted on inspection, which are predictive of intraabdominal injury. However, recent data suggest that the rate of intraabdominal injury with Chance fractures may previously have been overreported. Tyroch et al. reported only 26/79 (33%) of patients with Chance fracture as having intraabdominal injury.

A detailed neurologic exam must be performed by an orthopedic and/or neurosurgical physician. This entails a full motor and sensory exam, reflexes, rectal exam (including tone, sensation, and volition), and upper motor neuron signs such as clonus, Babinski reflex, and Hoffmann sign. Close attention should be paid to posterior spinal "step-off" and/or increased space between spinous processes. Likewise, palpation at the site of injury will often elicit pain. In the setting of spinal shock (temporary loss of reflexes caudal to the level of spinal cord injury), the bulbospongiosus reflex is useful in determining what phase of shock the patient is in. Ditunno et al. proposed four phases.[5]

The gold standard system with which spinal cord injuries are assessed and classified is that of the American Spinal Injury Association (ASIA). ASIA guidelines for examination and classification are strongly recommended for any suspected injury to the spine.

Spinal Imaging

Evaluation begins with an assessment of the bony anatomy, either using plain-film radiography or computed tomography (CT). On plain film, interspinous widening may be seen on both the anteroposterior (AP) and lateral views. Additionally, the lateral view may show some degree of segmental kyphosis. Any translation at the level of the injury on the AP or lateral views should be noted. Any translation is representative of significant instability.

If a high level of suspicion exists for a flexion-distraction injury based on plain film, mechanism of injury, or physical exam, a CT scan should be obtained to delineate the pattern of bony anatomy disruption further. Magnetic resonance imaging (MRI) is also typically obtained, especially if there is any evidence on physical examination of a neurologic deficit. The MRI is particularly sensitive in identifying compression of the neural elements and defining the integrity of the soft-tissue structures (i.e., intervertebral disk, facet capsules, interspinous and supraspinous ligaments, ligamentum flavum, and the thoracodorsal fascia). However, recent evidence suggests that in assessing the posterior ligamentous complex of the spine, specificity and positive predictive value are at times poor, ranging from 56% to 67% and 42% to 82%, respectively.[6,7] Hence, MRIs may be "over-read" and unnecessary surgery may occur. Injury morphology and neurologic status must be considered when devising a surgical plan.

 # Treatment

Nonoperative treatment is usually reserved for neurologically intact, primarily bony, flexion-distraction injuries with less than 15° of kyphosis. In these cases, patients may be treated with a simple extension-type cast or orthosis with 85% good to fair results expected.[8] Patients should be followed a minimum of 3 months with radiographs obtained at each interval visit to assess maintenance of sagittal alignment.

For injuries presenting with greater than 15° of kyphosis, neurologic deficit, or disruption of the posterior ligamentous complex, surgical stabilization is recommended.[8] The goal of surgery is to restore the posterior tension band. This can be usually be achieved with a posterior-only approach. The standard approach has been the stabilization of two levels above and two levels below the level of injury with a pedicle screw/rod construct; however, short-segment fixation can be used in flexion-distraction injuries in which there is minimal comminution and/or collapse of the anterior spinal column.[9] Injuries that involve significant comminution of the vertebral body have a flexion component with probable disruption of the posterior ligamentous complex. These injuries typically require both long-segment posterior stabilization and anterior corpectomy and fusion with use of a structural bone graft or interbody cage for anterior support.

It is vital to review the preoperative imaging studies prior to surgery to determine whether or not there are intervertebral disk or retropulsed vertebral body bone fragments that need to be decompressed at the time of surgery, either from a posterior, transpedicular approach or a combined anterior/posterior approach.

Outcomes

Surgical treatment yields satisfactory results in most cases. Finkelstein et al. reported that 88% of patients in which a short construct, spanning one motion segment, was used achieved minimal disability at minimum 20 months' follow-up.[10] In 2005, Tezer et al. reported on 48 patients treated surgically for thoracolumbar burst fractures associated with a flexion-distraction injury of the posterior elements. At mean follow-up of 70 months there was no loss of correction, a satisfactory reduction, and good stabilization with solid fusion achieved in all cases.[11]

Complications

Complications associated with the injury itself include epidural hematoma, neurologic injury, and kyphotic deformity. The most common complication associated with nonoperative management is progression of kyphosis. Complications of surgery include infection, instrumentation failure, pseudarthrosis, loss of correction, neurologic injury, and/or mortality.

Case Examples

Fig. 13.1A,B
Fig. 13.2A,B
Fig. 13.3A,B

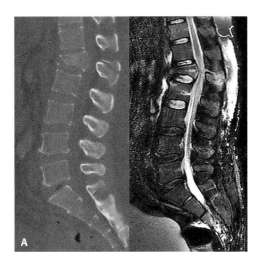

Fig. 13.1A Sagittal CT and MRI of L1 flexion-distraction injury at initial presentation. This injury was treated nonoperatively.

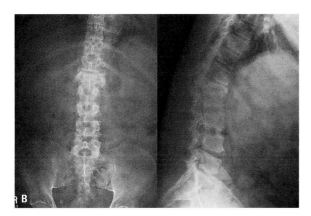

Fig. 13.1B AP and lateral radiographs obtained at follow-up visit showing significant thoracolumbar junctional kyphosis.

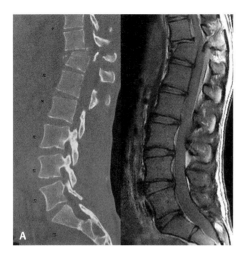

Fig. 13.2A Sagittal CT and MRI of T12 flexion-distraction injury at initial presentation.

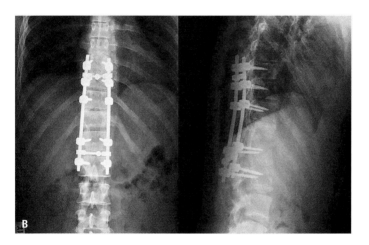

Fig. 13.2B Postoperative AP and lateral radiographs demonstrating a posterior-only approach with instrumented fusion from T9 through L2.

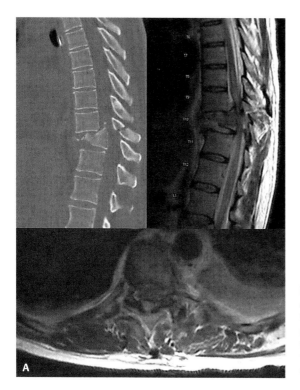

Fig. 13.3A Sagittal CT and sagittal/axial MRI of T10 flexion-distraction injury at initial presentation. Note the significant retropulsion of the vertebral body and spinal canal narrowing.

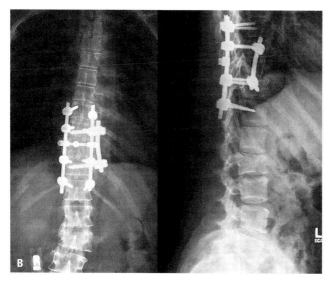

Fig. 13.3B Postoperative AP and lateral radiographs demonstrating an anterior and posterior approach with anterior corpectomy and graft placement, and posterior instrumented fusion from T8 through T12. Note the augmented lateral fixation as well.

References

1. Chance GQ. Note on a type of flexion fracture of the spine. Br J Radiol 1948;21(249):452
2. Vaccaro AR, Lehman RA, Jr., Hurlbert RJ, Anderson PA, Harris M, Hedlund R, et al. A new classification of thoracolumbar injuries: the importance of injury morphology, the integrity of the posterior ligamentous complex, and neurologic status. Spine 2005;30:2325–2333
3. Joaquim AF, Fernandes YB, Cavalcante RA, Fragoso RM, Honorato DC, Patel AA. Evaluation of the thoracolumbar injury classification system in thoracic and lumbar spinal trauma. Spine (Phila Pa 1976) 2011;36(1):33–36
4. Gumley G, Taylor TK, Ryan MD. Distraction fractures of the lumbar spine. J Bone Joint Surg Br 1982;64(5):520–525
5. Ditunno JF, Little JW, Tessler A, Burns AS. Spinal shock revisited: a four-phase model. Spinal Cord 2004;42(7):383–395
6. Rihn JA, Yang N, Fisher C, et al. Using magnetic resonance imaging to accurately assess injury to the posterior ligamentous complex of the spine: a prospective comparison of the surgeon and radiologist. J Neurosurg Spine 2010;12(4):391–396
7. Rihn JA, Fisher C, Harrop J, Morrison W, Yang N, Vaccaro AR. Assessment of the posterior ligamentous complex following acute cervical spine trauma. J Bone Joint Surg Am 2010;92(3):583–589
8. Anderson PA, Henley MB, Rivara FP, Maier RV. Flexion distraction and Chance injuries to the thoracolumbar spine. J Orthop Trauma 1991;5(2):153–160
9. Triantafyllou SJ, Gertzbein SD. Flexion distraction injuries of the thoracolumbar spine: a review. Orthopedics 1992;15(3):357–364
10. Finkelstein JA, Wai EK, Jackson SS, Ahn H, Brighton-Knight M. Single-level fixation of flexion distraction injuries. J Spinal Disord Tech 2003;16(3):236–242
11. Tezer M, Ozturk C, Aydogan M, Mirzanli C, Talu U, Hamzaoglu A. Surgical outcome of thoracolumbar burst fractures with flexion-distraction injury of the posterior elements. Int Orthop 2005;29(6):347–350

Suggested Readings

Chance GQ. Note on a type of flexion fracture of the spine. Br J Radiol 1948;21(249):452

> *In this seminal article, Dr. G. Q. Chance notes that in several of his thoracolumbar spine fracture cases, the vertebral body appears relatively incompressible and he notes that "something has to give way," referring the posterior bony structures, leading to the traditional definition of a "Chance" fracture.*

Joaquim AF, Fernandes YB, Cavalcante RA, Fragoso RM, Honorato DC, Patel AA. Evaluation of the thoracolumbar injury classification system in thoracic and lumbar spinal trauma. Spine (Phila Pa 1976) 2011;36(1):33–36

> *This article is a follow-up to the original article describing the Thoracolumbar Injury Classification and Severity Score (TLICS). TLICS in an attempt to address the shortcomings of previous methods of classification. This article shows that TLICS can reliably be used to predict surgical management.*

Tezer M, Ozturk C, Aydogan M, Mirzanli C, Talu U, Hamzaoglu A. Surgical outcome of thoracolumbar burst fractures with flexion-distraction injury of the posterior elements. Int Orthop 2005;29(6):347–350

> *In this article, Tezer reports on the outcomes of surgical treatment of thoracolumbar flexion-distraction injuries. At a mean of 70 months, there was no loss of correction, a satisfactory reduction, and good stabilization with solid fusion achieved in all cases. This article contributes to the rationale for surgical management.*

Vaccaro AR, Lehman RA, Jr., Hurlbert RJ, Anderson PA, Harris M, Hedlund R, et al. A new classification of thoracolumbar injuries: the importance of injury morphology, the integrity of the posterior ligamentous complex, and neurologic status. Spine 2005;30:2325–2333

> *This is the original article describing Thoracolumbar Injury Classification and Severity Score (TLICS), which, at the time, was a novel classification system for thoracolumbar spine injuries aiming to aid with the decisions in clinical management.*

Denis F. The three column spine and its significance in the classification of acute thoracolumbar spinal injuries. Spine 1983;8:817–831

> *Other classification systems that are more specific to flexion-distraction injuries have been described. Denis divided these injuries into four types: (A) one-level injury, primarily bone; (B) one-level injury, primarily soft tissue (i.e., ligamentous and disk); (C) two-level injury, primarily bone, through the posterior vertebral body; and (D) two-level injury, primarily soft tissue, through the posterior vertebral body.*

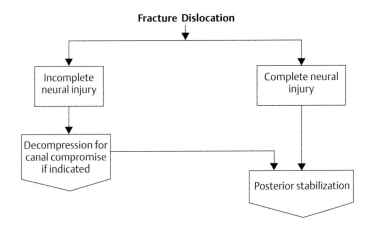

Fracture Dislocation

Incomplete neural injury

Complete neural injury

Decompression for canal compromise if indicated

Posterior stabilization

14

Thoracolumbar Fracture Dislocations

Moshe Yanko and Steven C. Ludwig

The thoracolumbar spine is a complex morphological structure that provides a challenging task regarding the evaluation and management of a traumatized patient. Fracture dislocations usually involve high-energy trauma and are associated with multisystem injuries. Diagnosis can be difficult because of the multiple distracting injuries. A patient might be physiologically unstable, preventing accurate history, physical examination, and radiological work-up. A thorough understanding of the complexities of thoracolumbar fracture dislocations is necessary. Management should therefore be conducted by a well-experienced multidisciplinary team.

The mechanical characteristics of the thoracolumbar junction place it as the most common site for spinal injuries. The thoracic spine is considered a stable segment because of the protective and stabilizing effects of the rib cage. The lumbar spine, as a mobile segment, creates a lever arm at this transitional zone. The L1 vertebra is the most common site of spinal fracture, and the T12 is the next most common site. Thoracolumbar fracture dislocations occur most frequently as a result of motor vehicle accidents and falls from heights. Both mechanisms involve high-energy impact and are frequently associated with spinal cord injury. Thoracolumbar fracture dislocations found in neurologically intact patients are those with spontaneous decompression of the spinal elements and widening of the spinal canal.

Classification

Several classification methods have been suggested over the years for thoracolumbar injuries. Unfortunately, no consensus exists among spine surgeons regarding the use of a single method with which to classify these injuries.

Denis Classification of Acute Thoracolumbar Spinal Injuries

With the advent of computed tomography (CT), Denis developed the "three column" concept in 1983. To this date, no one has validated the concept of the middle column. Denis defined four categories of major spinal injuries based on the mechanical forces at the time of impact: compression fractures, burst fractures, seat belt–type injuries (Chance fractures), and fracture dislocations. Fracture dislocations are defined as failure of all three columns under compression, tension, rotation, or shear. In his study, Denis classified three types of fracture dislocations: flexion-rotation, shear, and flexion-distraction injuries. The flexion-rotation type fracture was the most commonly observed.

AO Types

In the 1990s, the AO group suggested a different type of classification for spinal column injuries. This mechanistic classification system is based on the three basic functions of the normal and stable spine while resisting implied external forces: axial compression, axial distraction, and torsional forces. Three types of major injuries are as follows: Type A, compression; Type B, distraction; and Type C, rotation injuries. The AO classification demonstrates the severity of the injury, increasing instability, and risk of neurological compromise from Type A to C patterns. The groups are further divided into 27 total subtypes. This comprehensive and logical classification system has no specific advantage regarding fracture dislocations (Type C). However, with a more accurate and detailed description of the wide spectrum of injuries, it allows a more precise estimation of the severity of the fracture dislocation.

Thoracolumbar Injury Classification System

In 2005, Vaccaro et al. presented the Thoracolumbar Injury Classification and Severity Score (TLICS). This classification method was developed to serve more as an outcome-predictive tool and less as an injury morphology description method. This classification combines several factors regarding thoracolumbar injuries, including assessment of spinal stability, future deformity, and progressive neurological compromise.

One of the goals of the TLICS was to help spine surgeons in their clinical decision making. Three major variables were identified as critical in serving this purpose: (1) the morphology of the injury, (2) the integrity of the posterior ligamentous complex (PLC), and (3) the neurological status of the patient. Morphology refers to the three known types of injury forces affecting the human spine: compression, translation and/or rotation, and distraction. The PLC includes the supraspinous and interspinous ligaments, ligamentum flavum, and facet joint capsules. The role of this complex is to serve as a posterior tension band, and disruption of these structures usually requires surgical stabilization because of their poor healing ability. Information gathered from plain radiographs, CT scans, and MRI can categorize the PLC integrity as intact, indeterminate, or disrupted. Neurological status is the third element because of its important role in predicting prognosis and as a tool for treatment plan decision making. Four levels are considered: neurologically intact, nerve root injury, complete spinal cord injury, and incomplete spinal cord injury and cauda equina injury. An injury severity score is calculated by adding numeric values collected within each subgroup of the main three categories. A score of 3 or less indicates an injury that can be treated nonsurgically, a score of 5 or more indicates an injury for which surgery is recommended, and a score of 4 denotes a discretionary case, allowing clinical scenarios to bias the surgeon toward surgical or nonsurgical management. Although the usefulness of the TLICS is promising, long-term follow-up data regarding its prognostic value need to be collected and assessed.

Patient Management

The majority of patients diagnosed with thoracolumbar fracture dislocation have incurred multiple traumatic injuries. Treatment begins at the accident scene according to the Advanced Trauma Life Support (ATLS) guidelines. The patient should be immobilized and secured in a neutral position of the vertebral column, including a rigid cervical collar and a backboard. Detected hypotension can be caused by hemorrhage in addition to neurogenically mediated shock. Maintaining the mean arterial blood pressure above 85 mmHg is thought to maintain spinal cord perfusion and can improve neurological outcome. A full assessment of the chest and abdomen should be performed by a multidisciplinary trauma team to rule out any immediate life-threatening injuries. In the case of an unconscious patient, the medical team at the scene can provide additional information regarding mechanism of injury.

Physical examination of these patients should be handled with a systematic multidisciplinary team approach, taking into consideration all bodily systems. Examination of the vertebral column and the neurological examination should be performed under the assumption that an unstable injury is highly suspected until proven otherwise. The physical examination of an unconscious patient can be challenging, and in most cases, the only clues for spinal cord function can be obtained from emergency medical technician personnel on the scene with reports of spontaneous movements. Reaction to touch and/or painful stimuli might allow for assessment of spontaneous movements of the extremities. Additionally, asynchronous activity of normal chest motion versus diaphragmatic respiration might be a subtle clue of spinal cord injury. Signs of thoracic trauma, including ecchymosis, lacerations, abrasions, and step-off while palpating the spinous process, should alert the physician to a spinal column injury. A thorough motor and sensory neurological evaluation using the standard American Spinal Injury Association (ASIA) scoring method should be conducted. Additionally, the presence or absence of reflexes, including Babinski (upper motor neuron lesion), cremasteric (T12–L1), anal wink (S2, S3, S4), and bulbocavernosus (S3, S4) reflexes, should be assessed.

Any painful area on the thoracolumbar spine should be analyzed with anteroposterior and lateral radiographic views. In cases in which plain imaging findings are negative and in cases that require more thorough evaluation of the complexity of the thoracolumbar injury, CT scans can be obtained. Coronal and sagittal reconstructions can be helpful in gaining a better understanding of the bony injuries and can be used to assess the magnitude of bony canal compromise (**Fig. 14.1**). In patients with neurological deficits, MRI can be useful to determine the magnitude of soft-tissue canal compromise, such as hematoma, traumatic meningocele, and compromise by a herniated disk. In addition, MRI can assess whether the injury is at the cord, conus, or cauda equina level. From a prognostic standpoint, MRI can also assess edema of the spinal cord and conus medullaris. MRI can also provide additional information regarding discoligamentous disruptions at the site of the thoracolumbar dislocation.

Treatment

Fracture dislocations are unstable because of the magnitude of the spinal column disruption in addition to associated neurological deficits. Therefore, surgical treatment is recommended for most of these cases. When physiologically stable, the patient can be brought to the operating room. The goals of surgery are to improve or to preserve neurological function, to realign the spine, to stabilize the spine, to prevent post-traumatic deformity, and to enable early mobilization with aggressive rehabilitation.

The basic tenets of neurological recovery teach that patients with complete neurological deficits will achieve no significant gains in return of function. On the other hand, patients with incomplete deficits can make significant neurological gains with a decompressive and stabilization procedure. Decompression can be performed indirectly via fracture dislocation relocation or directly via an anterior approach. Alternatively, posterior decompression in the thoracolumbar spine can be performed through extracavitary or transpedicular decom-

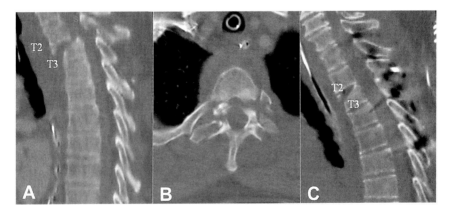

Fig. 14.1   T2–T3 flexion-rotation fracture dislocation that resulted in complete spinal cord injury. **(A)** Sagittal CT imaging. **(B)** Axial CT imaging. **(C)** With clear instability, spinal column was reduced and stabilized posteriorly.

pression. Stabilization of the spine with modern implants through an anterior and/or posterior approach enables a patient to begin the rehabilitation phase aggressively and reduces the need for postoperative bracing. Thus, fracture dislocations in patients who are neurologically intact typically require posterior reduction, stabilization, and fusion with pedicular instrumentation.

Additionally, patients with fracture dislocations who are neurologically complete require posterior reduction, stabilization, and fusion to facilitate mobilization and prevent delayed pain and sitting imbalance caused by post-traumatic thoracolumbar deformity. In rare cases of patients with incomplete thoracolumbar fracture dislocations, the spine typically is approached posteriorly first to reduce the spinal column dislocation. Postoperative CT is performed next, to assess the magnitude of persistent canal compromise. In the setting of a patient with incomplete deficit and persistent canal compromise, secondary anterior decompression and reconstruction place the neural elements in the best environment to recover function.

For the vast majority of fracture dislocations of the thoracolumbar spine, a posterior approach allows for reduction, stabilization, and potential decompression (e.g., extracavitary or transpedicular approach). However, in cases of significant comminution of the vertebral bodies, the mechanics of the vertebral body might not allow the spinal column to share the load with posteriorly directed stabilization and fusion. Thus, an additional anterior approach with corpectomy and reconstruction of the anterior column with structural bone grafts or other vertebral body replacement cages might be required.

Neurophysiologic monitoring of patients who are neurologically intact or who have incomplete deficits can safely assist with ensuring safe reduction of the fracture dislocation. Baseline and postposition potentials should be obtained before starting the procedure. Reductions of the fractures might require intraoperative distraction and compression maneuvers to unlock the dislocated facet joints. Considering that such maneuvers might require a significant amount of force on the spinal column through applied spinal instrumentation, alternative methods of reduction might be required. After placement of the pedicle screw implants above and below the level of dislocation, the surgeon can unlock the facet dislocation by excising the facet joints. This allows for a more controlled and gentle reduction maneuver. The gold standard for posterior stabilization includes the use of pedicle screws and rods. The goal is to restore the normal alignment of the vertebral column with adequate stability in all planes. By achieving control over the three columns of the spine, pedicle screws recreate a rigid construct within all degrees of freedom.

Newer surgical techniques have been developed for treating thoracolumbar trauma in recent years. Minimally invasive surgery is gaining popularity for treating such complex injuries. This technique uses percutaneously guided pedicle screws and rods, with reduction and realignment techniques similar to those implemented in open cases. This method cannot be used as posterior stabilization in cases in which direct anterior decompression of the neural elements is required. The benefits of minimally invasive techniques include reduction of paraspinal muscle injury, bleeding, infection, and pain. The downside of minimally invasive surgical techniques includes a long and steep learning curve, difficulties with reduction, and difficulties in achieving biological fusion.

Summary

With the continuing evolution of the delivery of medical care to patients with multiple traumatic injuries, more patients will survive their injuries. After initial stabilization via a multidisciplinary team approach, a systematic and accurate way of management is required to diagnose thoracolumbar injuries accurately and to treat properly. Defining the fracture type with proper plain and advanced imaging studies hastens diagnosis. Additionally, the use of a classification method allows surgeons to assess stability, communicate with other caregivers, determine treatment methods, and predict outcomes. Fractures that are considered unstable should be managed surgically when the general condition of the patient allows. Most patients with thoracolumbar fracture dislocations have associated neurological deficit. Conventional open techniques typically involve a posteriorly directed approach. However, in cases of incomplete neurological deficits and in cases of significant anterior column deficiency, anterior corpectomy and reconstruction might be required. Minimally invasive spine surgery as an option to treat thoracolumbar fracture dislocations has arrived. However, the superiority of minimally invasive techniques over conventional open techniques is yet to be determined.

Suggested Readings

Aebi M. Classification of thoracolumbar fractures and dislocations. Eur Spine J 2010;19(Suppl 1):S2–S7

> *The author compares the AO classification to other methods of classification of injuries of the thoracolumbar spine.*

Denis F, Burkus JK. Shear fracture-dislocations of the thoracic and lumbar spine associated with forceful hyperextension (lumberjack paraplegia). Spine (Phila Pa 1976) 1992;17(2):156–161

> *The authors describe the hyperextension mechanism of injury of the thoracolumbar spine in 12 patients who sustained shear fracture dislocation.*

Denis F. The three column spine and its significance in the classification of acute thoracolumbar spinal injuries. Spine (Phila Pa 1976) 1983;8(8):817–831

> *This study further develops the "three-column" concept in this retrospective study of 412 thoracolumbar injuries.*

Ferguson RL, Allen BL Jr. A mechanistic classification of thoracolumbar spine fractures. Clin Orthop Relat Res 1984;189(189):77–88

> *The authors present a mechanical description of thoracolumbar injuries and classification of the injuries into seven categories. The mechanical principles provide a better understanding of the instrumentation needed for spinal injury stabilization.*

Holdsworth F. Fractures, dislocations, and fracture-dislocations of the spine. J Bone Joint Surg Am 1970;52(8):1534–1551

> *This article defines spinal fractures based on the "two columns" concept and four basic mechanisms of injury: compression, flexion, extension, and flexion-rotation.*

Levine AM, Eismont FJ, Garfin SR, Zigler JE. Spine Trauma. Philadelphia, PA: WB Saunders; 1998

This is a profound overview of thoracolumbar injuries, including historic review, principles of management of the traumatized patient, and treatment methods.

Magerl F, Aebi M, Gertzbein SD, Harms J, Nazarian S. A comprehensive classification of thoracic and lumbar injuries. Eur Spine J 1994;3(4):184–201

This is a review of 1445 thoracolumbar injuries with classification based on the pathomorphological aspect (i.e., the AO classification).

Nicoll EA. Fractures of the dorso-lumbar spine. J Bone Joint Surg Br 1949;31B(3):376–394

This was one of the first descriptions of lumbar spine fractures in the modern medical literature. Nicoll differentiated between stable and nonstable thoracolumbar injuries.

Palmisani M, Gasbarrini A, Brodano GB, et al. Minimally invasive percutaneous fixation in the treatment of thoracic and lumbar spine fractures. Eur Spine J 2009;18(Suppl 1):71–74

A series of 51 patients with 64 fractures were treated with a minimally invasive technique. Satisfactory results were achieved for specific fracture types.

Rampersaud YR, Annand N, Dekutoski MB. Use of minimally invasive surgical techniques in the management of thoracolumbar trauma: current concepts. Spine (Phila Pa 1976) 2006;31(11, Suppl):S96–S102, discussion S104

This is an overview of concepts of minimally invasive surgical techniques for the management of thoracolumbar trauma.

Simpson AH, Williamson DM, Golding SJ, Houghton GR. Thoracic spine translocation without cord injury. J Bone Joint Surg Br 1990;72(1):80–83

This article describes fracture dislocations and conservative versus operative stabilization. It presents a series of 19 prospectively studied flexion-distraction thoracolumbar injuries (T11–L2) in patients between the ages of 20 and 33 years, with comparison of the different subgroups and management techniques.

Vaccaro AR, Lehman RA Jr, Hurlbert RJ, et al. A new classification of thoracolumbar injuries: the importance of injury morphology, the integrity of the posterior ligamentous complex, and neurologic status. Spine (Phila Pa 1976) 2005;30(20):2325–2333

This article presents a thoracolumbar injury classification system, including injury severity assessment, designed to assist in clinical management.

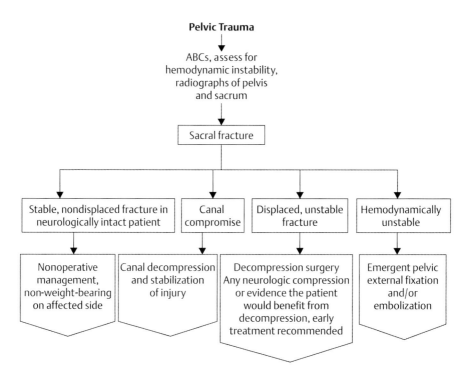

ABCs, airway, breathing, circulation

15

Sacral Fractures

Gregory Gebauer and D. Greg Anderson

Fractures of the sacrum make up ~1% of all spinal fractures. The sacrum is formed by the fusion of the caudal spinal segments. It forms the key link between the axial skeleton (pelvis) and the spine. It includes both bony and ligamentous components that serve as a solid weight-bearing platform, protecting the lumbosacral spine (L4–S1), sacral (S2–S4) nerve roots, and iliac vessels. Sacral fractures follow a bimodal distribution. Injuries in younger patients tend to involve high-energy trauma, such as falls or motor vehicle crashes. These fractures are often associated with injuries to the pelvic ring and with other associated traumatic injuries. Injuries resulting in pelvic ring instability and widening of the pelvic ring can result in significant blood loss and require emergent treatment. In contrast, older patients most commonly sustain insufficiency fractures of the sacrum as a result of osteoporosis and osteopenia. These fractures are notoriously difficult to diagnose and may require computed tomography (CT), bone scanning, or magnetic resonance imaging (MRI) to demonstrate the fracture.

Classification

Sacral fracture patterns include vertical fractures, transverse fractures, and U- or H-shaped fractures. Denis et al. described vertical fractures in relation to the sacral foramina. In the Denis classification system, a zone I fracture (**Fig. 15.1A**) involves the bone lateral to the foramina. It is the most common (50%) type of injury and has a low incidence of neurologic or bladder injury. Neurologic injury occurs in ~6% of Zone I injuries and often involves the L4 and L5 nerve roots. Zone II fractures (**Fig. 15.1B**) traverse the sacral foramina and account for ~34% of the vertical sacral fractures. These injuries have a higher incidence of neurologic injury (28%), which most commonly involves the L5, S1, and S2 nerve roots. A zone III injury (**Fig. 15.1C**) is medial to the sacral foramina and may involve the central spinal canal. Denis reported this pattern in 16% of sacral

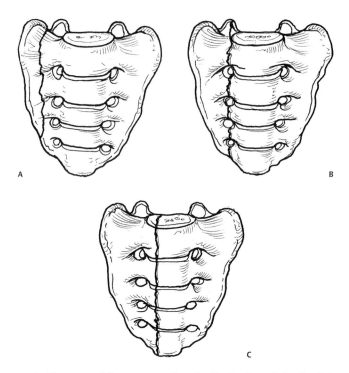

Fig. 15.1 Vertical fractures of the sacrum as described by Denis et al. Grading is based on the relationship of the fracture to the sacral foramina. **(A)** Zone I. **(B)** Zone II. **(C)** Zone III.

injuries and found the highest prevalence and severity of neurologic injuries. Bowel and/or bladder control or sexual function was impaired in 76% of the patients with a zone III injury.

Transverse fractures commonly occur in the area between S1 and S3 and are often associated with bladder dysfunction, especially if displaced. Any sacral or posterior pelvic fracture with displacement of 1 cm or greater is considered unstable.

U- and H-type fractures involve both a vertical and transverse component. These injuries are typically the result of high-energy trauma, more often than bony insufficiency. Insufficiency fractures are generally considered stable; however, U- or H-style fractures from high-energy trauma should be considered unstable until proven otherwise.

Diagnosis

Sacral fractures rarely occur in isolation. Therefore, it is essential to consider the possibility of a sacral fracture when patients have sustained high-energy trauma to the lower lumbar and pelvic regions. Vaccaro et al. discussed five basic principles when assessing a sacral injury. These include assessing for: (1) active bleeding, (2) an open fracture, (3) a neurologic injury, (4) fracture pattern, and (5) pelvic and spinal stability of skeletal injury. The physician should search for any signs of lacerations, bruising, tenderness, swelling, hematuria, and crepitus. In the setting of a severe pelvic ring disruption, severe soft-tissue injuries may be present and can be seen in the form of a palpable subcutaneous fluid mass, consistent with lumbosacral fascial degloving (Morel-Lavelle lesion). A rectal exam is mandatory to rule out internal lacerations and to assess rectal tone. In female patients, a vaginal exam must also be performed. A thorough neurologic exam is critical. It is important to assess the function of the lower sacral roots, rectal tone, and light touch and pinprick sensation along the perianal concentric dermatomes of S2 through S5, and elicitation of specific reflexes, including perianal wink and the bulbospongiosus and cremasteric reflexes. Pelvic ring stability should be evaluated manually.

Anterior-posterior, inlet, outlet, and lateral pelvic radiographs should be obtained. If an L5 transverse process fracture is found, there is a strong chance of an associated sacral fracture. In addition, avulsion fractures of the ischial spine, asymmetry of sacral foramina, or cephalad migration of the affected hemipelvis are findings suggestive of sacral injury with severe ligamentous disruption. CT is helpful when a posterior pelvic ring injury is suspected. A dedicated sacral CT with fine cuts and sagittal/coronal reformatting will help in detecting and understanding the fracture pattern. MRI is helpful in cases with neurologic deficits or when trying to assess for an insufficiency fracture.

Treatment

Patients with insufficiency fractures are generally treated nonoperatively. Treatment includes assistive devices for ambulation, pain medication, and physical therapy. A subset of patients refractory to nonoperative care may be considered for sacroplasty: the injection of polymethylmethacrylate (PMMA) or bone cement, similar to vertebroplasty.

For traumatic injuries, nonoperative management is indicated for nondisplaced and impacted sacral fractures in patients who are neurologically intact. This generally involves maintaining a restricted weight-bearing status on the affected side (non-weight-bearing or toe-touch) and allowing the fracture to heal.

Patients with major pelvic disruptions who have evidence of hemodynamic instability may require the application of a pelvic binder or clamp, an anterior external fixator, skeletal traction, and/or embolization to control pelvic bleeding. More definitive management, to reduce and stabilize the disruption by internal fixation to the pelvic ring and sacrum, is indicated when the patient stabilizes. Patients with displaced sacral fractures involving the spinal canal may require direct decompression in addition to reduction and internal fixation of the sacral fracture, although early surgery is associated with an increased risk of hemorrhage, wound-healing complications, and cerebrospinal fluid (CSF) leak. Those with evidence of sacral root stretch/avulsion fare best with early reduction and stabilization to allow an optimal environment for neural recovery. Stabilization of the sacrum and sacroiliac joints can be performed anteriorly or posteriorly. The most commonly performed procedure is the placement of iliosacral screws. When the fracture involves the foramina, fully threaded screws are generally used to avoid compression of the exiting nerves in the comminuted fracture site.

Outcome

The most important predictor of outcome is the neurologic status of the patient at the time of presentation. Following decompression/stabilization surgery, neurologic improvements in up to 80% of patients have been observed, although there is some degree of neurologic deficit. Denis et al. reported no improvement of bowel or bladder control in three patients in whom a transverse sacral fracture had been treated non-operatively. In contrast, all of five patients treated surgically had complete return of sphincter control. With instrumented procedures, Nork et al. reported successful results with percutaneous sacroiliac screw fixation in thirteen patients with Zone III injuries.

Complications

Nonunion, continued or worsened neurologic deficit, loss of bowel or bladder control, severe bleeding, infection, anesthesia-related complications, wound and hardware complications, dural tears with subsequent formation of a pseudomeningocele, and visceral damage are all possible.

Suggested Readings

Bayley E, Srinivas S, Boszczyk BM. Clinical outcomes of sacroplasty in sacral insufficiency fractures: a review of the literature. Eur Spine J 2009;18(9):1266–1271

> *In this meta-analysis of the results of sacroplasty, 15 papers including 108 patients were analyzed. Significant reduction in VAS pain scores was noted following sacroplasty (VAS 8.9 to 2.6).*

Cho CH, Mathis JM, Ortiz O. Sacral fractures and sacroplasty. Neuroimaging Clin N Am 2010; 20(2):179–186

> *This is an excellent review of the use of sacroplasty for treating sacral insufficiency fractures and metastatic tumors of the sacrum.*

Denis F, Davis S, Comfort T. Sacral fractures: an important problem. Retrospective analysis of 236 cases. Clin Orthop Relat Res 1988;227:67–81

> *This landmark retrospective study of 236 consecutive patients with sacral fractures in patients with 776 pelvic injuries describes the Denis classification system with typical injury patterns and projected outcomes.*

Kellam JF, McMurtry RY, Paley D, Tile M. The unstable pelvic fracture. Operative treatment. Orthop Clin North Am 1987;18(1):25–41

> *This overview of the importance of operative management of sacral fractures, and of the importance of obtaining an anatomic reduction, emphasizes the importance of appropriate preoperative evaluation, subsequent planning, and precise, technically skillful surgery done by an experienced surgeon.*

Lykomitros VA, Papavasiliou KA, Alzeer ZM, Sayegh FE, Kirkos JM, Kapetanos GA. Management of traumatic sacral fractures: a retrospective case-series study and review of the literature. Injury 2010;41(3):266–272

This is a review of the literature and presentation of a 16-patient case series. In this series, patients treated nonoperatively had better outcomes, which the authors attributed to the patients' having less severe initial injuries.

Nork SE, Jones CB, Harding SP, Mirza SK, Routt ML Jr. Percutaneous stabilization of U-shaped sacral fractures using iliosacral screws: technique and early results. J Orthop Trauma 2001; 15(4):238–246

This is a retrospective study of 442 patients with pelvic ring disruptions, thirteen with displaced U-shaped sacral fractures who underwent fracture stabilization via a fluoroscopically guided iliosacral screw. The authors concluded that percutaneous fixation diminishes potential blood loss and operative times and is an effective method of treatment.

Rommens PM, Vanderschot PM, Broos PL. Conventional radiography and CT examination of pelvic ring fractures. A comparative study of 90 patients. Unfallchirurg 1992;95(8):387–392

This retrospective review of 90 patients with pelvic ring fractures compared the interpretation of conventional X-ray films and CT images. The authors demonstrated that pelvic ring evaluation with films alone is inadequate, with fractures of the sacral body and lateral part of the sacrum being overlooked. CT imaging is necessary in combination with radiography to improve diagnosis of sacral injuries.

Routt ML Jr, Simonian PT, Swiontkowski MF. Stabilization of pelvic ring disruptions. Orthop Clin North Am 1997;28(3):369–388

This excellent review of pelvic ring injuries and their complications (including early hemorrhage, permanent nerve injury, and pelvic pain from deformity) discusses the treatment options for a disrupted pelvic ring as well as the treatment advantages and disadvantages.

Roy-Camille R, Saillant G, Gagna G, Mazel C. Transverse fracture of the upper sacrum. Suicidal jumper's fracture. Spine (Phila Pa 1976) 1985;10(9):838–845

This review of 13 patients with transverse fractures of the upper sacrum discusses fracture anatomy, presentation, and treatment options. The authors emphasize that sacral fractures are often missed in the setting of polytrauma, and that in the presence of perineal neurologic deficit or injury, appropriate exam and imaging are necessary.

Sabiston CP, Wing PC. Sacral fractures: classification and neurologic implications. J Trauma 1986;26(12):1113–1115

The authors divide sacral fractures into three categories, including sacral fractures in conjunction with pelvic fractures, isolated lower-segment sacral fractures, and upper-level sacral fractures. They recommend conservative treatment, as they feel that associated neurologic deficit improves spontaneously.

Strange-Vognsen HH, Lebech A. An unusual type of fracture in the upper sacrum. J Orthop Trauma 1991;5(2):200–203

This is an excellent review of the literature regarding sacral fractures. In addition, the authors define a fracture of the isolated upper sacrum and classify it as a special type—type 4 sacral fracture.

Schmidek HH, Smith DA, Kristiansen TK. Sacral fractures. Neurosurgery 1984;15(5):735–746

This review of sacral fracture patterns and their neurologic involvement discusses treatment options for sacral fractures and also correlates vertical sacral fractures and patterns of pelvic injury.

Vaccaro AR, Kim DH, Brodke DS, et al. Diagnosis and management of sacral spine fractures. Instr Course Lect 2004;53:375–385

This is an excellent overall review of diagnosis, imaging, and operative and nonoperative options for sacral fractures and the best overall treatment for the patient.

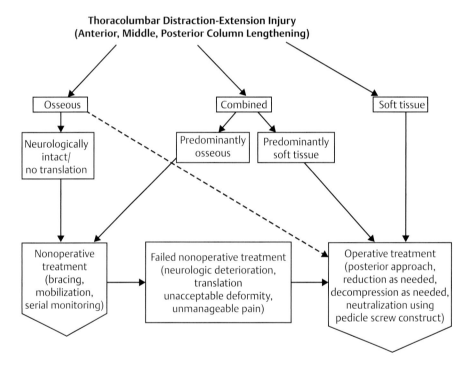

**Thoracolumbar Distraction-Extension Injury
(Anterior, Middle, Posterior Column Lengthening)**

Osseous

Neurologically
intact/
no translation

Combined

Predominantly
osseous

Predominantly
soft tissue

Soft tissue

Nonoperative
treatment
(bracing,
mobilization,
serial monitoring)

Failed nonoperative treatment
(neurologic deterioration,
translation
unacceptable deformity,
unmanageable pain)

Operative treatment
(posterior approach,
reduction as needed,
decompression as needed,
neutralization using
pedicle screw construct)

Note: Unless medical circumstances dictate otherwise, operative management is typically recommended for all patients with neurological deficits or if there is a loss of posterior column integrity.

16

Thoracolumbar Distraction-Extension Injuries

Y. Raja Rampersaud

Thoracolumbar distraction-extension injuries are uncommon. The mechanism of injury is the opposite of the more common flexion-distraction injuries and involves hyperextension. The extension moment causes tensile failure (distraction) of the vertebral body as well as tensile or compressive failure of the posterior elements. This injury pattern is most common in patients with stiff or kyphotic thoracolumbar spines; for example, those with ankylosing spondylitis (AS) and diffuse idiopathic skeletal hyperostosis (DISH).[1–5] These injures are most commonly seen at the thoracolumbar junction, although injuries in the mid-thoracic and lumbar spine are occasionally seen. Most occur as a result of low-energy trauma, such as a fall, although injuries from high-energy trauma can result in significant translation of the spine. The risk of neurologic injury varies but neurologic injury is much more likely to occur in the presence of spinal translation.

Classification

Distraction-extension injures are specifically described within the context of a classification system by Ferguson and Allen.[3] The authors reported one such injury in their series of 54 patients with thoracolumbar injuries. This particular mechanism of injury is not mentioned in the original Denis (or subsequent modifications) thoracolumbar injury classification system.[6] Distraction-extension injuries represent a B3 distraction injury in the Magerl (AO Group) thoracolumbar classification system, where only three such injuries out of 1445 (0.21%) were identified.[7] From a practical standpoint, it is simplest to think of this uncommon mechanism of injury as a reverse flexion-distraction injury, which can be morphologically sub-classified as follows: (1) osseous (injury to bone only), (2) soft-tissue (purely soft-tissue injury, such as transdiskal and ligamentous injuries), and (3) combination (osseous and soft-tissue injuries). Furthermore, the presence or absence of translation (subluxation/dislocation = grossly unstable) must be noted.

Workup

History

Because of the rarity of these injuries, the diagnosis may be easily overlooked. In addition, they are often due to minor trauma, where suspicion for a significant spinal injury is typically low. Consequently, a high index of suspicion for this injury should be maintained in kyphotic elderly patients complaining of back pain following minor or major thoracolumbar trauma.

Spinal Imaging

The presence of anterior vertebral column widening (i.e., distraction) on plain radiographs, computed tomography (CT), or magnetic resonance imaging (MRI) confirms the diagnosis of an extension-distraction mechanism of injury (**Fig. 16.1**). However, the transverse nature of this injury, concomitant degenerative changes, osteoporosis, and the difficulties visualizing the posterior elements on plain radiographs, as well as the propensity for the more stable injuries to reduce in flexion, may render this injury undetectable on plain radiographs. Consequently, CT with sagittal and coronal reformats (a transverse plane of fracture is easy to miss on axial slices) and MRI are the imaging modalities of choice.

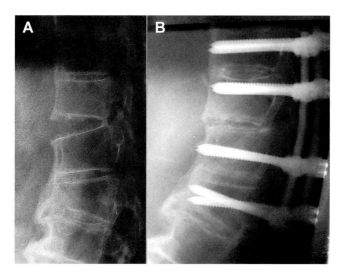

Fig. 16.1 **(A)** Lateral plain radiograph of the midthoracic spine, showing unstable fracture through ankylosed intervertebral elements without neurologic compromise. **(B)** Posterior fusion with pedicle screw instrumentation provides stable fixation.

Treatment

If a distraction-extension injury is suspected or diagnosed, then maintenance of the patient's normal alignment (for example, similar to cervical fractures in AS) should be pursued (i.e., maintain a patient-specific neutral position). For the neurologically intact patient with a purely or predominantly (anterior and middle column) osseous injury, nonoperative treatment with bed rest and progressive mobilization in a thoracolumbar orthosis that maintains a neutral or slightly flexed posture can be successful. (Note that extension braces commonly used for other thoracolumbar fractures are contraindicated.) In general, neurologic injury and/or evidence of posterior vertebral element injury or vertebral translation requires operative management. A patient with purely or predominantly soft-tissue injuries will also benefit from operative management because of the low likelihood of healing.

Using the recently described Thoracolumbar Injury Classification System and Severity Score (TLICS) from the Spine Trauma Study Group (STSG), which assigns points according to fracture morphology, neurologic status, and the integrity of the posterior column, most of these injuries will score at least seven points (four points for the extension/distraction morphology and three points for the posterior complex disruption), strongly suggesting surgery, four points being the cutoff point, even in the absence of neurologic deficit.[8] In a recent evidence-based review process by the STSG that assessed the question "Does surgical treatment improve the outcome of patients with AS or DISH with hyperextension fractures of the thoracolumbar spine?" a strong recommendation for operative treatment was supported.[9]

Patient medical factors must be strongly considered with these injuries because most patients are older and have multiple comorbidities. In most cases, operative management consists of a posterior approach, decompression or reduction as needed, and a neutralization segmental construct of appropriate length to provide adequate stability and enable rapid mobilization and rehabilitation. Pedicle screws are typically preferred, as they are best suited to reverse and resist the extension moment of these injuries (**Fig. 16.1**).

Outcomes

Although very limited data exist, the overall outcome for neurologically intact patients with this injury is very favorable. As with other injuries, the outcome following neurologic injury is multifactorial and is largely dependent on the degree of neurologic impairment at presentation.

Complications

Patients with the presence of a stiff/ankylosed and kyphotic thoracolumbar spine are at risk of increasing extension deformity or translation during transportation, transfers, or recumbency with "flat" positioning. These patient are particularly at risk during operative stabilization of their injuries, where typical prone, "belly free," positioning may significantly worsen an unstable distraction-extension injury. Therefore, appropriate bolstering to maintain and support patients in their specific pre-morbid spinal alignment (if it is known) is necessary.

References

1. Burkus JK, Denis F. Hyperextension injuries of the thoracic spine in diffuse idiopathic skeletal hyperostosis. Report of four cases. J Bone Joint Surg Am 1994;76(2):237–243
2. Dorr LD, Harvey JP Jr, Nickel VL. Clinical review of the early stability of spine injuries. Spine (Phila Pa 1976) 1982;7(6):545–550
3. Ferguson RL, Allen BL Jr. A mechanistic classification of thoracolumbar spine fractures. Clin Orthop Relat Res 1984;189(189):77–88
4. Ghavam C, Kirkpatrick JS. Extension-distraction fracture of the first lumbar vertebra. Spine (Phila Pa 1976) 1995;20(9):1080–1083
5. Hitchon PW, From AM, Brenton MD, Glaser JA, Torner JC. Fractures of the thoracolumbar spine complicating ankylosing spondylitis. J Neurosurg 2002;97(2, Suppl):218–222
6. Denis F. The three-column spine and its significance in the classification of acute thoracolumbar spinal injuries. Spine (Phila Pa 1976) 1983;8(8):817–831
7. Magerl F, Aebi M, Gertzbein SD, Harms J, Nazarian S. A comprehensive classification of thoracic and lumbar injuries. Eur Spine J 1994;3(4):184–201
8. Rihn JA, Anderson DT, Harris E, et al. A review of the TLICS system: a novel, user-friendly thoracolumbar trauma classification system. Acta Orthop 2008;79(4):461–466
9. Hedlund R, Verlaan JJ. Thoracolumbar hyperextension injuries in the stiff spine. In: Vaccaro AR, Fehlings MG, Dvorak MF, eds. Spine and Spinal Cord Trauma: Evidence-Based Management. New York, NY: Thieme; 2011:391–399

Suggested Reading

Burkus JK, Denis F. Hyperextension injuries of the thoracic spine in diffuse idiopathic skeletal hyperostosis. Report of four cases. J Bone Joint Surg Am 1994;76(2):237–243

> *The authors conclude that these injuries in this patient population are unstable, and they recommend operative treatment.*

Hedlund R, Verlaan JJ. Thoracolumbar hyperextension injuries in the stiff spine. In: Vaccaro AR, Fehlings MG, Dvorak MF, eds. Spine and Spinal Cord Trauma: Evidence-Based Management. New York, NY: Thieme; 2011:391–399

> *This systematic review provides the most comprehensive look at the literature related to this topic and provides the insight and treatment recommendations of a multinational group of spine trauma experts (Spine Trauma Study Group). In the stiff spine, these injuries are considered unstable, with a high potential for translation and catastrophic neurological injury. Surgical stabilization is generally recommended.*

Hitchon PW, From AM, Brenton MD, Glaser JA, Torner JC. Fractures of the thoracolumbar spine complicating ankylosing spondylitis. J Neurosurg 2002;97(2, Suppl):218–222

> *The predisposition of the ankylosed spine to extension fractures (9 out of 11 patients) is reported. Over 50% were neurologically impaired, and 9 underwent operative intervention.*

III Cervical Degenerative/ Metabolic Disease

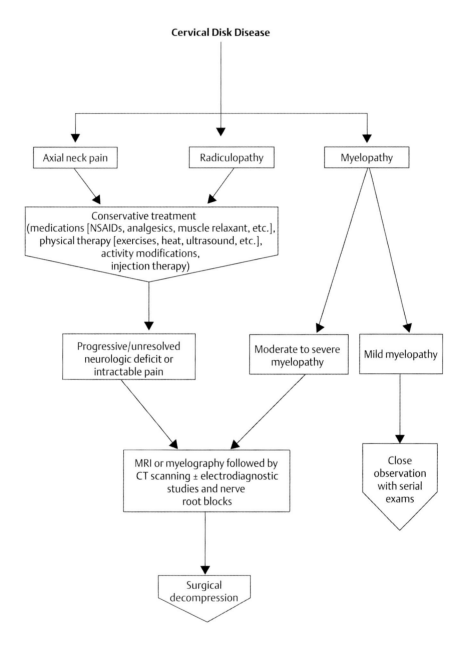

Cervical Disk Disease

Axial neck pain

Radiculopathy

Myelopathy

Conservative treatment
(medications [NSAIDs, analgesics, muscle relaxant, etc.],
physical therapy [exercises, heat, ultrasound, etc.],
activity modifications,
injection therapy)

Progressive/unresolved
neurologic deficit or
intractable pain

Moderate to severe
myelopathy

Mild myelopathy

MRI or myelography followed by
CT scanning ± electrodiagnostic
studies and nerve
root blocks

Close
observation
with serial
exams

Surgical
decompression

CT, computed tomography; MRI, magnetic resonance imaging;
NSAIDs, nonsteroidal anti-inflammatory drugs

17

Cervical Disk Degeneration

Kanit Chamroontaneskul

Cervical disk degeneration is commonly a matter of gradual, age-related deterioration of the intervertebral disks, but the condition is also affected by lifestyle, genetics, cigarette smoking, nutrition, and physical activity. Some people with disk degeneration develop symptoms, while others who also have disk degeneration remain asymptomatic. The reason for these differences is unclear. Most symptomatic disk degeneration occurs at the C5–C6 and C6–C7 levels, followed by the C4–C5 level. Two general types of symptoms are seen: axial neck pain, often due to disk degeneration itself, and neurologic symptoms due to a disk herniation resulting in compression of the nerve roots or the spinal cord.

The normal aging process begins with disk desiccation, resulting in a decrease in the water content of the nucleus pulposus and weakening of the annulus fibrosus. With desiccation, the disk loses height and may bulge or permit the extrusion of nuclear material into the spinal canal or neural foramen, leading to compression of the neural structures. As the degenerative process progresses in conjunction with the more global process of cervical spondylosis, osteophytes develop along the posterior aspects of the uncovertebral joint, facet joint, and vertebral body. As the segment collapses, the ligamentum flavum can buckle inward, compromising the space available for the neural elements.

Classification

Cervical disk disease has been categorized by Odom et al. into four groups: (1) unilateral soft disk protrusion with nerve root compression, (2) foraminal spur or hard disk formation with nerve root compression, (3) central soft disk protrusion with spinal cord compression, and (4) transverse ridging from cervical spondylosis with spinal cord compression.

Workup

History

Cervical disk disease may present with general nonspecific symptoms, including axial neck pain, stiffness, loss of motion, and shoulder girdle pain. Posterior neck pain, worse with head extension and rotation, suggests a discogenic or facetogenic component, and posterior neck muscle pain, worse with head flexion, suggests a more common myofascial etiology. Neurologic symptoms may include radiculopathy or, less commonly, myelopathy.

Radiculopathy presents as radiating pain into the arm(s), numbness, motor weakness, and posterior shoulder pain. Myelopathy presents with symptoms of arm and leg dysfunction, including weakness, numbness, and clumsiness in the hands, walking difficulties, and frequent falls.

Physical Examination

Patients with discogenic neck pain without nerve root involvement demonstrate a normal neurologic examination, decreased cervical range of motion, pain exacerbation with axial compression, and pain alleviation with neck distraction. Myofascial tenderness or trigger points, which may be primary in origin or secondary to other pathologic processes, are commonly palpable.

Physical examination of the patient with radiculopathy may reveal weakness or decreased sensation along the affected dermatome. A Spurling test is often positive (increased radicular symptoms with neck rotation, lateral bending toward the affected side, and extension). Common physical findings due to myelopathy include hyperreflexia, spasticity, clonus, and pathologic reflexes (Hoffmann sign and Babinski reflexes).

Spinal Imaging

Because of a high rate of asymptomatic changes present on radiologic studies, any radiologic findings that reveal degenerative changes must be correlated with the patient's symptoms. Initial evaluation should include plain radiographs, which may show disk space narrowing, osteophyte formation, possible metastatic disease, spinal deformity, and spine instability. Magnetic resonance imaging (MRI) is the standard diagnostic test for evaluation of the spine because of its excellent resolution in differentiating soft tissue, such as disk, ligament, and neural elements (**Fig. 17.1**). However, MRI is less adequate in visualizing the neural foramen and in assessing hard disk pathology or ossification of the posterior longitudinal ligament (OPLL). In these cases, myelography followed by computed tomography (CT) scanning is useful. Electrodiagnostic studies and nerve root blocks may play a role in evaluating or localizing neurologic lesions. Provocative cervical diskography has been controversial but may identify a symptomatic disk, assisting in evaluation of patients with inconclusive diagnostic tests and presurgical fusion planning.

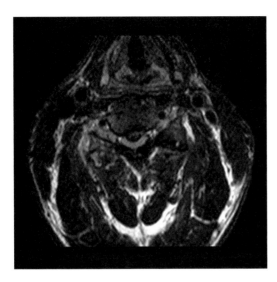

Fig. 17.1 Axial MRI T2 view of the C4–5 level showing the flattening of the spinal cord and myelomalacia secondary to cervical disk degeneration and herniation.

 Treatment

Nonoperative

The initial treatment of symptomatic cervical disk degeneration is supportive, including rest, activity modification, medications (nonsteroidal anti-inflammatory drugs or NSAIDs, analgesics, muscle relaxants, and antidepressants), intermittent soft collar immobilization, and physical therapy. Cervical traction may be beneficial in some patients with radicular pain. Selective nerve root injections with local anesthetic agents with or without steroids may serve a diagnostic and therapeutic role. Most patients with cervical disk disease will respond to a multifaceted nonoperative treatment approach. However, up to one-third of patients with radicular symptoms may fail to improve and may benefit from surgical intervention. In contrast, patients with myelopathy will generally continue to be symptomatic and may experience progressive deterioration over time.

Operative Treatment

The indications for surgical treatment in patients with cervical disk disease include persistent or recurrent radicular pain unresponsive to appropriate conservative measures for 6–8 weeks, progressive or persistent neurologic deficit, and cervical myelopathy in the setting of significant neurocompressive lesion from imaging studies.

Operative treatment for axial neck pain without evidence of radiculopathy or myelopathy is controversial and is used only in selective cases that fail all conservative treatments. However, some studies have demonstrated a substantial decrease in pain and improved function after anterior cervical decompression and fusion (ACDF) for axial neck pain.

Outcome

A majority of patients with axial neck pain and cervical radiculopathy will experience improvement in symptoms, at least initially, with conservative treatment. In patients with progressive or unresolved neurodeficit and intractable radicular pain, adequate surgical decompression usually achieves good results. Cervical spine surgery, however, is less reliable for relief of axial pain than for radicular pain. In patients with myelopathy, surgical decompression usually can arrest myelopathic progression, but recovery of neural function is variable, depending on severity of spinal cord dysfunction. The result is more favorable in early mild to moderate spinal cord dysfunction.

Complications

Complications include failure to improve, persistent pain, adverse reactions to NSAIDs, narcotics, and all the general complications related to cervical spine surgery.

Suggested Readings

Garvey TA, Transfeldt EE, Malcolm JR, Kos P. Outcome of anterior cervical discectomy and fusion as perceived by patients treated for dominant axial-mechanical cervical spine pain. Spine (Phila Pa 1976) 2002;27(17):1887–1895, discussion 1895

This retrospective study reports significant pain relief and good outcome in patients who underwent ACDF for chronic axial neck pain.

Okada E, Matsumoto M, Ichihara D, et al. Aging of the cervical spine in healthy volunteers: a 10-year longitudinal magnetic resonance imaging study. Spine (Phila Pa 1976) 2009;34(7):706–712

This study clarifies the normal aging process of cervical spine and correlation between progression of disc degeneration and development of clinical symptoms.

Peolsson A. Investigation of clinically important benefit of anterior cervical decompression and fusion. Eur Spine J 2007;16(4):507–514

This study reports the clinically relevant change after ACDF.

Rao RD, Currier BL, Albert TJ, et al. Degenerative cervical spondylosis: clinical syndromes, pathogenesis, and management. J Bone Joint Surg Am 2007;89(6):1360–1378

This is an excellent review of clinical presentation, pathogenesis, and treatment options for cervical spondylosis.

Sambrook PN, MacGregor AJ, Spector TD. Genetic influences on cervical and lumbar disc degeneration: a magnetic resonance imaging study in twins. Arthritis Rheum 1999;42(2):366–372

This study suggests an important influence on variation in intervertebral disk degeneration.

Walraevens J, Liu B, Meersschaert J, et al. Qualitative and quantitative assessment of degeneration of cervical intervertebral discs and facet joints. Eur Spine J 2009;18(3):358–369

This study proposes a scoring system to describe and quantify cervical disk degeneration and to evaluate the relationship between degeneration and biomechanic parameters.

Zeidman SM. Evaluation of patients with cervical spine lesions. In: Clark CR, ed. The Cervical Spine. 4th ed. Philadelphia, PA: Lippincott-Raven; 2005:149–165

This chapter provides a detailed description of clinical presentation, physical examination, and evaluation of patients with cervical disk problems.

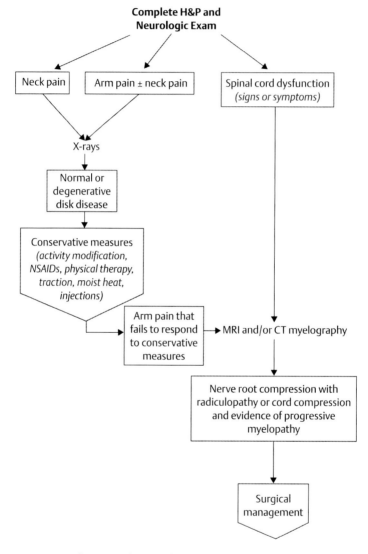

CT, computed tomographic; H&P, history and physical exam; MRI, magnetic resonance imaging; NSAIDs, nonsteroidal anti-inflammatory drugs

18

Cervical Radiculopathy

Gregory Gebauer and D. Greg Anderson

Cervical disk degeneration is a normal part of aging and is found in ~85% of individuals by the seventh decade of life. Although most people do not have major symptoms resulting from the degenerative process, a subset develop neck or arm pain and may require medical intervention. The term *radiculopathy* denotes the constellation of symptoms caused by compression and/or inflammation of a nerve root, including radiating arm pain, sensory changes and/or motor loss. Nonsurgical treatment is the mainstay of treatment for most patients with neck pain and is the initial treatment offered to patients with symptoms of radiculopathy. Those who fail to respond and have continued severe radicular symptoms are candidates for surgical intervention. The usual underlying pathology involves compression of the neural elements by a combination of herniated disk material and/or osteophytes secondary to spondylosis. The pathophysiology of cervical disk degeneration involves dehydration of the nucleus pulposus and weakening and fissuring of the annulus fibrosus. This combination may allow herniation of nuclear material into the spinal canal or neural foramen. Additionally, the specialized uncovertebral joints of Luschka may form bony osteophytes that compress the cervical nerve roots as they enter the neural foramen.

 Workup

History

Patients with cervical radiculopathy will classically present with complaints of pain radiating from the cervical region and down the arm along a particular dermatomal distribution. There are often associated symptoms of sensory changes (numbness or tingling) or weakness. The pain is often described as sharp, shooting, lancinating, or numbing. There is frequently associated pain along the medial border of the scapula.

Physical Examination

A complete spinal and neurologic physical examination should be performed. Affected patients will commonly exhibit decreased range of motion and avoid neck positions (extension and/or rotation) that aggravate the pain. It is common to note minor changes in strength and sensation that are related to the affected nerve root. The reflex arc of the affected nerve root is generally depressed. A Spurling test (cervical extension, rotation, and lateral bending toward the affected side) or axial compression will usually reproduce or worsen the radicular pain. Axial traction generally lessens radicular pain. A differential diagnosis should be considered, including shoulder pathology, brachial plexopathy, peripheral nerve entrapment, or coronary artery disease.

Spinal Imaging

Plain radiographs will often demonstrate disk space narrowing and osteophyte formation. Magnetic resonance imaging (MRI) is the most useful study in patients with radiculopathy and can be used to show disk herniation, foraminal narrowing, and neural element compression. Computed tomography (CT) with myelography can be utilized in patients unable to undergo MRI.

Treatment

In the absence of major neurologic loss, conservative measures should be pursued initially. Conservative care includes activity modification, anti-inflammatory drugs, gentle active exercises, cervical traction, and spinal injections. Acute radiculopathies often respond to conservative measures, although the potential for recurrent symptoms exists. Indications for surgical management for cervical radiculopathy generally include severe pain despite 6 to 12 weeks of conservative therapy or progressive/severe neurologic deficits.

Surgical intervention can be pursued with one of four available treatment approaches: anterior cervical discectomy and fusion (ACDF), anterior foraminotomy, anterior cervical discectomy and artificial disk replacement, or posterior cervical foraminotomy. Each approach has certain advantages and disadvantages. At the current time, the ACDF approach is the most common surgical procedure done for cervical radiculopathy worldwide.

Outcome

Up to two-thirds of those with radiculopathy obtain improvement with conservative measures. Patients failing to respond have a high success rate for surgery, with rates of arm pain relief in many studies ranging from 85% to 95%.

Complications

Complications of treatment include recurrent symptoms (with nonoperative care or foraminotomies), swallowing problems, vocal cord paralysis, and adjacent segment degeneration.

Suggested Readings

Boden SDWS. Nonoperative management of cervical disc disease. In: Camins MB, O'Leary PF, eds. Disorders of the Cervical Spine. Baltimore, MD: Williams & Wilkins; 1992:157–164

This is a good review of the history, clinical examination, and management of cervical disk disease.

Davidson RI, Dunn EJ, Metzmaker JN. The shoulder abduction test in the diagnosis of radicular pain in cervical extradural compressive monoradiculopathies. Spine (Phila Pa 1976) 1981;6(5):441–446

This study describes patients with cervical radiculopathies who experienced relief of their symptoms with abduction of the shoulder.

Heller JG. The syndromes of degenerative cervical disease. Orthop Clin North Am 1992;23(3): 381–394

This study describes the patho-anatomic changes in the cervical spine that lead to clinical radicular and myelopathic symptoms.

Jenis LG, An HS. Neck pain secondary to radiculopathy of the fourth cervical root: an analysis of 12 surgically treated patients. J Spinal Disord 2000;13(4):345–349

This article describes the results of surgical intervention in a series of patients with radicular neck pain from involvement of the C4 nerve root.

Swezey RL, Swezey AM, Warner K. Efficacy of home cervical traction therapy. Am J Phys Med Rehabil 1999;78(1):30–32

This article describes the treatment and outcome of cervical radiculopathy with traction.

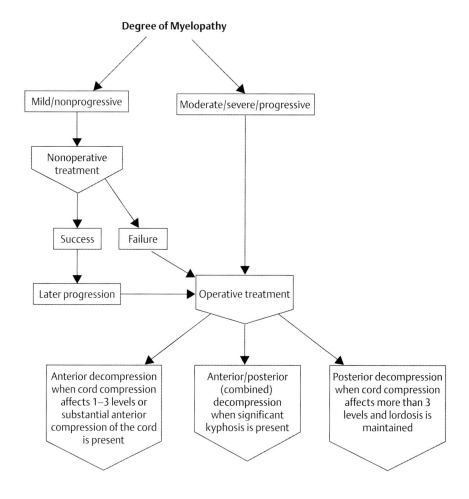

19

Cervical Myelopathy: Anterior Approach

Gregory Gebauer, Alan S. Hilibrand, and Maurice Goins

Myelopathy is a constellation of symptoms resulting from spinal cord dysfunction due to compression on the spinal cord. Symptoms are often vague and tend to progress over time. The spinal cord can be compressed from anterior structures, such as disk herniations or osteophytes, or from posterior structures, including the facet joints and ligamentum flavum. While mild cases can be treated with observation, most cases require surgical decompression. Anterior, posterior, and combined approaches can be used depending on the location of the compression, extent of disease, number of levels involved, posture of the cervical spine, and other patient and disease related factors.

In its normal state, the cervical spine is in lordotic posture as a result of the anterior disk height being slightly greater than the posterior disk height. The disk functions to dissipate the energy of vertical forces, but with aging it sustains weakening of the annular fibers, leading to posterior protrusion, loss of disk height, and redundancy of the ligamentum flavum, which encroaches on the spinal canal and decreases the space available for the spinal cord. In addition, decreased disk height can lead to loss of the normal lordotic curvature and development of a kyphotic posture. This causes the spinal cord to be further draped over anterior structures and can lead to increased pressure on the cord.

Biomechanically, disk degeneration transfers stress to the vertebral endplates, resulting in the formation of osteophytes along the margins of the disk space and behind the uncovertebral joints. By age 50, at least half of patients will have radiographic evidence of spondylosis. Although most will remain asymptomatic, in some individuals these may contribute to further compression of the spinal canal.

Classification

Cervical myelopathy is graded from 0 to V using the Nurick classification. This classification takes ambulatory ability into account in determining the grade (**Table 19.1**).

 Workup

Symptoms of cervical spondylotic myelopathy are often vague and may include neck pain or stiffness, numbness and tingling, loss of fine finger dexterity, and gait disturbances. Changes in dexterity may manifest as difficulty buttoning shirts or manipulating small objects and/or changes in handwriting. Patients may complain of gait unsteadiness and may appear to have a wide-based or waddling style of gait. In severe cases, bowel and/or bladder function may be affected.

Clinical findings in myelopathy often include a wide-based gait, difficulty with tandem gait, upper and/or lower extremity weakness, hyperreflexia, intrinsic hand muscle wasting, and the presence of abnormal reflexes, such as Babinski reflex, Hoffmann sign, inverted radial reflex, ulnar escape sign, and ankle clonus. Initial radiographic assessment begins with evaluation of plain radiographs, including anteroposterior (AP), lateral, and flexion-extension lateral views (**Fig. 19.1A,B**). Observed changes may include spondylosis, loss of lordosis, or subluxations.

Patients with symptoms of myelopathy require advanced imaging, such as magnetic resonance imaging (MRI) or computed tomography (CT) myelogram, to assess compression of the spinal cord. MRI is generally ordered first because it is noninvasive and demonstrates cord compression and changes in spinal cord parenchyma (**Fig. 19.2**). Increased signal intensity in spinal cord parenchyma on T2 images may represent spinal cord edema and/or myelomalacia and is considered to be a sign of significant compression.

Table 19.1 The Nurick Classification

Grade 0	Root signs and symptoms, no cord involvement
Grade I	Signs of cord involvement, normal gait
Grade II	Mild gait involvement, able to be employed
Grade III	Gait abnormality prevents employment
Grade IV	Able to ambulate only with assistance
Grade V	Chair-bound or bedridden

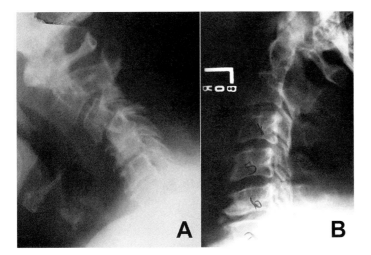

Fig. 19.1 **(A)** Flexion plain radiograph demonstrating instability in a severely spondylotic cervical spine with motion. **(B)** Extension plain radiograph showing osteophytes located on the posterior surface of the vertebral bodies, illustrating how they can lead to compression of the spinal cord.

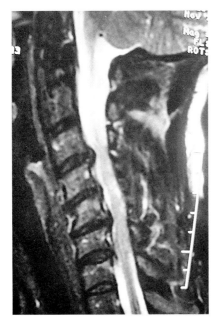

Fig. 19.2 Sagittal cervical MRI demonstrating spinal cord impingement and signal intensity in the spinal cord.

Treatment Options

Treatment of cervical myelopathy is geared toward preservation of neurologic function. In the early stages of myelopathy, careful observation and treatment of neck pain with gentle and nonsteroidal anti-inflammatory drugs (NSAID) can be used. Care should be taken to observe any signs of neurologic progression. Patients should be instructed to avoid activities at high risk for neck injuries. Patients should be carefully re-examined at intervals, looking for changes in spinal cord functioning.

Surgery is generally considered in those patients with progressive symptoms or in patients with moderate to severe myelopathy leading to a decrease in function. The primary goal of surgery is to prevent further declines in neurologic function, although functional improvement may be achieved following decompression in patients with early to moderate myelopathy. Even older patients have the potential to improve following adequate decompression.

Surgery should be designed to decompress the spinal cord and nerve roots via an anterior, posterior or combined anterior/posterior approach. Anterior decompression is preferred when the site of cord compression affects one to three levels or substantial anterior compression of the cord is present (**Fig. 19.3**). The advantages of anterior surgery include less postoperative pain (due to the decreased muscle dissection required), the ability to address compression from anterior structures (such as large disk herniations) directly, and the ability to restore the normal lumbar lordosis. The disadvantages of anterior surgery include increased risk of dysphagia, particularly in older patients, and an increased

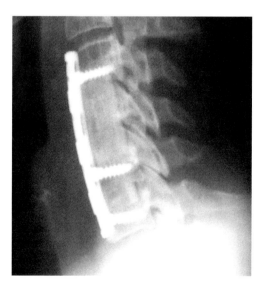

Fig. 19.3 Lateral radiograph shows an implanted plate and screws that are commonly used in anterior cervical fusion procedures. The strut graft can be seen, as well as the corpectomy graft.

pseudarthrosis risk when addressing multiple levels. In addition, when addressing multiple levels, exposure through a cosmetically appealing transverse incision can be difficult, and a less appealing oblique incision may be required. During an anterior approach, the esophagus and trachea are retracted laterally to expose the anterior spine. The disks and/or vertebral bodies are removed as necessary and the operated segments are typically stabilized by using bone graft, either autograft harvested from the patient or cadaveric allograft. Alternatively, metal or polyetheretherketone (PEEK) cages have also been used. Surgical implants, such as metallic plates and screws, are used as an adjunct to secure the implanted graft(s) and to stabilize the segment until the bone graft consolidates. Recently, the use of cervical disk arthroplasty has also been suggested for one-level disease, with results that appear to be clinically equivalent to traditional decompression and fusion.

Posterior approaches involve the removal of the lamina and often involve fusions as well. The advantages of a posterior approach include the ability to address many levels at one time and the decreased risk of pseudarthrosis compared with multilevel anterior surgery. The disadvantages include increased postoperative pain, increased risk of infection, and increased blood loss. In addition, posterior surgery alone should not be performed in patients with fixed kyphotic posture, as these patients will tend to have continued progression of their kyphotic deformity, leading to increased disability, pain, and further neurologic decline. These patients may require either anterior surgery alone or combined anterior and posterior surgery.

Outcomes

With anterior decompression for moderate myelopathy, ~90% of patients will experience significant improvement of neurologic function. Patients with severe neurologic deficits prior to surgery generally experience less improvement in symptoms. Patients who achieve a solid fusion have better outcomes than those who develop nonunion. In comparing anterior procedures to posterior procedures, Wada et al. showed no difference in neurologic recovery at the ten-year follow-up time point, although those treated with anterior corpectomy did experience more axial neck pain.

Complications

Complications of all cervical spine procedures include neurologic injury, inadequate decompression with persistent symptoms, and dural tears with cerebrospinal fluid (CSF) leaks. Complications more likely with anterior procedures include vertebral artery injury, nonunion, hardware failure, dysphagia, dysphonia, and graft dislodgement. Complications that may result from a posterior procedure include the development of instability (if laminectomy is performed without a fusion), wound infection, development of axial neck pain, and hardware failure.

Suggested Readings

Bolesta MJ, Rechtine GR II, Chrin AM. Three- and four-level anterior cervical discectomy and fusion with plate fixation: a prospective study. Spine 2000;25(16):2040–2044, discussion 2045–2046

> *This study evaluates the outcomes of multilevel anterior cervical discectomy and fusion (ACDF) with hardware and shows that such patients show an unacceptably high rate of nonunion of bone graft.*

Emery SE, Bohlman HH, Bolesta MJ, Jones PK. Anterior cervical decompression and arthrodesis for the treatment of cervical spondylotic myelopathy. Two to seventeen-year follow-up. J Bone Joint Surg Am 1998;80(7):941–951

> *This study evaluates ACDF surgery with significant follow-up and gives some general statistics regarding success rates of the procedure.*

Heller JG, Edwards CC II, Murakami H, Rodts GE. Laminoplasty versus laminectomy and fusion for multilevel cervical myelopathy: an independent matched cohort analysis. Spine 2001; 26(12):1330–1336

> *This study compares two posterior procedures, laminectomy and laminoplasty, and shows that laminoplasty has both higher recovery rates and decreased complication rates.*

Koakutsu T, Morozumi N, Ishii Y, et al. Anterior decompression and fusion versus laminoplasty for cervical myelopathy caused by soft disc herniation: a prospective multicenter study. J Orthop Sci 2010;15(1):71–78

> *The authors compared 30 patients treated with ACDF and 30 patients treated with laminoplasty for soft disk herniations causing myelopathy. The patients had equivalent outcomes at 1 year.*

Matsuda Y, Shibata T, Oki S, Kawatani Y, Mashima N, Oishi H. Outcomes of surgical treatment for cervical myelopathy in patients more than 75 years of age. Spine 1999;24(6):529–534

> *This study shows that although outcomes for patients older than 75 years are generally poorer than those for younger patients, adequate recovery is made that allows the patients to return to independent living.*

Riew KD, Buchowski JM, Sasso R, Zdeblick T, Metcalf NH, Anderson PA. Cervical disc arthroplasty compared with arthrodesis for the treatment of myelopathy. J Bone Joint Surg Am 2008;90(11):2354–2364

> *The authors compared 106 patients who had undergone ACDF and 93 who had had a cervical disk replacement for the treatment of single-level myelopathy. They reported equivalent outcomes at 1 year.*

Vaccaro AR, Falatyn SP, Scuderi GJ, et al. Early failure of long segment anterior cervical plate fixation. J Spinal Disord 1998;11(5):410–415

> *The authors observed a high rate of failure when anterior plates were used to stabilize three-level corpectomy/strut graft constructs and recommended an adjunct posterior stabilization procedure in this setting.*

Wada E, Suzuki S, Kanazawa A, Matsuoka T, Miyamoto S, Yonenobu K. Subtotal corpectomy versus laminoplasty for multilevel cervical spondylotic myelopathy: a long-term follow-up study over 10 years. Spine 2001;26(13):1443–1447, discussion 1448

> *This study compares anterior and posterior procedures over a long follow-up of 10 years. It reports that the recovery rates are comparable for the two approaches, but axial pain is decreased with anterior procedures.*

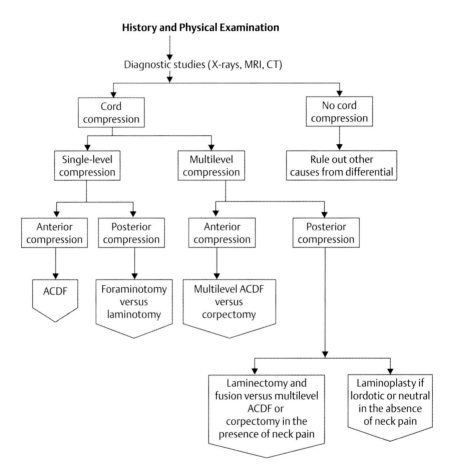

History and Physical Examination

Diagnostic studies (X-rays, MRI, CT)

Cord compression

No cord compression

Single-level compression

Multilevel compression

Rule out other causes from differential

Anterior compression

Posterior compression

Anterior compression

Posterior compression

ACDF

Foraminotomy versus laminotomy

Multilevel ACDF versus corpectomy

Laminectomy and fusion versus multilevel ACDF or corpectomy in the presence of neck pain

Laminoplasty if lordotic or neutral in the absence of neck pain

ACDF, anterior cervical discectomy and fusion; CT, computed tomography; MRI, magnetic resonance imaging

20

Cervical Myelopathy: Posterior Approach

Andrew K. Simpson, Stewart Kerr, and Andrew P. White

Cervical spondylotic myelopathy is the most common cause of spinal cord dysfunction in older individuals. The onset of symptoms, however, can be insidious. The stepwise progression of the disease is slow and may be difficult to predict. Since the natural history of the disease is variable, management can be challenging.

Surgical intervention has been shown to prevent neurologic deterioration and to provide superior outcomes as compared with conservative management.[1] Because surgery can reliably halt the progression of disease, but typically not reliably reverse symptoms or reliably restore pre-disease function, there is significant interest in determining the factors that would predict which patients are likely to have progressive neurologic decline. Thus, current research efforts are focused on elucidating the anatomic, physiologic, and genetic features that influence the development of progressive myelopathy in patients who have spinal cord compression.

Classification

The Nurick classification, a 6-point scale from 0 (root signs but no cord involvement) to V (chair-bound or bedridden), is the most commonly utilized system for categorizing the degree of myelopathy.[2] A modified Nurick classification system has also been utilized in which grade 0 identifies patients with no symptoms and grades I through VI correspond to the classic grading system.[3] The Japanese Orthopedic Association has also developed a scoring system for cervical myelopathy, termed the JOA score, based on degree of motor and sensory dysfunction in the extremities and urinary dysfunction. This system is more complex and specific than the Nurick classification and consequently is less commonly utilized.

Workup

A careful history is imperative in the evaluation of myelopathy, as the symptoms of cord compression are often vague and can relate to difficulty with ambulation and extremity dysfunction, which patients may not necessarily relate to spinal disease. For instance, loss of upper-extremity dexterity and decreased fine motor skills will manifest as difficulty manipulating small objects, as in buttoning shirts, or difficulty with handwriting or typing. Patients may also note difficulty with balance or bowel/bladder dysfunction. When taking a history, family members may be helpful in corroborating subtle changes in gait or dexterity of which patients themselves may be unaware.

The physical examination of patients with myelopathy is paramount for both diagnosis and surgical decision making. Clinical symptomatology and the severity of myelopathy are widely variable among patients with identical imaging studies. Furthermore, clinical manifestations, rather than imaging findings, dictate the need for surgical intervention.

Patients with cervical spondylotic myelopathy demonstrate upper motor neuron findings in the lower extremities and mixed upper and lower motor neuron findings in the upper extremities. For instance, C5–C6 pathology may cause flaccid weakness of the deltoid and biceps with concomitant spasticity of the triceps, wrist flexors, and lower extremities. Patients who demonstrate lower motor neuron signs in the lower extremities should be evaluated for lumbar spine pathology, as lumbar and cervical stenosis are associated and can occur in conjunction.

The most common initial signs and symptoms of cervical myelopathy are: (1) gait abnormalities, (2) upper-extremity clumsiness, (3) spasticity of the extremities (lower more frequent than upper), (4) multisegmental sensory involvement, (5) Hoffmann sign, and (6) Lhermitte sign. Gait dysfunction is most often characterized by a broad-based, shuffling gait resultant from lower extremity spasticity and proprioceptive deficits. Upper-extremity examination is likely to reveal a mixed picture of flaccid and spastic weakness, whereas lower-extremity examination is often characterized by spasticity, hyperreflexia, positive Babinski sign, and clonus.

Spinal Imaging

The initial diagnostic imaging evaluation of cervical myelopathy should consist of plain radiographs of the cervical spine, including anteroposterior (AP), lateral, and flexion-extension films. Cervical myelopathy can result from both primary congenital cervical stenosis and acquired cervical stenosis, each of which has unique radiographic findings. Congenital cervical stenosis is relatively rare and results from abnormal development of the vertebral column. Patients with congenital stenosis are predisposed to spinal cord injury from minor trauma. Acquired cervical stenosis, or cervical spondylosis, refers to the more common pathology of age-related changes to the cervical spine. The AP diameter of the spinal canal can be assessed on lateral radiographs and Pavlov's ratio (AP diameter of the canal over that of the vertebral body) calculated. A value less than 0.8 is associated with neurologic changes and worse outcome. In the case of congenital stenosis, decreased canal diameters occur at the level of the mid-vertebral body (developmental segmental sagittal diameter), whereas in cervical spondylosis, decreased canal diameters are seen near the endplates secondary to encroachment of the intervertebral disk and osteophytes into the spinal canal (spondylotic segmental sagittal diameter). Flexion-extension radiographs are helpful for assessing dynamic changes, such as spondylolisthesis, which can result in positional symptomatology and demonstrate potential dynamic instability. This is of particular importance, as these patients demonstrate particularly good outcomes with surgical decompression and fusion.[4]

The current gold standard imaging technique for evaluation of patients with cervical spondylosis is magnetic resonance imaging (MRI), as it provides multiplanar images that visualize neural elements, intervertebral disks, and ligamentum flavum, accurately identifying the location(s) of cord compression. Furthermore, MRI can detect the presence of signal change (myelomalacia) within the spinal cord, which may be associated with more severe cord compression and may have prognostic significance. A sagittal MRI demonstrating multilevel spondylosis and associated myelomalacia is demonstrated in **Fig. 20.1**. Ossification of the posterior longitudinal ligament (OPLL), an entity that can result in cervical myelopathy independent of other spondylotic changes, is best seen on computed tomography (CT) studies, but can also be characterized on MRI in many cases. CT and CT myelography are useful in assessing bony structures, including the neural foramen, though they are less commonly utilized with the availability of MRI.

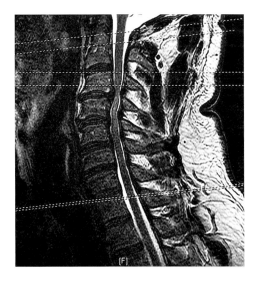

Fig. 20.1   Sagittal T2 MRI demonstrating multilevel cervical stenosis and associated myelomalacia.

Treatment

The treatment of cervical myelopathy is aimed at the preservation of neurologic function. Nonsurgical treatment options can provide symptomatic relief, such as analgesics, anti-inflammatory medications including steroids, and antispasmodic agents, but in the presence of significant myelopathy, radiculopathy, and/or neurogenic claudication, surgical intervention is warranted.

One challenging aspect of treating patients with myelopathy has been determining which patients are likely to progress and thus merit early surgical intervention. Recently, three risk factors for progression have been elucidated: (1) MRI cord changes (multilevel high-intensity changes on T2 and low-intensity changes on T1), (2) concordant radiculopathy, and (3) electromyography changes. The role of electrophysiological evaluation in these patients remains undefined as of yet, but given recent data, electromyography (EMG) may serve as an important tool in following patients with cervical spondylosis and determining who will benefit most from surgery in the future. Surgical decompressions can be performed via anterior, posterior, or combined approaches.

Posterior approaches for cervical decompression are classically utilized for patients with multilevel cord compression with preserved lordosis. The maintenance of lordosis is imperative when considering posterior decompression, as this allows the cord to migrate posteriorly or "float" away from the anterior compression once the posterior elements are modified or removed. In addition, postoperative kyphotic deformity and instability are more likely to occur after posterior decompression in patients who do not demonstrate adequate preoperative lordosis.

Posterior cervical spine decompression can be performed through laminectomy or laminoplasty. Traditionally, laminectomy alone was performed in these patients as removal of the entire dorsal portion of the spinal canal. Laminectomy alone provides excellent decompression, but long-term follow-up studies of these patients have demonstrated several major complications, including instability, postoperative kyphotic deformity, and late neurologic deterioration. During 2002–2012 in particular, studies have demonstrated significant advantages of laminectomy with fusion or laminoplasty over laminectomy alone, specifically better neurologic recovery (strength and gait), decreased pain, and decreased incidence of major complications.[5] **Figure 20.2** demonstrates anteroposterior and lateral plain radiographs of a patient following multilevel laminectomy with fusion. In patients with multilevel cervical myelopathy, laminectomy with fusion and laminoplasty have also demonstrated favorable results over anterior surgery (multilevel anterior decompression and fusion [ACDF]) with greater postoperative neurologic recovery, better range of motion, and lower complication rates, although systematic reviews have demonstrated greater postoperative pain with posterior decompressions (**Fig. 20.2**).[6,7]

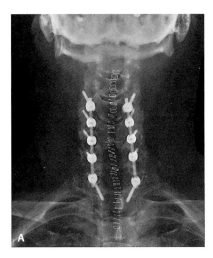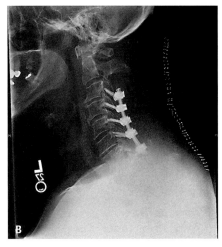

Fig. 20.2   Cervical spine radiographs of patient following posterior multilevel laminectomy and fusion. **(A)** AP. **(B)** Lateral.

Outcomes

Multilevel laminectomy with fusion has demonstrated favorable results. Kumar et al. and Gok et al. evaluated patients with an average follow-up greater than 2 years and similarly found rates of neurologic recovery of 76% and 81%, respectively.[8,9] Results after laminoplasty for multilevel cervical myelopathy have also been encouraging. Wang et al. reported on 204 patients who underwent laminoplasty and followed them on average for 16 months.[10] Laminoplasty prevented further neurologic decline in all but three patients, and neurologic improvement was demonstrated in 56% of patients, half of whom had improvement greater than or equal to two Nurick classification grades. Kawaguchi et al. followed laminoplasty patients for a 10-year period and found a similar functional recovery rate (58%), which was maintained over the 10-year period.[11]

Complications

Complications associated with posterior approaches for cervical myelopathy decompression include nerve root traction or neuropraxia injury (most commonly to C5), dural sac injury, postoperative infection, and loss of lordosis or late kyphotic deformity. Laminectomy with fusion inherently has slightly higher rates of graft complications, but it seems to have more predictable neurologic recovery as compared with laminoplasty.

References

1. Sampath P, Bendebba M, Davis JD, Ducker TB. Outcome of patients treated for cervical myelopathy. A prospective, multicenter study with independent clinical review. Spine 2000; 25(6):670–676
2. Nurick S. The natural history and the results of surgical treatment of the spinal cord disorder associated with cervical spondylosis. Brain 1972;95(1):101–108
3. O'Brien MF, Peterson D, Casey AT, Crockard HA. A novel technique for laminoplasty augmentation of spinal canal area using titanium miniplate stabilization. A computerized morphometric analysis. Spine 1996;21(4):474–483, discussion 484
4. Dean CL, Gabriel JP, Cassinelli EH, Bolesta MJ, Bohlman HH. Degenerative spondylolisthesis of the cervical spine: analysis of 58 patients treated with anterior cervical decompression and fusion. Spine J 2009;9(6):439–446
5. Heller JG, Edwards CC II, Murakami H, Rodts GE. Laminoplasty versus laminectomy and fusion for multilevel cervical myelopathy: an independent matched cohort analysis. Spine 2001;26(12):1330–1336
6. Edwards CC II, Heller JG, Murakami H. Corpectomy versus laminoplasty for multilevel cervical myelopathy: an independent matched-cohort analysis. Spine 2002;27(11):1168–1175
7. Cunningham MR, Hershman S, Bendo J. Systematic review of cohort studies comparing surgical treatments for cervical spondylotic myelopathy. Spine 2010;35(5):537–543
8. Kumar VG, Rea GL, Mervis LJ, McGregor JM. Cervical spondylotic myelopathy: functional and radiographic long-term outcome after laminectomy and posterior fusion. Neurosurgery 1999;44(4):771–777, discussion 777–778
9. Gok B, McLoughlin GS, Sciubba DM, et al. Surgical management of cervical spondylotic myelopathy with laminectomy and instrumented fusion. Neurol Res 2009;31(10):1097–1101
10. Wang MY, Shah S, Green BA. Clinical outcomes following cervical laminoplasty for 204 patients with cervical spondylotic myelopathy. Surg Neurol 2004;62(6):487–492, discussion 492–493
11. Kawaguchi Y, Kanamori M, Ishihara H, Ohmori K, Nakamura H, Kimura T. Minimum 10-year followup after en bloc cervical laminoplasty. Clin Orthop Relat Res 2003;411(411): 129–139

Suggested Readings

Bednarik J, Kadanka Z, Dusek L, et al. Presymptomatic spondylotic cervical myelopathy: an updated predictive model. Eur Spine J 2008;17(3):421–431

This recent article elucidates the predictive factors of progressive neurologic decline in patients with spondylotic cervical myelopathy.

Cunningham MR, Hershman S, Bendo J. Systematic review of cohort studies comparing surgical treatments for cervical spondylotic myelopathy. Spine 2010;35(5):537–543

This thorough review article identifies and compares the outcomes of the various surgical options for treatment of cervical spondylotic myelopathy.

Nurick S. The natural history and the results of surgical treatment of the spinal cord disorder associated with cervical spondylosis. Brain 1972;95(1):101–108

This classic article examines the natural history of cervical spondylotic myelopathy.

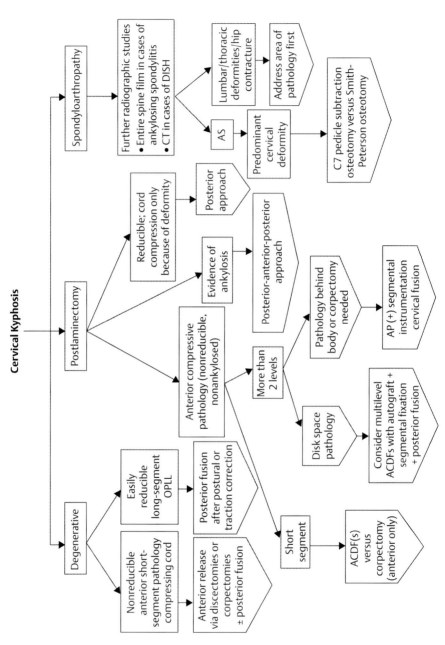

ACDF, anterior cervical discectomy and fusion; AP, anteroposterior; AS, ankylosing spondylitis; CT, computed tomography; DISH, diffuse idiopathic skeletal hyperostosis; OPLL, ossification of the posterior longitudinal ligament

21

Cervical Kyphosis

Todd J. Albert

Lordosis is the normal cervical posture, with the weight-bearing axis falling posterior to the vertebral bodies of C3 to C7, and this posture is important for proper head positioning and horizontal gaze. In the normal state, nearly two-thirds of the compressive load of the neck is borne by the posterior elements (**Fig. 21.1**). Certain conditions result in progressive loss of cervical lordosis and may lead to kyphosis. Examples of such conditions include cervical spondylosis, cervical trauma, cervical laminectomy, ankylosing spondylitis (AS), and diffuse idiopathic skeletal hyperostosis (DISH).

Classification

Cervical kyphosis is best classified as degenerative, post-traumatic, iatrogenic, or related to spondylarthropathy (AS/DISH) (**Fig. 21.2**). Degenerative kyphosis occurs because of sequential loss of disk height, which makes up around 15% of anterior column height in the normal cervical spine. Loss of intervertebral height leads to loss of cervical lordosis, shifting the compressive load from the posterior to the anterior column, and ultimately results in a kyphotic alignment. Traumatic injury may result in anterior column compression, posterior element tension failure, or both. Iatrogenic kyphosis most often occurs following a cervical laminectomy and is more common in the setting of underlying preoperative kyphosis or in the immature spine. Kyphosis related to spondylathropathy occurs as the spine ossifies and stiffens, shifting the weight-bearing axis anteriorly and leading to a progressive sagittal imbalance.

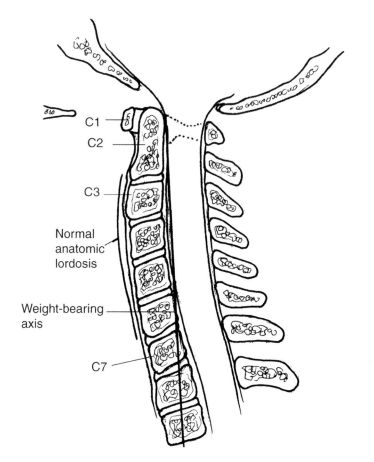

Fig. 21.1   The weight-bearing axis should fall posterior to the vertebral bodies of C3–C7 because of the normal anatomic lordosis of the cervical spine.

Workup

History

Evaluation of cervical kyphosis requires a thorough history to elucidate the cause of deformity, such as personal or family history of a spondylarthropathy or symptoms suggestive of an undiagnosed spondylarthropathy, history of cervical laminectomy, or neck and/or arm pain consistent with degenerative disease.

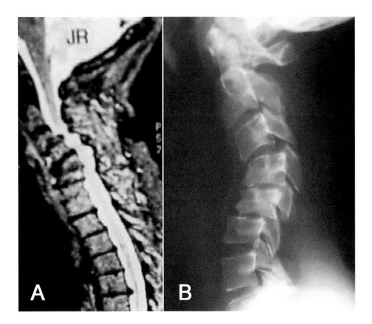

Fig. 21.2 **(A)** Sagittal MRI shows degenerative kyphosis with loss of the disk height. **(B)** Lateral plain radiograph of postlaminectomy kyphosis resulting from an overly aggressive facet resection with decreased posterior column stability.

Physical Examination

Examination should include assessment of the gross alignment of the head and neck, the degree of forward tilt, the degree of flexibility of the deformity, and the presence of radiculopathy or myelopathy. Sagittal alignment should be characterized by viewing the standing patient from the side, and photographs may be helpful for surgical planning. Range-of-motion testing in extension, flexion, side bending, and rotation helps to define a rigid or fixed deformity.

Evaluation of the nerve roots and spinal cord requires motor, reflex, and sensory testing of the C3–T1 nerves. Special tests necessary to rule out "upper tract signs" include Romberg sign, Babinski reflex, and Hoffmann sign, which may be associated with spinal cord compression.

Spinal Imaging

Imaging should include anteroposterior (AP), lateral, flexion/extension, and oblique radiographs, with careful attention paid to sagittal alignment, evidence of instability on the flexion/extension views, and facet ankylosis (best seen on oblique views). In patients with AS who present with cervical kyphosis, an entire-spine lateral radiograph that includes the head will enable measurement of the chin-brow vertical angle (**Fig. 21.3**), which quantifies the overall kyphosis of the head on the torso and is useful in planning reconstructive surgery.

Magnetic resonance imaging (MRI) helps to assess alignment, nerve or spinal cord compression, and signal change within the spinal cord (**Fig. 21.4**). Patients with DISH should be evaluated for the presence of ossification of the posterior longitudinal ligament. Computed tomography (CT) best demonstrates this ossification; post-myelogram CT is highly useful in defining cord compression due to ossification. Similarly, CT scan is often beneficial in defining fracture anatomy after cervical trauma. In certain special situations, vertebral artery characterization may be necessary via conventional angiography or magnetic resonance (MR) arteriography to plan the surgical approach for decompression and instrumentation.

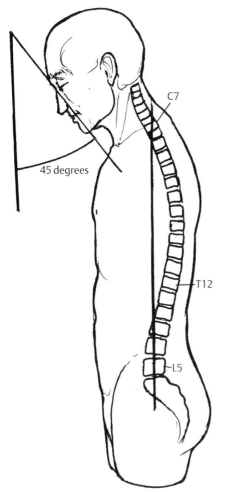

Fig. 21.3 The chin-brow vertical angle is used to measure the overall kyphosis of the head on the torso. It is calculated by drawing one line from the eyebrow to the chin and a second line vertically, and then measuring the angle formed by the intersection of the two lines.

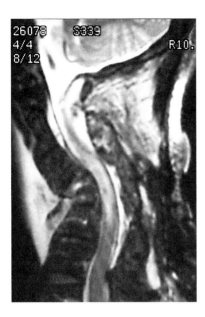

Fig. 21.4 Sagittal MRI demonstrates signal change of the spinal cord as it drapes over the vertebral bodies of a kyphotic cervical spine.

Treatment

Treatment of cervical kyphosis depends on the etiology, stability, stiffness, overall sagittal alignment, and location and severity of spinal cord compression. The goals of treatment are to obtain neural decompression, stability, and sagittal plane alignment. The approach can be anterior alone, posterior alone, or anterior and posterior. Patients may or may not require a decompression, and consideration should be given to the need for releases prior to deformity correction if any degree of ankylosis is evident on preoperative imaging.

In cases of flexible, correctible kyphosis where cord compression is predominantly due to the deformity, a posterior fusion after postural or traction correction with or without decompression is appropriate. If the same deformity is rigid, an anterior release via either discectomy or corpectomy is necessary to achieve sagittal correction and to obtain decompression. In the setting of postlaminectomy kyphosis, a high rate of graft failure has been reported with anterior-only approaches. Therefore, an anterior and posterior approach is generally required to provide correction and support of the unstable and often stiff deformity. For all surgery to correct cervical kyphosis, loupe or microscope magnification, illumination, and excellent spinal cord monitoring are helpful to prevent neurologic injury.

In cases of chin-on-chest deformity seen in patients with severe AS, osteotomy of the cervicothoracic junction is often necessary. Preoperatively, hip flexion contractures, lumbar deformity, and degree of hip arthritis in these patients must be analyzed. We prefer to perform cervicothoracic osteotomy with the patient in the seated position using a posterior-only approach, full decompression of the C8 nerves, and removal of the C7 pedicle. If a pedicle subtraction approach is attempted, we also remove the pedicle of T1. Postoperatively, these patients are immobilized in a halo vest or cast.

Outcome

The outcome of decompression and correction of cervical myelopathy with kyphosis is dependent on the severity of the myelopathy, the absence or presence of cord damage, and the intraoperative ability to obtain a generous decompression, correction of sagittal alignment, and adequate fixation. The goal of myelopathy surgery is to arrest progression of neurologic disability. In most cases, patients are able to gain improvement in balance, strength, and sensation, but patients who are elderly, infirm, or severely myelopathic (e.g., have lost the ability to walk) will have less reliable outcomes. After healing of the fusion, there is little restriction on activity. The rate of junctional degeneration and need for further surgery ranges from 3.4% to 5% per year. Patients with postlaminectomy kyphosis have higher rates of graft failure and overall higher complication rates. Patients who undergo osteotomy for severe deformity, such as those with AS, often have very gratifying results and improvements in their quality of life and overall function, provided that the correction is sufficient to enable horizontal gaze.

Complications

Infection rates are low with anterior surgery, but somewhat higher with posterior surgery. Neurologic deterioration, while uncommon (less than 1%), remains the biggest concern in these complex procedures. Other complications include swallowing dysfunction (2–15%), recurrent laryngeal or superior laryngeal nerve palsies, and pseudarthrosis (2–30% depending on number of segmental levels, graft surfaces, and graft type). Problems with AS osteotomies done with the patient in the sitting position include air embolism, neurologic injury, C8 nerve palsy, failure of fusion, and translation of the osteotomy.

Suggested Readings

Albert TJ, Vaccaro A. Postlaminectomy kyphosis. Spine 1998;23(24):2738–2745
    This is a review of the pathogenesis and treatment of this disorder.

Breig A, el-Nadi AF. Biomechanics of the cervical spinal cord. Relief of contact pressure on and overstretching of the spinal cord. Acta Radiol Diagn (Stockh) 1966;4(6):602–624
    This is an important analysis of a potential mechanism of spinal cord damage in kyphosis related to vascular compromise.

Cusick JF, Pintar FA, Yoganandan N. Biomechanical alterations induced by multilevel cervical laminectomy. Spine 1995;20(22):2392–2398, discussion 2398–2399

> *This article discusses the biomechanics and alterations in stability after laminectomy.*

Kaptain GJ, Simmons NE, Replogle RE, Pobereskin L. Incidence and outcome of kyphotic deformity following laminectomy for cervical spondylotic myelopathy. J Neurosurg 2000;93(2, Suppl):199–204

> *A series of patients who had undergone laminectomy for cervical spondylotic myelopathy showed that kyphosis may develop in up to 21%, with progression of the deformity twice as likely in patients with a straight spine as demonstrated by preoperative radiographic studies.*

Simmons EH. Kyphotic deformity of the spine in ankylosing spondylitis. Clin Orthop Relat Res 1977;128(128):65–77

> *The author presents a large series of cervicothoracic osteotomies for AS with technical notes, outcomes, and complications.*

Zdeblick TA, Bohlman HH. Cervical kyphosis and myelopathy. Treatment by anterior corpectomy and strut-grafting. J Bone Joint Surg Am 1989;71(2):170–182

> *This is an excellent review of treatment of kyphotic myelopathy with anterior corpectomy and strut grafting.*

Classification

There are four different patterns of OPLL that can be identified. The first pattern is continuous, in which the ossification proceeds in a flowing, uninterrupted fashion along the posterior border of the vertebral border of the vertebral body, spanning the retrovertebral space. The second pattern is noncontinous ossification, which appears only adjacent to each vertebral body and is often referred to as segmental. The third type is localized, where only one area of ossification is identified adjacent to a single vertebra. The forth type is "mixed" and contains features of each of these aforementioned three types.

Workup

History

OPLL of the cervical spine may present with a spectrum of findings. Many patients are asymptomatic and are unaware that they have OPLL. The natural history of the disease in these individuals is unknown; however, it is known that even patients who are asymptomatic are at higher risk of spinal cord injury following a trauma. When OPLL causes symptoms, the initial presentation can be that of neck pain, arm pain, and/or weakness. Patients may also report symptoms of cervical myelopathy, including loss of dexterity or clumsiness of the hands and difficulty walking. With increasing ossification of the PLL, patients may begin to notice a decrease in range of motion of the neck. Among the majority of these patients who present with myelopathy, the severity of the symptoms can be graded using the Japanese Orthopedic Association (JOA) scoring system.

A detailed history obtained from the patient at the time of initial presentation should clarify the spectrum and duration of symptoms. Key complaints include myelopathic symptoms, such as difficulties with dexterity and manipulating small objects, worsening handwriting, problems with balance and gait, and alterations in bowel/bladder function. In addition, radicular patterns of sensory loss or motor weakness may be identified.

Physical Examination

A careful physical exam should elucidate any signs of myelopathy as well, such as disturbance in gait, loss of manual dexterity, and the presence of hyperreflexia, especially in the lower extremities. Abnormal reflexes may also be present, such as Hoffmann sign, Babinski reflex, reversed radial reflex, finger-escape sign, or sustained ankle clonus. Although these findings are classically associated with spinal cord compression, some patients with extensive cord compression due to OPLL nevertheless exhibit few of these findings. This may be due to the very slow growth of OPLL over time.

Spinal Imaging

The presence of OPLL can be confirmed with radiographic evaluation. Plain radiographs are commonly used in the initial assessment. The four different patterns of OPLL (continuous, segmental, localized, and mixed) can be identified on lateral radiographs. Narrowing of the spinal canal can be seen on radiographs in areas where the ossification is significant. It can be seen anywhere from the levels of C2 to C6. OPLL can also be seen at the thoracic and lumbar levels, most commonly at the levels T4 to T7 and L1–L2. Below the level of the conus medullaris, OPLL is rarely clinically significant.

Computed tomography (CT) is the most useful radiographic modality in evaluating OPLL. It is particularly effective in defining the extent of the ossification and the resulting stenosis. Myelography is often used as an adjunct with CT scans to provide better definition of the neural elements and the compressive effects placed on these structures. However, myelography is an invasive procedure and carries with it risks of infection, dye allergy, and spinal headache if a cerebrospinal fluid (CSF) leak occurs.

Magnetic resonance imaging (MRI) is able to define the neural elements while remaining noninvasive and precluding the need for patient radiation. MRI is also able to identify subtle parenchymal changes within the spinal cord and nerve roots. However, the typical lesions in OPLL are not well defined on T1- or T2-weighted scans, thus making MRI a poor test for diagnosing OPLL.

Treatment

Nonoperative management of OPLL is appropriate for those patients with neither symptoms nor physical findings of cervical myelopathy. These patients, whose only complaint is usually neck pain, may be helped with a course of physical therapy and anti-inflammatory medications. In addition, a judicious trial of cervical traction may benefit patients who present with radicular complaints. However, traction is not appropriate for patients with progressive myeloradiculopathy. Operative treatment is generally recommended for patients with any degree of significant myelopathy or radicular symptoms unresponsive to nonoperative measures. These patients usually have a JOA score of 12 or lower (maximum score of 17). The fundamental goal may be best achieved through an anterior, posterior, or combined decompressive procedure.

Although most patients with myelopathy are safely decompressed via an anterior approach, anterior decompressive procedures in the presence of OPLL have an additional high risk of dural injury due to adherence of the OPLL to the dura anteriorly. As a result, many prefer a posterior decompression in patients with severe OPLL, especially when it occurs in a continuous fashion. Posterior approaches provide an indirect decompression of the spinal cord via cervical laminectomy, which is usually performed in conjunction with a fusion procedure, or laminoplasty. Cervical laminectomy involves complete removal of the cervical lamina across the involved segments. Laminoplasty entails enlargement of the spinal canal by hinging the lamina open on one side and securing it in an open position.

Outcome

Houten and Cooper showed in their retrospective review that cervical laminectomy with fusion not only halted the progression of disease but also showed significant improvement in JOA scores in 97% of patients. Excellent recovery rates have also been reported for laminoplasty. Laminoplasty has been shown in at least one comparative study to be superior to laminectomy and fusion, although that study was not specific to patients with OPLL. However, Hirabayashi et al. have shown laminoplasty to be at least as effective as laminectomy in treating OPLL. Cervical kyphosis precludes the use of posterior surgery because the spinal cord is not able to shift away from the anterior compressive lesions.

Complications

Decompressive surgical treatment of cervical spinal cord compromise, whether performed anteriorly or posteriorly, carries inherent risk present in all surgery, such as infection, bleeding, deep vein thrombosis/pulmonary embolism, and complications from anesthesia. Specific risks with cervical surgery may be damage to nearby anatomic structures, such as the trachea, esophagus, and great vessels within the neck. Anterior, posterior, or circumferential decompressive procedures performed on or around the spinal cord in particular carry specific risks, such as paralysis, CSF leak, nerve damage leading to paresthesia or motor deficits, continuation of symptoms, axial pain, and reduced neck range of motion. Hilibrand et al. demonstrated that patients with OPLL have a significantly higher risk of neurophysiologic changes and possible spinal cord injury than other patients undergoing cervical spine decompressive procedures. Intraoperative neurophysiologic monitoring may allow early recognition of an impending neurologic injury. Early recognition of these insults may allow early institution of intraoperative maneuvers, which may curtail or reverse evolving spinal cord injuries.

A complication unique to patients with long-standing cord compression due to OPLL and severe spondylosis is the presence of thinning or complete erosion/absence of the dura. This absence of dura is usually recognized after the ossified longitudinal ligament has been removed. It is often discrete and well demarcated, with the spinal cord and nerve roots being clearly visible through the remaining arachnoid layer. This can ultimately result in CSF leakage or a CSF fistula. The limited exposure often precludes a direct repair and requires an alternative technique, such as the use of sealants (such as fibrin glue), fascial grafts, or even subarachnoid drains.

Suggested Readings

Chikuda H, Seichi A, Takeshita K, et al. Acute cervical spinal cord injury complicated by pre-existing ossification of the posterior longitudinal ligament: a multicenter study. Spine 2011; 36(18):1453–1458

> *The authors retrospectively reviewed 453 patients with spinal cord injury and found OPLL in 106 (23%) of the patients. Of the injuries in patients with OPLL, 94 out of 106 occurred without bony injury. Only 25% of patients were aware of the diagnosis of OPLL prior to the injury. Most injuries were incomplete. Patients with gait dysfunction prior to the injury did better with surgical treatment. The study was conducted in Japan, which has a higher incidence of OPLL.*

Epstein NE. Circumferential cervical surgery for ossification of the posterior longitudinal ligament: a multianalytic outcome study. Spine 2004;29(12):1340–1345

> *This study reports the results for combined anterior and posterior procedures. It demonstrates that patients show the greatest improvements 1 year following surgery.*

Epstein NE. Identification of ossification of the posterior longitudinal ligament extending through the dura on preoperative computed tomographic examinations of the cervical spine. Spine 2001;26(2):182–186

> *This article evaluates the ability of CT to predict involvement of dura in the ossified lesion.*

Heller JG, Edwards CC II, Murakami H, Rodts GE. Laminoplasty versus laminectomy and fusion for multilevel cervical myelopathy: an independent matched cohort analysis. Spine 2001; 26(12):1330–1336

> *This study compares two posterior procedures, laminectomy and laminoplasty, and shows that laminoplasty has both higher recovery rates and lower complication rates.*

Hilibrand AS, Schwartz DM, Sethuraman V, Vaccaro AR, Albert TJ. Comparison of transcranial electric motor and somatosensory evoked potential monitoring during cervical spine surgery. J Bone Joint Surg Am 2004;86-A(6):1248–1253

> *The authors of this study showed that transcranial electric motor evoked potential appeared to be a better modality than conventional somatosensory evoked potential, for monitoring patients during spinal surgery, especially those patients with OPLL.*

Hirabayashi K, Toyama Y, Chiba K. Expansive laminoplasty for myelopathy in ossification of the longitudinal ligament. Clin Orthop Relat Res 1999;359(359):35–48

> *This study compares laminoplasty to laminectomy and shows that similar success is seen with either procedure, and although an advantage of laminoplasty has been theorized, it has not yet been shown.*

Houten JK, Cooper PR. Laminectomy and posterior cervical plating for multilevel cervical spondylotic myelopathy and ossification of the posterior longitudinal ligament: effects on cervical alignment, spinal cord compression, and neurological outcome. Neurosurgery 2003;52(5): 1081–1087, discussion 1087–1088

> *This study shows that laminectomy has a high rate of success while having lower complication rates than anterior surgery.*

Japanese Orthopedic Association. Scoring system for cervical myelopathy. J Orthop Sci 1994; 68:490–503

> *This article by the JOA reports a method with which to score cervical myelopathy, thus enabling objective comparison between cases and studies.*

Kobashi G, Washio M, Okamoto K, et al.; Japan Collaborative Epidemiological Study Group for Evaluation of Ossification of the Posterior Longitudinal Ligament of the Spine Risk. High body mass index after age 20 and diabetes mellitus are independent risk factors for ossification of the posterior longitudinal ligament of the spine in Japanese subjects: a case-control study in multiple hospitals. Spine 2004;29(9):1006–1010

> *This study demonstrates a link between OPLL and weight gain and diabetes mellitus, and suggests that these may be risk factors for the disease.*

Li H, Dai LY. A systematic review of complications in cervical spine surgery for ossification of the posterior longitudinal ligament. Spine J 2011;11(11):1049–1057

> *The authors performed a meta-analysis that included 27 studies with 1,558 patients. They found that the rate of complications following surgery was 21.8%, including an 8.3% risk of neurologic injury. The overall rate of complication did not vary with regard to approach (anterior vs. posterior); however, C5 palsy was more common with a posterior approach, and CSF leak, hoarseness, dysphagia, implant complications, and dyspnea were more common with anterior surgery.*

Matsunaga S, Yamaguchi M, Hayashi K, Sakou T. Genetic analysis of ossification of the posterior longitudinal ligament. Spine 1999;24(10):937–938, discussion 939

> *This study shows that OPLL has a definite genetic link.*

Onishi E, Sakamoto A, Murata S, Matsushita M. Risk factors for acute cervical spinal cord injury associated with ossification of the posterior longitudinal ligament. Spine 2011 Aug 18. [Epub ahead of print]

> *The authors reviewed patients with OPLL and spinal cord injury, OPLL and myelopathy, and normal controls to identify risk factors for spinal cord injury in patients with OPLL. They identified advanced age, mixed/segmental OPLL, and ossification of the anterior longitudinal ligament as risk factors for spinal cord injury. Spinal stenosis was not an essential risk factor.*

Smith MD, Bolesta MJ, Leventhal M, Bohlman HH. Postoperative cerebrospinal-fluid fistula associated with erosion of the dura. Findings after anterior resection of ossification of the posterior longitudinal ligament in the cervical spine. J Bone Joint Surg Am 1992;74(2):270–277

> *The authors of this study concluded that given the higher risk of dural tears with anterior surgery for OPLL, the surgical plan should always include preparation for a dural tear.*

Sugimori K, Kawaguchi Y, Ohmori K, Kanamori M, Ishihara H, Kimura T. Significance of bone formation markers in patients with ossification of the posterior longitudinal ligament of the spine. Spine 2003;28(4):378–379

> *This study shows that certain markers may indicate the presence of OPLL and that a hyperostotic state exists in OPLL patients.*

Wu JC, Chen YC, Liu L, et al. Conservatively treated ossification of posterior longitudinal ligament increases risk of spinal cord injury: A nationwide cohort study. J Neurotrauma. 2011 Oct 12. [Epub ahead of print]

> *The authors compared 265 patients with conservatively treated OPLL and an age-matched cohort of 5,339 patients with no OPLL. They found statistically higher rates of spinal cord injury among the OPLL cohort (4.81 vs. 0.18 per 1000 person-years), resulting in a 32-times increased risk of spinal cord injury.*

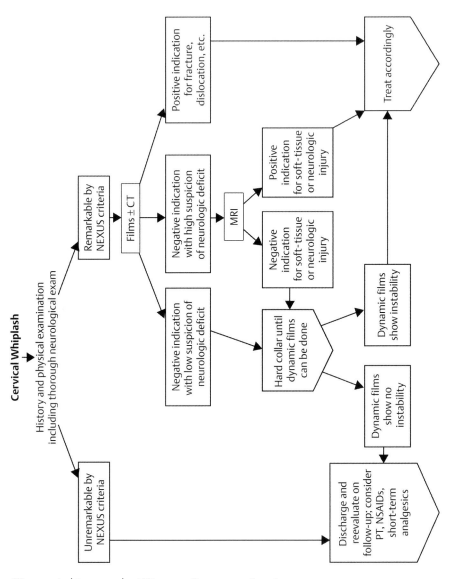

Cervical Whiplash

History and physical examination including thorough neurological exam

Remarkable by NEXUS criteria

Unremarkable by NEXUS criteria

Films ± CT

Positive indication for fracture, dislocation, etc.

Negative indication with high suspicion of neurologic deficit

Negative indication with low suspicion of neurologic deficit

MRI

Positive indication for soft-tissue or neurologic injury

Negative indication for soft-tissue or neurologic injury

Hard collar until dynamic films can be done

Dynamic films show instability

Dynamic films show no instability

Treat accordingly

Discharge and reevaluate on follow-up; consider PT, NSAIDs, short-term analgesics

CT, computed tomography; MRI, magnetic resonance imaging; NEXUS, National Emergency X-Radiography Utilization Study; NSAIDs, nonsteroidal anti-inflammatory drugs; PT, physical therapy

23

Cervical Whiplash

Brett A. Braly, Antonia F. Chen, Ishaq Y. Syed, and Joon Y. Lee

Whiplash is defined as an injury caused by a flexion-extension energy mechanism that is usually the direct result of a motor vehicle collision (MVC). Crowe first used the term "whiplash" in 1928, although injuries fitting the pattern of whiplash can be found in documents as early as the 17th century.[1] The resultant injury can be manifested by multiple complaints, and common to all is often the lack of objective evidence supporting any pathology.

In the United States, it is estimated that whiplash is diagnosed in 3 of every 1000 people every year. Studies have indicated that 15–40% of people involved in a MVC will complain of acute neck pain. The majority of whiplash cases resolve uneventfully, though 5–7% of patients will complain of permanent disability.[2] Although whiplash is a common diagnosis, special care should be taken to evaluate for other causes of patients' complaints.

Whiplash is a popular medicolegal subject. The societal cost to the United States has been estimated at 4.5–29 billion dollars per year.[3,4] Many studies have evaluated the effect of medicolegal variables on a patient's recovery.

Mechanism

Whiplash injury is the result of a low-velocity flexion-extension stress on the cervical spine. Fifty percent of cases can be related to rear-end MVCs at low speeds. The whiplash event has been shown to last fewer than 500 milliseconds.[5] Energy is transferred from the bullet vehicle to the struck vehicle, through the frame and seat to the body of the patient. The body of the patient moves in concordance with the seat and the patient's head lags behind, causing the head to go into extension and act as though on a whip. Once the head contacts the head restraint, a forward momentum is applied causing the flexion mechanism.

The forward momentum can be affected by the height of the headrest. A low headrest acts as a fulcrum about which the neck can whip. Raising the headrest has been shown to decrease the number of claims of whiplash secondary to car manufacturing. Studies have shown that a collision from a velocity of 8.7 mph is necessary to damage a struck vehicle, while a collision with an increase of only 2.5 mph can produce complaints of neck pain in subjects. Furthermore, subjects not wearing seatbelts during airbag deployment were 1.7 times more likely to sustain major cervical injury than those wearing seatbelts.[6]

The resultant energy affects the structures of the spine in specifically described manners. The facet joints each show compression posteriorly, combined with distraction anteriorly. The annulus fibrosus of the disk, as well as ligamental constraints, may also be disrupted in the injury. Studies of the kinematics of the facet joint have shown that there is a multitude of possible injury patterns associated with a whiplash event. These may include capsular strain and/or tears, bony impingement, synovial fold pinching, and direct-impact injury. Any of these may result in contusion, intra-articular hemorrhage, and damage to subchondral bone, any of which may result in pain.[7]

Presentation

Presentation after a whiplash injury can include complaints of neck pain, stiffness, headache, back pain, and parasthesias of the upper limbs. Pain described within 24 hours of an accident has been related to the more symptomatic one-third of patients who develop whiplash-associated disorder (WAD).

Multiple studies have tried to evaluate the prognostic symptoms and signs associated with a rapid recovery from a whiplash injury. Ozegovic reviewed 2335 patients with traffic-related WAD and showed that postcollision neck pains, as well as depressive symptomatology, affected a patient's ability for, and timing of, return to work.[8] This indicates that there may be a psychologic component associated with recovering from WAD. Other psychologic complaints include impaired concentration, somatoform disorder, forgetfulness, post-traumatic stress disorder, and driving anxiety.[9–11] The psychological response to a WAD may be as marked as a structural injury and should be appropriately addressed.

Workup

Natural History

The natural history of WAD has been well studied. It has been estimated throughout the literature that 50% of patients who initially complain of WAD will go on to full recovery by 2 years, while 4.5% remain permanently disabled. Gargan and Bannister have developed a classification system that can be used to predict the prognosis for WAD.[9] Based on complaints in the first 3 months postinjury, 70% of patients' outcomes can be predicted. Poor prognostic factors include: rapid onset and severity of neck pain, hospital admission, radiation, headache, neurologic deficit, stiffness, and tenderness. Depressive symptoms may be noticed at 6 weeks postinjury.[12] Preinjury psychiatric disease, older age, lower educational status, part-time employment, and preinjury complaints of neck or back pain have also been shown to confer a worse prognosis. Female sex is a poor prognostic factor, and an estimated two-thirds of women experience sufficient pain from WAD to take time off from work.[13,14]

Gargan et al. reported on psychological test scores following whiplash injuries and showed that, while testing was initially normal in 82% of patients, by 2 years postinjury, 69% of patients had abnormal test results.[9] The conclusion from this study was that psychological disturbance may be a sequela of enduring a WAD.

A positive prognostic factor that reduces the return to work time is self-employment status, although timing to full asymptomatic recovery is unchanged. Gozzard et al. found that 7% of patients who suffered from WAD had not returned to work, with the strongest predictor of disability being the intensity of symptoms.[15]

It has been shown that injured workers do worse than others with similar injuries, and whiplash is no different. Litigation has also been sought as a prognostic factor. Swartzman et al. noted that patients with active litigation claims secondary to WAD complained of worse pain than those with completed claims, though there were no differences in function or employment status.[16] Regional governments may influence the rates and recoveries from whiplash, as well. In 1987, Victoria, Australia, required that subjects reporting WADs pay the first 317 Australian dollars of medical care out of pocket. This decreased the rate of reported whiplash by 68%, though chronic disability from whiplash remained unchanged at ~10%.[17]

Imaging

Multiple imaging modalities have been used to further identify the pathology of WAD (**Fig. 23.1**). No imaging modality has been shown to be effective for detecting WAD. A 10-year follow up of magnetic resonance imaging (MRI) in both WAD and asymptomatic patients showed no statistical correlation between MRI findings (disk signal change, foraminal stenosis, disk protrusion and narrowing) and neck pain in WAD patients.[18] MRI should be used in specific cases when nerve root impingement is thought to be the result of disk herniation.[19]

Treatment

The first step to evaluate a patient with acute neck pain suspected to be due to WAD is to ensure that a more serious injury does not exist. A thorough history and physical exam and possible imaging modalities may be needed as part of the workup. In case whiplash is the correct diagnosis, the initial treatment should consist of education and reassurance. It is imperative that patients resume normal daily activities despite discomfort. Patients who remain active have better outcomes than those who limit or avoid activities altogether.[20,21] Medical treatment with nonsteroidal anti-inflammatory drugs (NSAIDs) and intravenous steroids has also been shown to decrease symptoms and shorten return to work time.[22,23] It is currently thought that cervical orthoses add little if any benefit and may result in a poorer prognosis than if not used at all.[23]

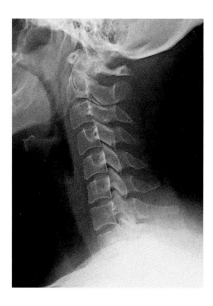

Fig. 23.1 Loss of cervical lordosis consistent with muscle spasm, which is frequently seen after whiplash trauma.

There is little difference in managing a patient with chronic WAD and those with chronic cervical neck pain. Physical therapy and stretching modalities can be tried as first-line treatment. Medial branches of the cervical dorsal rami innervate the cervical facet joints; anesthetizing this pathway provides temporary relief for the discomfort of WAD. Facet blocks have resulted in pain relief but have a high recurrence rate, at around 50% within a week.[24] This information may be used to direct patients toward radiofrequency neurotomy (RFN). RFN can be beneficial to patients with facet-mediated pain, as well as those with facet joint-mediated cervicogenic headache.[24] Although RFN is also temporary, the relief is usually longer than facet blocks and lasts an average of 270–400 days. Once symptoms begin to return in a patient after RFN, the procedure can be repeated as needed. Radiofrequency ablation is not currently a standard of treatment and may be reserved for specific patients on a case-by-case basis.

References

1. Crowe H. A new diagnostic sign in neck injuries. Calif Med 1964;100:12–13
2. Radanov BP, Sturzenegger M, Di Stefano G. Long-term outcome after whiplash injury. A 2-year follow-up considering features of injury mechanism and somatic, radiologic, and psychosocial findings. Medicine (Baltimore) 1995;74(5):281–297
3. Chapple D, Walker R. Initial management of whiplash injuries. J Bone Joint Surg Br 2000; 28B(3, suppl):274–278
4. Cassidy JD, Carroll LJ, Côté P, Lemstra M, Berglund A, Nygren A. Effect of eliminating compensation for pain and suffering on the outcome of insurance claims for whiplash injury. N Engl J Med 2000;342(16):1179–1186
5. McConnel W, Howard R, Guzman H, et al. Analysis of human test subject kinematic responses to low velocity rear end impacts. 37th Stapp Car Crash Conference Proceedings. San Antonio, TX: Society of Automotive Engineers; 1993;21–30

6. Donaldson WF III, Hanks SE, Nassr A, Vogt MT, Lee JY. Cervical spine injuries associated with the incorrect use of airbags in motor vehicle collisions. Spine 2008;33(6):631–634
7. Stemper BD, Yoganandan N, Gennarelli TA, Pintar FA. Localized cervical facet joint kinematics under physiological and whiplash loading. J Neurosurg Spine 2005;3(6):471–476
8. Ozegovic D, Carroll LJ, Cassidy JD. What influences positive return to work expectation? Examining associated factors in a population-based cohort of whiplash-associated disorders. Spine 2010;35(15):E708–E713
9. Gargan M, Bannister G, Main C, Hollis S. The behavioural response to whiplash injury. J Bone Joint Surg Br 1997;79(4):523–526
10. Guez M. Chronic neck pain: an epidemiological, psychological and spect study with emphasis on whiplash-associated disorders. Acta Orthop Scand 2006;77(320):1–33
11. Gargan MF, Bannister GC. Long-term prognosis of soft-tissue injuries of the neck. J Bone Joint Surg Br 1990;72(5):901–903
12. Carroll LJ, Cassidy JD, Côté P. Frequency, timing, and course of depressive symptomatology after whiplash. Spine 2006;31(16):E551–E556
13. Cobo EP, Mesquida ME, Fanegas EP, et al. What factors have influence on persistence of neck pain after a whiplash? Spine 2010;35(9):E338–E343
14. Murray PA, et al. The Cost of Long Term Disability from Road Traffic Accidents: Four Year Study: Final Report. London, UK: HMSO; 1993:1–58. Transport Research Laboratory, Project Report 45
15. Gozzard C, Bannister G, Langkamer G, Khan S, Gargan M, Foy C. Factors affecting employment after whiplash injury. J Bone Joint Surg Br 2001;83(4):506–509
16. Swartzman LC, Teasell RW, Shapiro AP, McDermid AJ. The effect of litigation status on adjustment to whiplash injury. Spine 1996;21(1):53–58
17. Gibson T, Bogduk N, Macpherson J, et al. The accident characteristics of whiplash associated chronic neck pain. J Musculoskeletal Pain 2000;8:87–95
18. Matsumoto M, Okada E, Ichihara D, et al. Prospective ten-year follow-up study comparing patients with whiplash-associated disorders and asymptomatic subjects using magnetic resonance imaging. Spine 2010;35(18):1684–1690 [Epub ahead of print]
19. Pettersson K, Hildingsson C, Toolanen G, Fagerlund M, Björnebrink J. Disc pathology after whiplash injury. A prospective magnetic resonance imaging and clinical investigation. Spine 1997;22(3):283–287, discussion 288
20. Schnabel M, Ferrari R, Vassiliou T, Kaluza G. Randomised, controlled outcome study of active mobilisation compared with collar therapy for whiplash injury. Emerg Med J 2004;21(3):306–310
21. Borchgrevink GE, Kaasa A, McDonagh D, Stiles TC, Haraldseth O, Lereim I. Acute treatment of whiplash neck sprain injuries. A randomized trial of treatment during the first 14 days after a car accident. Spine 1998;23(1):25–31
22. Gunzberg R, Spalski M. Whiplash Injuries: Current Concepts in Prevention, Diagnosis and Treatment at the Cervical Whiplash Syndromes. Philadelphia, PA: Lippincott-Raven; 1998.
23. Pettersson K, Toolanen G. High-dose methylprednisolone prevents extensive sick leave after whiplash injury. A prospective, randomized, double-blind study. Spine 1998;23(9):984–989
24. Barnsley L, Lord SM, Wallis BJ, Bogduk N. The prevalence of chronic cervical zygapophysial joint pain after whiplash. Spine 1995;20(1):20–25, discussion 26

Suggested Reading

Rooker J, Bannister M, Amirfeyz R, Squires B, Gargan M, Bannister G. Whiplash injury: 30-year follow-up of a single series. J Bone Joint Surg Br 2010;92(6):853–855

Twenty-two patients were followed for a mean of 30 years after whiplash injuries. As previously shown, roughly 50% showed full recovery. Psychological issues were noted in those with persistent disability. By 30 years, 45% of the patients followed were disabled more by knee pain than by neck pain.

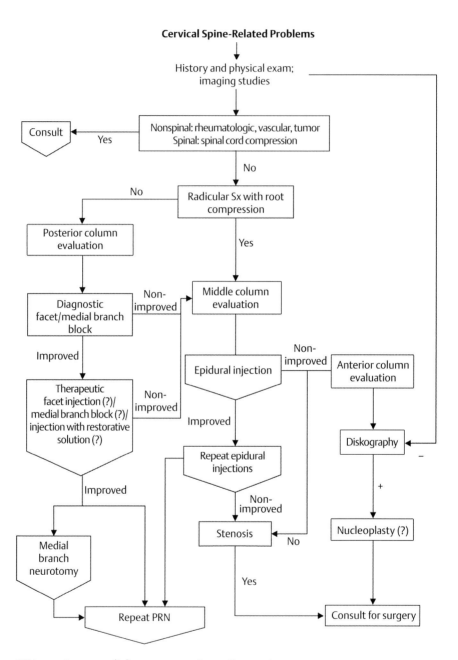

Cervical Spine-Related Problems

History and physical exam; imaging studies

Nonspinal: rheumatologic, vascular, tumor
Spinal: spinal cord compression

Consult ← Yes

No

Radicular Sx with root compression

No

Posterior column evaluation

Yes

Middle column evaluation

Diagnostic facet/medial branch block

Non-improved

Epidural injection

Non-improved

Anterior column evaluation

Improved

Therapeutic facet injection (?)/ medial branch block (?)/ injection with restorative solution (?)

Non-improved

Improved

Diskography

Repeat epidural injections

Improved

−

+

Non-improved

Nucleoplasty (?)

Medial branch neurotomy

Stenosis ← No

Improved

Repeat PRN

Yes

Consult for surgery

PRN, percutaneous radiofrequency neurotomy; Sx, symptoms

24

Cervical Diagnostic and Therapeutic Injections and Procedures

Richard Derby, Irina L. Melnik, and Kwan Sik Seo

Chronic neck pain in the adult general population has 26% to 71% lifetime prevalence, contributing to significant socioeconomic impact. The etiology of neck pain is complex. To ensure accuracy in the diagnosis and in the selection of appropriate treatment, it is recommended to use an algorithmic approach with correlation between history, physical exam, imaging tests, and confirmatory diagnostic or therapeutic procedures. It is important to exclude nonspinal causes, rheumatologic disease, infection, and tumor as well as cord compression (myelopathy or large disk herniations) in the early stages. Differential diagnosis should also exclude proximal compression of the brachial plexus (as with thoracic outlet syndrome) or distal nerve compression caused by entrapment syndromes that can mimic root compression, as well as the shoulder complex. Once other sources of pain have been mostly eliminated from the differential diagnosis, structure-specific spine injections may help to establish diagnosis in over 80% of cases and may significantly increase the efficacy of treatment.

Posterior Column

Chronic axial neck pain related to cervical zygapophyseal (facet) joints and supporting capsules may account for 36% of patients, with prevalence increasing to 60% after a whiplash-type injury. Imaging tests and clinical examination, including localized pain during palpation and increase in neck pain with extension, are not very specific and reliable. There are two diagnostic procedures available to confirm the diagnosis: one is intra-articular facet joint injection, which can be associated with potentially higher neurovascular complications, and another is a medial branch block (MBB). MBB is an indirect but simple and safe way of assessing facet joint–mediated pain, with a low (3.9%) rate of inadvertent intravascular penetration reported. In order to block pain from one facet joint, at least two medial branches have to be anesthetized. Because of high false-positive rates (38%) with uncontrolled MBBs, patients who respond initially to blocks with lidocaine should subsequently undergo confirmatory blocks with bupivacaine. Complete or definite (>80%) relief of pain following a block of two adjacent medial branches identifies the symptomatic joint (**Fig. 24.1A**). Partial relief may mean that the blocked joint is not painful and that the adjacent joint that was partially blocked is symptomatic, or it could mean that the blocked joint is symptomatic but another joint or a different structure is also symptomatic. Some reports describe prolonged pain relief after MBBs with moderate evidence for therapeutic utility.

Therapeutic approaches include intraarticular facet injection of corticosteroid (**Fig. 24.1B**) combined with local anesthetic, especially with acute pain or when intraarticular inflammation is suspected. Although not validated in the general patient population, older patients often have chronic pain secondary to intraarticular inflammation, and therapeutic corticosteroid facet joint injections can be used on an occasional basis for pain control. Another common treatment modality is radiofrequency neurotomy (RFN). In this procedure, a Teflon-coated electrode with an exposed tip is inserted close to and parallel to a medial branch of a spinal nerve, and a high-frequency electrical current is applied to the electrode with concentration around the exposed tip, heating and coagulating the immediately surrounding tissue, including the target nerve. RFN is not a permanent treatment, and the medial branch nerves will usually regenerate in 6 to 18 months, but the procedure can be repeated if necessary. It has been reported that repeated procedures provide equal effectiveness for a mean duration of 10 months. Alternative approaches include pulsed radiofrequency, with less than 42°C temperature at the tip of the electrode applied in a pulsed manner to a medial branch, which may decrease pain for several months with no well-established mechanism of action. However only RFN at 80°C showed positive outcomes in randomized controlled trials in well-selected patients. Since neurotomies are considered to be palliative procedures, some physicians advocate

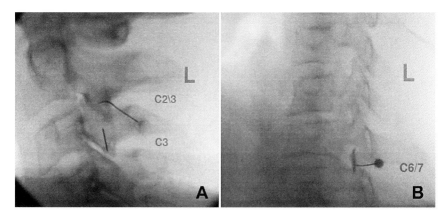

Fig. 24.1 **(A)** Fluoroscopy showing a facet injection at C2–C3 and medial branch block at C3. **(B)** Fluoroscopy showing a transforaminal epidural steroid injection at C6–C7.

the injection of hypertonic solutions into the ligamentous structures of the posterior column, theoretically to promote both added tissue desensitization and connective tissue repair, or injections of "restorative solutions."

Middle Column

Middle column pain is typically a result of inflammation or epidural and dural tissue irritation. It can be a result of static/dynamic stenosis, protruding or herniated disks, uncinate osteophytes with neuroforaminal stenosis, postlaminectomy syndrome, or nerve root inflammation. In most cases the structural abnormalities can be seen on a cervical magnetic resonance imaging (MRI) scan, and once they correlate with the clinical presentation consistent with middle column structure inflammation or nerve root compression, a therapeutic epidural injection of corticosteroids can be performed as a primary interventional procedure. Diagnostic accuracy of cervical selective nerve root blocks has not been established. Although the transforaminal approach (**Fig. 24.2A**) is the most selective route for delivering local anesthetic and corticosteroids to the site of inflammation, it has been associated with substantial risk. This approach has become controversial, because injection of particulate corticosteroids into the vertebral artery can cause cerebellar infarcts, and injection into a radicular artery can cause cord infarction. Neurologic complications, which have been discussed in several recent review articles, can be minimized with the use of nonparticulate steroids, injection of a test dose bolus of short-acting local anesthetic, use of live digital subtraction fluoroscopy, and avoidance of excessive sedation.

Many interventionalists currently prefer the interlaminar route using a single-needle technique because the risk of injecting into the vertebral or radicular artery is remote (**Fig. 24.2B**). However, injection into the spinal cord or compression of the spinal cord by a hematoma or abscess may rarely occur.

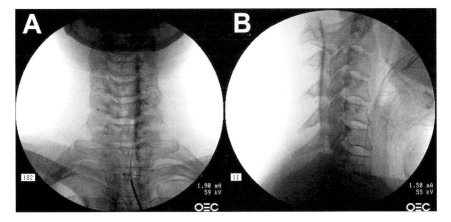

Fig. 24.2   Interlaminar epidural steroid injection with catheter at right C6–C7. (**A**) Anteroposterior view. (**B**) Lateral view.

Manchikanti L, Dunbar EE, Wargo BW, Shah RV, Derby R, Cohen SP. Systematic review of cervical discography as a diagnostic test for chronic spinal pain. Pain Physician 2009;12(2): 305–321

> *This is a systematic review, evaluating validity and usefulness of cervical provocative diskography in managing and diagnosing discogenic pain. Despite paucity of literature and a small number of studies that performed the test utilizing IASP criteria, as well as methodologic discrepancies, it showed that diskography may be a useful tool for evaluationg chronic cervical pain without disk herniation, radiculitis or stenosis, with the strength of evidence as Level II-2 for diagnostic accuracy. The prevalence of cervical discogenic pain was found to be between 16% and 20% based on IASP criteria, requiring a concordantly painful disk and two negative control disks, one above and one below the affected level .*

Manchikanti L, Helm S, Singh V, et al.; ASIPP. An algorithmic approach for clinical management of chronic spinal pain. Pain Physician 2009;12(4):E225–E264

> *The authors propose an algorithmic approach, addressing how to diagnose and manage spinal pain and how to choose appropriate diagnostic or therapeutic interventional technique. In managing pain of cervical origin, if radiculitis is suspected, it is advisable to proceed with epidural injections. In a case of chronic neck pain without disk herniation or radiculopathy, facet joints are entertained first, because of they are a more common cause, accounting for 40–50% of cases, while discogenic pain accounts for ~20% of patients based on the United States literature, with more rare need for cervical diskography.*

Yin W, Bogduk N. The nature of neck pain in a private pain clinic in the United States. Pain Med 2008;9(2):196–203

> *This is a retrospective audit of 143 patients to determine the prevalence of different causes of neck pain. In a private practice clinic, a patho-anatomic diagnosis for chronic neck pain can be established in over 80% patients, given that when the diagnosis was not clinically evident, patients underwent investigation using structure-specific diagnostic blocks and diskography. Among the 46% of patients who completed investigations, the prevalence of facet joint pain was 55%, discogenic pain was 16%, lateral atlanto-axial joint pain was 9%, and undetermined in 32%. Invasive tests are useful in the diagnostic process. Morphological changes on MRI do not correlate with diskography and thus are not diagnostic of cervical discogenic pain.*

IV Thoracic Degenerative/ Metabolic Disease

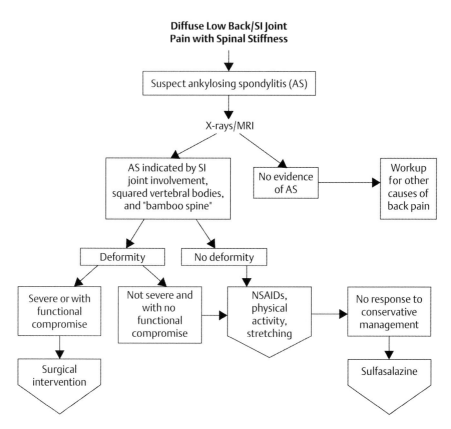

Diffuse Low Back/SI Joint Pain with Spinal Stiffness

Suspect ankylosing spondylitis (AS)

X-rays/MRI

AS indicated by SI joint involvement, squared vertebral bodies, and "bamboo spine"

No evidence of AS

Workup for other causes of back pain

Deformity

No deformity

Severe or with functional compromise

Not severe and with no functional compromise

NSAIDs, physical activity, stretching

No response to conservative management

Surgical intervention

Sulfasalazine

MRI, magnetic resonance imaging; NSAIDs, nonsteroidal anti-inflammatory drugs; SI, sacroiliac

25

Ankylosing Spondylitis

Tony Tannoury and Jeffery Thomas P. Luna

Ankylosing spondylitis (AS) is a seronegative inflammatory autoimmune disease of unknown etiology and is one of the spondylarthritides commonly associated with HLA-B27.[1-6] This disease manifests around the third or fourth decade and is more common among Western societies. The worldwide prevalence has been determined to be 0.9%.[2,5] The disease affects an average of 350,000 persons in the United States and around 600,000 in Europe, primarily white males.[3] Diagnosis of AS is often delayed and can take an average of 3–11 years from the onset of symptoms[3,4] The end result of the disease is early retirement and severe functional impairment in ~30% of the affected population.[7]

AS is also known as Bekhterev disease, as it was originally described and published by the Russian neurophysiologist Vladmir Bekhterev (or Bechterew). Significant contributions were made by Pierre Marie and Adolph Strumpell.[1,8]

Classification

AS has been classified and described based on the Rome and New York diagnostic criteria,[9-11] established solely on clinical and radiologic manifestations. These criteria, originally established in 1961 and 1966, respectively, have been modified over subsequent years to improve sensitivity and specificity (**Table 25.1**).

Etiology and Pathophysiology

The precise etiology of AS is unknown. A strong genetic linkage has been confirmed and established with the major histocompatibility human leukocyte antigen (HLA) HLA-B27, but unavailability of routine biopsy makes it highly unlikely for the disease to be diagnosed at an earlier stage. Carriers of HLA-B27 have a 16% greater risk of acquiring the disease than noncarriers, and the proba-

Table 25.1 The Modified New York Classification Criteria for Ankylosing Spondylitis

Clinical Criteria	– Low back pain for a minimum 3 months, relieved by exercise but not rest
	– Limited sagittal and frontal plane lumbar spinal motion
	– Decreased chest expansion contrary to age and sex
Radiological Criteria	– Bilateral sacroiliitis, grade 2–4
	– Unilateral sacroiliitis, grade 3–4

Source: van der Linden S, Valkenburg HA, Cats A. Evaluation of diagnostic criteria for ankylosing spondylitis. A proposal for modification of the New York criteria. Arthritis Rheum 1984;27:361–368.

bility of having AS is increased by 10 times after testing positive for HLA-B27.[6,12] Besides the HLA-B27 genetic linkage, it has been hypothesized that involvement of the IL-23 signaling pathway could be a determinant in the development of AS. Inflammatory mediators involved in the disease process usually are CD4 and CD8 helper T lymphocytes, along with tumor necrosis factor (TNF)-α and transforming growth factor (TGF)-β.[8,12]

Pathogenesis of the disease is immune mediated and begins where articular cartilage, ligaments, and other structures attach to the bone (enthesis). Involvement of the sacroiliac joint is considered a hallmark for the disease and a requirement for diagnosis. The axial skeleton is involved to a variable extent. Sacroiliitis along with synovitis, mucoid marrow, subchondral granulation tissue, enthesitis, and chondroid differentiation are usually found and accompanied by fibrocartilage regeneration and ossification of the eroded joint margins. This ultimately results in complete joint fusion.[5,9,10,13]

In the spine, inflammatory granulation tissue at the junction of the annulus fibrosus and vertebral bone leads to the formation of a syndesmophyte, which gradually progresses, along with diffuse osteoporosis and squaring of vertebrae, and finally results in bony ankylosis (**Fig. 25.1A,B**).[8,9,14] This ultimately results in the characteristic "bambooing" of the spine seen on radiographs.

The spinal column becomes very rigid and brittle and highly susceptible to injury. Any fracture should be considered to involve both spinal columns and to be highly unstable.[15]

Clinical Presentation

Patients with AS usually present with one of the following complaints:

- Dull, aching, deep, and insidious-onset pain in the neck or lower lumbar region as well as gluteal region
- Spinal deformity: inability to look straight forward, chin-to-chest deformity, tipping forward
- Spinal fracture
- Spinal stenosis, leg weakness, neurologic claudication

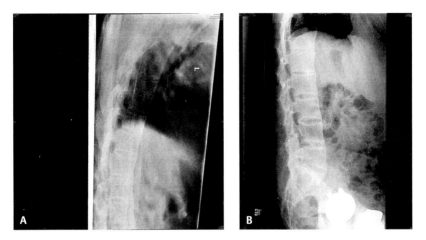

Fig. 25.1   **(A)** Thoracic spine ankylosis. **(B)** Lumbar spine ankylosis and loss of lumbar lordosis.

Seventy percent of patients with AS report daily pain and stiffness, 20% of patients display signs and symptoms of emotional problems, 47% present with physical disability, and 60% of patients present with fatigue.

Articular sites of AS usually involve the proximal, large joints (sacroiliac, hip, and shoulder joints), but peripheral joints may be involved as well. Bony tenderness at various locations (costovertebral junction, spinous process, iliac crests, ischial tuberosities, tibial tubercles, heels, and greater trochanter) may accompany lower back pain or stiffness or can be a primary complaint. Shoulder and hip involvement occurs in ~50% of the patients who also have involvement of more distal joints. Spinal involvement usually involves flattening of the normal lumbar lordosis and an increasingly smooth thoracic kyphosis, with the head and neck thrust forward. This increased kyphosis may lead to a "chin-on-chest" deformity and may make it difficult or impossible for the patient to look straight ahead (**Fig. 25.1A,B**).[9,11,16–18] The level of deformity must be assessed clinically by either chin-brow angle, occiput-to-wall distance, or hip flexion contracture. Other measurements of spinal mobility, especially fingertip-to-floor distance, lateral spine flexion, modified Schober's index, and tragus-to-wall distance, may be performed to evaluate disease status.[9]

One of the most serious presentations of patients with AS is spinal fractures. Fractures commonly occur with a distraction-extension pattern and may be the result of relatively minor injuries. Even though they appear benign (**Fig. 25.2A,B**), these fractures can be highly unstable, with high rates of catastrophic neurologic injuries. Epidural hematomas are often present and can lead to further neural compression. Wedging of the thoracic vertebrae is common and leads to accentuated kyphosis. Rarely, traumatic disk degeneration and secondary dislocation has been observed with highly ossified AS spine fractures.

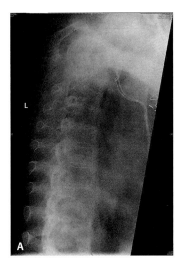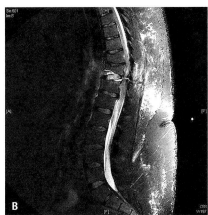

Fig. 25.2   (A) Thoracic radiographs showing what can be perceived as minor stable fracture. **(B)** MRI, T2-weighted images showing a highly unstable extension injury to the thoracic spine seen in **(A)**.

Imaging

The earliest radiographic changes seen in AS are blurring of the cortical margins of the subchondral bone, erosions and sclerosis. Imaging the lumbar spine reveals straightening due to loss of lordosis and reactive sclerosis. Marginal syndesmophytes are visible on plain radiographs. Spinal osteoporosis along with spondylodiskitis, ligament ossification, and involvement of the facet joints may be evident on plain radiographs or computed tomography (CT). CT scans with sagittal reconstruction have been recommended to assess the level of the lesion as well as any concomitant spinal cord lesions or epidural hematoma. Dynamic magnetic resonance imaging (MRI) with fat saturation is now being used to detect the early intraarticular inflammation, cartilage changes, and underlying bone marrow edema in sacroiliitis.[9,18]

For patients with AS who sustain traumatic injuries, radiographs should be critically analyzed. It should be assumed that every fracture of the spinal column is a bicolumnar injury, and MRI and/or CT scanning should be performed (**Fig. 25.2A,B**)[19,20]

Treatment

The treatment modalities should be tailored to address the presenting complaints as just illustrated.

Nonsurgical Management

This is the primary treatment of patients with chronic neck and back pain with or without mild or moderate spinal deformity. It is primarily based on optimal utilization of nonpharmacologic as well as pharmacologic treatment modalities. Nonpharmacologic modalities focus on patient education and regular exercise. Genetic counseling and patient support groups are useful in further educating the patient on the disease.[21] Regular exercises through physical therapy should focus on maintaining posture and improving range of motion to avoid the long-term outcome of flexion deformity of the spine.

Pharmacological treatment modalities, especially nonsteroidal anti-inflammatory drugs (NSAIDs), have long been considered the cornerstone of intervention for AS. They have been shown to reduce pain and stiffness rapidly within 48–72 hours. Phenylbutazone and indomethacin were among the first NSAIDs to be used; however, recently emphasis has shifted to cyclooxygenase-2 (COX-2) inhibitors. With the use of celecoxib and etoricoxib, 70–80% patients have reported a better outcome. However, continuous therapy with NSAIDs has not been shown to decrease the development of spinal deformity. Oral steroids are not used for long term because of potential adverse effects. Sulfasalazine has been reported to be effective in some patients with peripheral involvement along with coexisting inflammatory bowel disease.[20,22]

Promising results have been shown with anti-TNF medications (infliximab, adalimumab, etanercept) in outcomes of the disease either clinically, radiologically, or in terms of laboratory measures. Infliximab is given as 3–5 mg/kg body weight, repeated 2 weeks after, followed by 6 weeks, and then at 8-week intervals.[20,22,23] Significant improvements have been reported in both objective and subjective indicators of the disease.[9] Extraskeletal manifestations also need to be treated appropriately. Osteoporosis is a frequent manifestation of AS, and use of bisphosphonates has been reported in the past for managing osteoporosis. Some recent studies have shown the effectiveness of anti-TNF agents in increasing bone mineral density after 6 months of treatment.

Surgical Management

Surgical treatment is usually reserved for the treatment of significant spinal stenosis, spinal deformities, and fractures.

Spinal Deformities

Management of AS-related deformities is associated with a significantly high rate of complications due to the location of the deformities, the diffuse nature of ankylosis, and the patient's overall health status.[24] Multiple and incremental corrective osteotomies based on the posterior elements, such as wide facetectomy, Smith-Peterson, or Ponte osteotomies, are not applicable for patients with AS, as they rely on an open disk space for anterior column mobility. Any osteotomy used for AS has to involve both the anterior and posterior spinal columns.

When the cervicothoracic junction is affected, patients with abnormal chin-brow angle or chin-on-chest deformity can have significant impairment in both looking straight[25] and swallowing. This severe kyphosis is best addressed at the C7 level, since the vertebral arteries enter the spine rostral to it (90% of the time) and there are no rib attachments. Corrective osteotomy via either a posterior approach or a combined posterior-anterior approach is the definitive treatment.[4,26] The possibility of neurologic complications with the anterior approach is relatively high, compared with the posterior approach.[4,26–28] Opening-wedge osteotomy has been associated with development of permanent neurologic complications.[28,29] 33% of the instrumentation failure cases have been reported.

Osteotomies at the thoracic or lumbar spine are also technically challenging, but complications have been noted to be relatively rare with posterior-based closing-wedge osteotomies.[30–33]

Traumatic Conditions

The majority of traumatic injuries seen in patients with AS fit the extension-distraction pattern and are commonly due to the patients' falling forward.[34] These injuries can be extremely unstable, and dislocations can occur even as the patient lies in bed. Due to the pre-existing kyphotic deformity, the weight of the patient's head and upper body may cause increased extension of the injury unless these areas are properly supported. Immobilization of the spine should reflect the preinjury posture. Fusion and increased stiffness at the cervicothoracic junction makes fractures at C7–T1 common.[22] The cervical spine should not be forced into neutral position to fit the cervical collar.[35] Patients with thoracolumbar injuries are best placed on their side in bed or supine with good support under the head and shoulders (**Fig. 25.3A,B**).

Surgical stabilization of AS fractures should take into account the presence of long ankylosed segments above and below the fracture. This would concentrate the physiologic stresses at the fracture level and stabilizing construct. Therefore, rigid, long-segment and multiple-point fixations are recommended. In the cervical spine, anterior and posterior fixation[36] or long posterior fixation constructs are recommended (**Fig. 25.4A,B**).

Thoracolumbar fractures are best stabilized using long-segment pedicle screw fixation.[37] Percutaneous screw fixation with or without focal decompression can be very helpful in minimizing the surgical time, blood loss, and postoperative wound complications.

Epidural hematoma and delayed neurological deterioration are a real concern in patients with AS.[27,38]

Patients with AS who have spinal stenosis are at risk of developing cauda equina syndrome. This should be treated as a surgical emergency and treated with emergent decompression.[36]

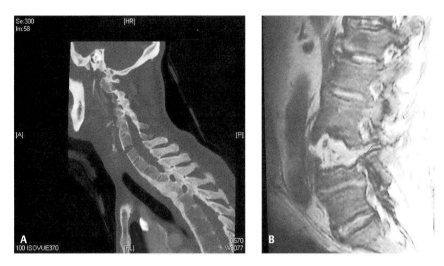

Fig. 25.3 **(A)** Radiograph showing a three-column injury of the cervical spine. **(B)** MRI: T2-weighted images demonstrating an extension-pattern three-column injury of the lumbar spine.

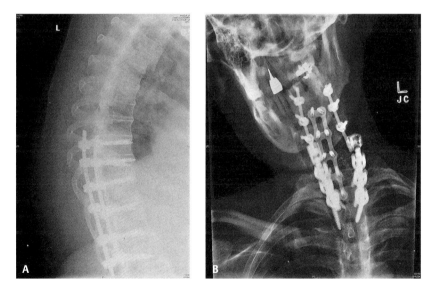

Fig. 25.4 **(A)** Patient of **Figs. 25.2A,B** stabilized posteriorly with pedicle screws. **(B)** Radiographs of the patient in **Fig. 25.3A** stabilized with anterior and posterior instrumentations.

Harrop JS, Sharan A, Anderson G, et al. Failure of standard imaging to detect a cervical fracture in a patient with ankylosing spondylitis. Spine 2005;30(14):E417–E419

> *Fractures should be evaluated in any AS patients with severe pain or a spinal cord injury following any degree of trauma despite the presence of initial negative imaging findings. Present imaging modalities (MRI, CT, plain radiographs, and bone scans) are limited in assessing for spinal fractures in patients with metabolic bone disease.*

Mehdian SMHMD, Arun R. A safe controlled instrumented reduction technique for cervical osteotomy in ankylosing spondylitis. Spine 2011;36(9):715–720

> *Cervical osteotomy in AS is a major operative undertaking with serious neurologic risks. A severe cervicothoracic kyphotic deformity (CTKD) compromising frontal visual field is best addressed by performing a cervical osteotomy. A lumbar extension osteotomy in this instance can improve forward vision to some extent but is not sufficient to restore horizontal gaze. The site of election for this osteotomy is preferred at C7/T1 because: The spinal canal is wide here, and cord, nerve roots, and vertebral artery are favorably placed. The C8 nerve roots are more mobile, and damage to the C8 nerve roots is less detrimental to hand function. The vertebral arteries pass anterior to the transverse process of C7 before entering the foramen; therefore, the risk of kinking on neck extension during the osteotomy is low. Using malleable rods provides for temporary stabilization by avoiding sagittal translation during the extension maneuver, and they also serve as an accurate template for contouring the definitive titanium rods. Rod contouring is very critical in AS patients undergoing instrumentation after the osteotomy. The rods have to fit into the screw heads easily without any persuasion, as screw pullout in the osteoporotic spine is quite frequent.*

Campagna R, Pessis E, Feydy A, et al. Fractures of the ankylosed spine: MDCT and MRI with emphasis on individual anatomic spinal structures. AJR Am J Roentgenol 2009;192(4):987–995

> *Vertebral artery injury is a well-known complication of cervical spinal injury and fracture. Dissection or thrombosis can occur. MRI or CT angiography should be performed to improve imaging sensitivity. Chronic persistent motion of isolated nonfused levels can lead to complete destruction of the diskovertebral junction, mimicking infectious spondylodiskitis. A fluid-like appearance can mimic spinal abscess, tumor necrosis, and avascular osteonecrosis and must not delay the diagnosis of trauma-related fracture.*

Wu CT, Lee ST. Spinal epidural hematoma and ankylosing spondylitis: case report and review of the literature. J Trauma 1998;44(3):558–561

> *Epidural hematoma should be suspected during the workup of any neurological deterioration. MRI scan is mandatory despite obvious fracture on radiographs and or CT scans.*

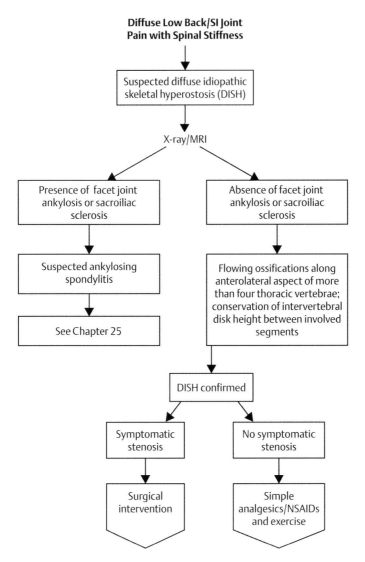

Diffuse Low Back/SI Joint Pain with Spinal Stiffness

↓

Suspected diffuse idiopathic skeletal hyperostosis (DISH)

X-ray/MRI

Presence of facet joint ankylosis or sacroiliac sclerosis

Absence of facet joint ankylosis or sacroiliac sclerosis

Suspected ankylosing spondylitis

Flowing ossifications along anterolateral aspect of more than four thoracic vertebrae; conservation of intervertebral disk height between involved segments

See Chapter 25

DISH confirmed

Symptomatic stenosis

No symptomatic stenosis

Surgical intervention

Simple analgesics/NSAIDs and exercise

MRI, magnetic resonance imaging; NSAIDs, nonsteroidal anti-inflammatory drugs; SI, sacroiliac

26

Diffuse Idiopathic Skeletal Hyperostosis

Kornelis A. Poelstra

Diffuse idiopathic skeletal hyperostosis (DISH), or Forestier disease, is a fairly common (up to 28% of elderly patients) degenerative disorder of unknown etiology, affecting mostly older patients (45 to 85 years old) and men (65%) more than women. It was first described in 1950 as a disorder characterized by spinal stiffness, osteophytosis, and "flowing" new bone formation along the margins of the thoracic spine (**Fig. 26.1A**). The anterior longitudinal ligament (ALL) is usually most involved. Although the disease is more prevalent in certain families, no clear genetic association with the human leukocyte antigen (HLA) system has been identified, and no relationships have been found with either rheumatoid arthritis or ankylosing spondylitis (AS), with which it is often confused. DISH can be associated with type II diabetes, obesity, biliary stones, atheromatous vascular disorders, hypertension, and lipid and purine metabolism disorders.

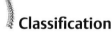 Classification

DISH is characterized by ossification of the ligamentous insertions (fibro-osteosis) and ossification/calcification of tendons, ligaments, and fascia in both the axial and the appendicular skeleton. This is caused by invasion of blood vessels into cartilage and differentiation of pluripotent cells into osteoblasts. The most common symptoms of DISH are spinal rigidity and decreased joint mobility with occasional dysphagia from esophagus compression (**Fig. 26.1B**). Pain and nerve root irritation due to narrowing of the vertebral foramina rarely occur, but spinal cord compression secondary to ossification of the posterior longitudinal ligament (OPLL; see Chapter 22) can cause myelopathy. The diagnostic criteria for DISH include (1) flowing ossifications along the anterolateral aspect of at least four thoracic vertebrae, (2) absence of (**Fig. 26.1A**) facet-joint ankylosis or sacroiliac sclerosis (these criteria belong to AS; see Chapter 25), and (3) conservation of intervertebral disk height between involved segments.

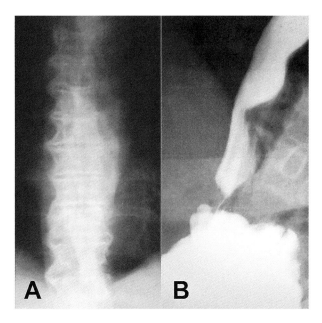

Fig. 26.1 **(A)** Characteristic chest X-ray finding of "flowing" bone on the right side of the thoracic spinal column. **(B)** Dysphagia due to a large diffuse idiopathic skeletal hyperostosis–anterior osteophyte compressing the esophagus.

 Workup

History

Most patients are asymptomatic or have short episodes of "periarthritis" due to activation of the enthesopathy process. For the spine, patients usually have a history of stiffness upon forward bending and mild to moderate pain in the mid-back region. Complaints are fairly nonspecific, but radiographic findings may be dramatic. DISH is often discovered incidentally and is predominantly a radiographic diagnosis.

Spinal Imaging

The T7 to T11 levels are most frequently involved, and the changes are often visible even on a chest radiograph. Extraarticular ankyloses take the form of flowing candle wax in DISH, as opposed to the vertically oriented osteophytes in the "bamboo spine" that form intraarticular ankyloses in AS (see Chapter 25). Disk space narrowing is minimal, and the facet joints are usually preserved. A bone scan generally shows increased uptake and can raise the suspicion of a malignancy. Axial computed tomography (CT) cuts show a thin radiotransparent band between the calcified ALL and the vertebral body wall on the right side of the anterior spine.

Treatment

Because no specific drug therapy has been discovered, simple analgesics or nonsteroidal anti-inflammatory drugs (NSAIDs) are usually prescribed.

Outcome

Improved flexibility and activities of daily living were successfully maintained for up to 2 years after the end of an active rehabilitation program. Cases associated with symptomatic stenosis may require surgical decompression.

Complications

Patients suffering from DISH are at high risk for spinal fractures. Delayed diagnosis is frequent because the trauma is often trivial. Hyperextension injuries occur most frequently through an entire vertebral body or through a disk space in between the ankylosed segments; the incidence of neurologic compromise is relatively high. The long lever arm that develops as a consequence of the ankylosis of multiple vertebral elements causes fractures to displace easily. Back and neck pain after minor trauma in a patient with DISH need to be worked up with a high index of suspicion for fracture. Involved areas need to be imaged (**Fig. 26.2A,B**) with either CT or magnetic resonance imaging (MRI) to rule out global spinal instability, because this is usually underrepresented on plain radiographs.

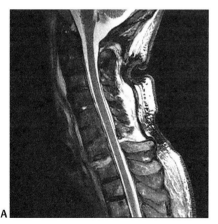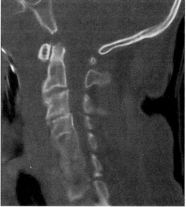

Fig. 26.2   Sagittal **(A)** MRI and **(B)** CT reconstruction in DISH patient after motorcycle accident showing three-column bone injury at the cervico-thoracic junction with minimal soft-tissue damage. These patients are at extreme risk of becoming paralyzed if the diagnosis is missed. Halo immobilization is strongly recommended pending surgical stabilization.

Pseudarthrosis develops and spinal instability may result, with increased risk for spinal cord or nerve root compression. Decompression and instrumentation of the involved elements may become complicated by subsequent fractures above or below the construct (stress-riser) because of the lack of mobile motion segments.

Suggested Readings

Belanger TA, Rowe DE. Diffuse idiopathic skeletal hyperostosis: musculoskeletal manifestations. J Am Acad Orthop Surg 2001;9(4):258–267

This is an excellent and the most complete depiction of the disease and its presentation in the spine and other musculoskeletal tissues.

Cammisa M, De Serio A, Guglielmi G. Diffuse idiopathic skeletal hyperostosis. Eur J Radiol 1998; 27(Suppl 1):S7–S11

This description and radiologic classification of DISH offer modality advice (CT or MRI) for detecting associated findings/complications of the disease better.

Caron T, Bransford R, Nguyen Q, Agel J, Chapman J, Bellabarba C. Spine fractures in patients with ankylosing spinal disorders. Spine 2010;35(11):E458–E464

This retrospective, consecutive 112-patient series review identified high rates of spinal cord injury and subsequent morbidity and mortality rates in this challenging patient group.

Mata S, Hill RO, Joseph L, et al. Chest radiographs as a screening test for diffuse idiopathic skeletal hyperostosis. J Rheumatol 1993;20(11):1905–1910

This study found reliability and validity of chest radiograph for diagnosing DISH: 97% specific; 91% pos/neg predictive; kappa 0.93 between radiologists.

Olivieri I, D'Angelo S, Palazzi C, Padula A, Mader R, Khan MA. Diffuse idiopathic skeletal hyperostosis: differentiation from ankylosing spondylitis. Curr Rheumatol Rep 2009;11(5): 321–328

Distinguishable clinical and radiological characteristics between AS and DISH are outlined and implications for treatment are rendered.

Resnick D, Niwayama G. Diffuse idiopathic skeletal hyperostosis (DISH): ankylosing hyperostosis of Forestier and Rotes-Querol. In: Resnick D, ed. *Diagnosis of Bone and Joint Disorders.* 3rd ed. Vol 3. Philadelphia: WB Saunders; 1995:1436–1495

This article presented the original description of DISH and distinguishing (radiologic) diagnostic criteria.

Sarzi-Puttini P, Atzeni F. New developments in our understanding of DISH (diffuse idiopathic skeletal hyperostosis). Curr Opin Rheumatol 2004;16(3):287–292

This review of clinical, pathogenetic, and therapeutic insights into DISH is an excellent overview of the basic science behind the osteophyte/bone formation.

Weinfeld RM, Olson PN, Maki DD, Griffiths HJ. The prevalence of diffuse idiopathic skeletal hyperostosis (DISH) in two large American Midwest metropolitan hospital populations. Skeletal Radiol 1997;26(4):222–225

This is a random review of 2364 chest radiographs for DISH of four levels or more: >50 years, males:females = 25%:15%; >80 years, males:females = 28%:26%.

Kandziora F, Verlaan JJ, Oner FC. Reviewer's comment concerning "Spinal fractures in patients with ankylosing spinal disorders: a systematic review of the literature on treatment, neurological status and complications" (L. A. Westerveld et al. Ms-no: ESJO-D-08-00152R1). Eur Spine J 2009;18(2):157–164

> *This is an excellent review of 93 recent papers on ankylosing disease of the spine, its increasing incidence, and the complications associated with the trauma and subsequent treatment.*

Whang PG, Goldberg G, Lawrence JP, et al. The management of spinal injuries in patients with ankylosing spondylitis or diffuse idiopathic skeletal hyperostosis: a comparison of treatment methods and clinical outcomes. J Spinal Disord Tech 2009;22(2):77–85

> *This 30-patient review identifies, for diagnoses of both AS and DISH, high incidence of spinal cord injury due to injury in the subaxial spine, with greater than 30% complication rate during treatment. Stable fractures do not necessarily require operative intervention but can be immobilized. Halo vest immobilization is associated with significant mortality and needs to be avoided.*

Clinical Signs and Symptoms of Thoracic Disk Herniation

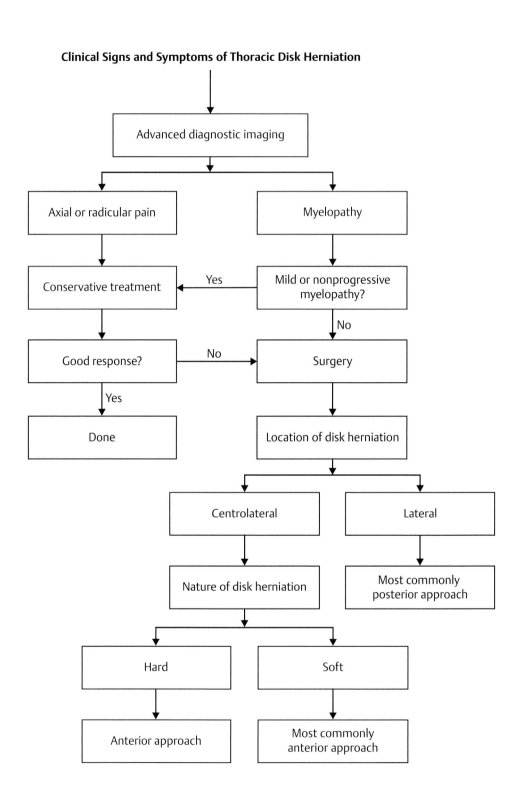

27

Thoracic Disk Herniation

Matthew G. Zmurko

Thoracic disk herniations are less frequent than cervical and lumbar herniations because the thoracic spine has increased stability provided by the thoracic rib cage. The majority of thoracic disk herniations occur below T8 as the thoracic spine transitions into the more mobile lumbar spine. Like disk herniations in the cervical and lumbar regions, most thoracic disk herniations respond to non-operative management.

Classification

Thoracic disk herniations are classified according to their location and nature. The location is centrolateral if the majority of the herniation is medial to the lateral margin of the thecal sac. It is a lateral disk herniation if the majority is lateral to the thecal sac. The nature of the disk herniation may be described as soft or hard. Soft disk herniations usually occur in the younger population and result from acute and often traumatic injuries. Hard disk herniations are more chronic in nature and result from the degenerative process, which may lead to calcification of the disk. Calcified disks are associated with a higher incidence of intradural herniations.

Workup

History

Thoracic disk herniations present with a wide range of symptoms that often mimic other pathologic conditions. Often these patients have undergone extensive medical workups to rule out cardiac, pulmonary, and/or gastric abnormalities. It is during these workups that diagnostic imaging may show an incidental thoracic disk herniation.

Patients typically present with axial pain, radicular pain, or myelopathy. Axial pain is the most common symptom. Thoracic radiating pain typically follows a dermatomal distribution anterolaterally around the chest wall. Myelopathic symptoms present in a multitude of ways. Often patients may present with difficulty ambulating because of a sense of heaviness or weakness in the lower extremities, increased spasticity, or changes in proprioception. Bowel or bladder dysfunction is not uncommon in symptomatic thoracic disk herniations.

Physical Examination

Examination begins with a thorough inspection of the patient's posture and gait pattern. Myelopathic patients can present with a wide range of gait patterns due to their loss of proprioception, increased spasticity, and generalized weakness of the lower extremities. Percussion of the thoracic spine may reproduce radicular symptoms. Sensory level identification is an important localizer of symptoms, as motor examination of the thoracic innervated muscles is less specific in the thoracic spine (**Table 27.1**).

The presence or absence of pathologic reflexes is an important component of the examination. The Romberg sign is useful to elicit changes in proprioception. Ankle clonus, Babinski reflex, and/or superficial abdominal reflex may indicate the potential for an upper motor neuron lesion or compression of the thoracic spine. The presence of abnormal reflexes is a good indication to proceed with further diagnostic imaging of the thoracic spine.

Spinal Imaging

Magnetic resonance imaging (MRI) is the gold standard, as it is noninvasive and provides excellent soft-tissue resolution. MRIs are helpful in evaluating intrinsic cord edema suggestive of myelomalacia, which may result from compression of the spinal cord. MRIs may have difficulty in differentiating calcified disks from soft disks and may overestimate the degree of spinal cord compression. Therefore, it is not unreasonable to also obtain a computed tomography (CT) scan or CT myelogram to clarify this information further (**Fig. 27.1**). CT scans may make it easier to localize the level of disk involvement by counting up from the sacrum or from the most inferior rib.

Table 27.1 Corresponding Sensory Dermatomes of the Thoracic Spine

Thoracic level	Level of corresponding sensory level
T4	Nipple line
T7	Xiphoid process
T10	Umbilicus
T12	Inguinal crease

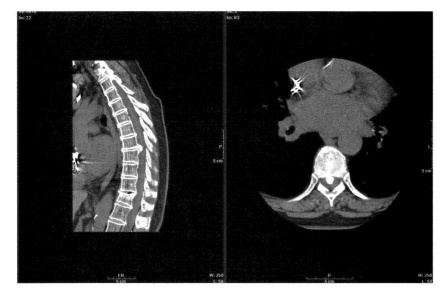

Fig. 27.1   Sagital and axial CT images of a calcified centrolateral disk at the T7–T8 level.

Treatment

Nonoperative treatment is used for the majority of patients with axial or radicular pain complaints due to a thoracic disk herniation. It may also be initiated for patients with mild and nonprogressing myelopathy. Nonoperative treatment encompasses a wide range of modalities, including oral medications, physical therapy, and selective nerve root blocks. Narcotic and muscle relaxant usage should be carefully monitored and limited to short periods of time. Nonoperative measures should be tried for a minimum of 2 months before surgical intervention is considered.

Accepted surgical indications for thoracic disk herniations are myelopathy and intractable radicular and axial pain that are not responsive to nonoperative treatment modalities. The primary objective of surgical intervention is to achieve decompression of the spinal cord and/or nerve root. Surgical approaches to the thoracic spine vary and depend upon location and nature of the thoracic disk herniation, patient's health, and surgeon training and preference.

Posterior laminectomies have historically been associated with high rates of complications and are not recommended. Posterolateral approaches, which include transpedicular, transfacet pedicle-sparing costotransversectomy and microendoscopic keyhole diskectomies, may be employed for soft lateral disk herniations and limited centrolateral disk herniations. Anterior and lateral approaches are suggested for hard calcified centrolateral disk herniations. Fusions are recommended for the anterolateral approaches and transfacet approaches to prevent the development of postoperative instability and deformity. The literature reports approximately a 10% rate of significant operative complications that is consistent between the different surgical approaches, with each approach having its own particular risks.

 Outcome

Studies show the outcomes for treatment of thoracic disk herniations are dependent upon the duration and severity of the patient's symptoms. The vast majority of myelopathic patients who require surgical intervention improve. Aizawa et al. noted that neurological improvement for thoracic myelopathy was not as good as that for cervical myelopathy. It is theorized that this may result from delay in diagnosis, poor vascularity in the thoracic spine, or greater compression in the thoracic spine due to smaller canal area.

Suggested Readings

Aizawa T, Sato T, Sasaki H, et al. Results of surgical treatment for thoracic myelopathy: minimum 2-year follow-up study in 132 patients. J Neurosurg Spine 2007;7(1):13–20

> *This retrospective study reviewed surgical outcome for patients with thoracic myelopathy and found patients with shorter duration of myelopathy improved.*

Ayhan S, Nelson C, Gok B, et al. Transthoracic surgical treatment for centrally located thoracic disc herniations presenting with myelopathy: a 5-year institutional experience. J Spinal Disord Tech 2010;23(2):79–88

> *This retrospective study of the transthoracic approach showed improvement or stabilization of myelopathic symptoms in the majority of patients.*

Bransford R, Zhang F, Bellabarba C, Konodi M, Chapman JR. Early experience treating thoracic disc herniations using a modified transfacet pedicle-sparing decompression and fusion. J Neurosurg Spine 2010;12(2):221–231

> *This is a good review of the literature and a description of a transforaminal thoracic interbody fusion technique to treat disk herniations in the thoracic spine.*

Sheikh H, Samartzis D, Perez-Cruet MJ. Techniques for the operative management of thoracic disc herniation: minimally invasive thoracic microdiscectomy. Orthop Clin North Am 2007;38(3):351–361, abstract vi

> *The authors describe minimally invasive microdiscectomy technique for thoracic disk herniations. They do not recommend this technique to treat calcified centrolateral disk herniations.*

V Lumbar Degenerative/ Metabolic Disease

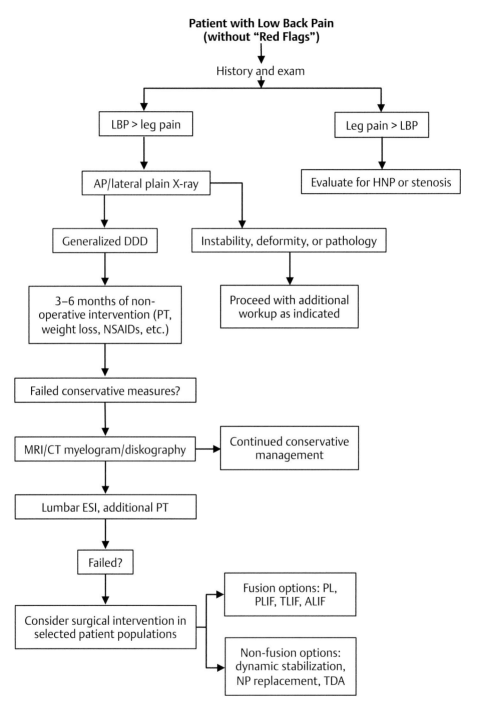

ALIF, anterior lumbar interbody fusion; AP, anteroposterior; CT, computed tomography; DDD, degenerative disk disease; ESI, epidural steroid injection; HNP, herniated nucleus pulposus; LBP, low back pain; MRI, magnetic resonance imaging; NP, nucleus pulposus; NSAIDs, nonsteroidal anti-inflammatory drugs; PL, posterolateral; PLIF, posterior lumbar interbody fusion; PT, physical therapy; TDA, total disk arthroplasty; TLIF, transforaminal lumbar interbody fusion

28

Lumbar Disk Disease and Low Back Pain

Brian C. Werner and Adam L. Shimer

Lumbar degenerative disk disease (DDD) and low back pain (LBP) are common conditions, with more than 12 million Americans diagnosed each year, and 70% to 85% of adults affected by LBP at some point during their lifetimes. The sequelae of DDD are among the leading causes of functional incapacity and a common source of chronic disability in the working years. Diagnostic options and surgical interventions for LBP due to lumbar DDD without radicular symptoms are controversial, and clinicians are left without clear evidence as to the best avenues for accurately diagnosing and effectively managing this common and debilitating condition. This chapter reviews the workup of the patient with discogenic LBP, including physical examination, imaging, and special diagnostic studies, and presents available treatment options for the condition, including current nonsurgical and surgical interventions as well as future biologic options.

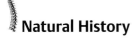

Natural History

LBP due to DDD is believed to be a result of the loss of normal structure and function of the intervertebral disk. Although lumbar DDD is a recognized cause of LBP, it is important to note that disk degeneration can occur in the absence of back pain or other symptoms in over 30% of individuals by age 30, in 50% of individuals by age 50, and nearly 100% of 80-year-old individuals.[1] The etiology of degenerative disk changes is multifactorial and can be related to aging, wear and tear, environmental factors, such as nutrition and cigarette use, or even genetics. In a degenerating disk, over time, the collagen structure of the annulus fibrosus weakens and the proteoglycan content decreases. These physiologic changes lead to a decrease in the water content of, and nutritional supply to, the disk, making it more susceptible to mechanical stresses. This progresses to altered spinal biomechanics, which, combined with release of neural mediators and neurovascular ingrowth into the disk, generate LBP.[2] Continued degeneration of an affected disk can lead to secondary problems, such as degenerative spondylolisthesis, lumbar stenosis, and facet arthrosis, which are not the focus of this chapter.

Workup

History and Clinical Presentation

The clinical presentation of a patient with discogenic LBP is variable. An acute or insidious onset can be described, and a variety of alleviating and aggravating factors are often implicated. Differentiating between acute and chronic LBP is important because the natural history, treatment, and prognosis are different. Lower-extremity radicular symptoms are typically absent, unless there is an associated disk herniation or foraminal stenosis. Claudication symptoms are likewise generally absent unless concomitant spinal stenosis is also present. It is imperative to differentiate discogenic LBP from the aforementioned entities before proceeding with diagnostic and therapeutic measures.[3] Screening for secondary gain issues and inconsistencies is also important. The goal of the history and exam in a patient with LBP is to determine a likely etiology, evaluate treatments already rendered, and rule out serious pathology ("red flags"), such as neural compromise, trauma, neoplasm, and infection.

Physical Examination

Patients with primarily discogenic LBP usually have an unremarkable physical examination. Regardless, a thorough exam should still be performed. The patient should be observed closely while walking and during movement to and from the examination table, which may reveal an antalgic gait and guarding during transfers. A meticulous neurological exam usually will not reveal any focal findings. Provocative tests, such as the straight leg raise and femoral stretch test, are usually negative. There may be limited range of motion of the lumbar spine, with greater pain typically in flexion. "Red flag" symptoms, such as bowel or bladder changes, fevers, night sweats, or unexplained weight loss, should be absent with this diagnosis.

Radiographic Imaging

Upright plain anteroposterior (AP) and lateral radiographs, including flexion and extension views, should be the first study used in the evaluation of the lumbar spine. These radiographs should be evaluated for coronal and sagittal alignment, as well as for the presence of degenerative changes, including osteophyte formation, foraminal narrowing, disk space narrowing, endplate sclerosis, and vacuum phenomenon within the disk.

Magnetic resonance imaging (MRI) is the imaging modality of choice for evaluation of spinal soft tissues and disk detail. MRI must be used carefully as an adjunct to the clinical presentation, history, and physical examination, as 30% of asymptomatic individuals show degenerative disk changes on MRI.[1] MRI, however, is not initially indicated in the majority of patients presenting with LBP due to DDD. If there is concern for malignancy, infection, or if red flag or neurologic symptoms are present, MRI should be obtained. For LBP due to DDD that is unresponsive to reliable nonsurgical intervention after 3 to 6 months, MRI can be a useful diagnostic adjunct. Signs of degeneration, endplate changes, presence or absence of annular tears, Modic changes, or the presence of high-intensity zones all can be evaluated on an MRI.[4] Unfortunately, the low sensitivity and specificity of these MRI findings limit their usefulness.

Other Diagnostic Studies

Diskography is a potentially helpful adjunct in the diagnostic algorithm for LBP due to DDD, as it is the only diagnostic modality that involves direct stimulation of the potentially offending disk. Diskography must involve a low-pressure injection, must involve abnormal morphology (extravasation), must reproduce the patient's usual pain, and should be nonpainful at control levels to be considered a reliable test. As diskography relies on the patients' subjective reporting of their pain, it is limited in its diagnostic reliability, leading to significant debate and controversy over its effectiveness. Furthermore, it has been demonstrated that abnormal psychometric testing further skews diskographic results.[5] Accordingly, diskography is largely considered an available diagnostic tool but not an initial or confirmatory diagnostic test.

 Treatment

Nonsurgical

The mainstay of treatment for patients with chronic LBP due to DDD is nonsurgical management. After an appropriate diagnostic workup ruling out serious pathology, including neoplasm, trauma, and infection, and in the absence of any neurologic or motor deficits, a 6-month regimen of active physical therapy, behavioral modification (i.e., smoking cessation), weight loss, and nonsteroidal anti-inflammatory drugs (NSAIDs) should be instituted.[6] Care should be taken to evaluate imaging studies for correlative pathology that could account for the pain, such as segmental instability, pars interarticularis defects, or deformity, rather than just generalized DDD. Approximately 90% of individuals with LBP due to generalized DDD will have resolution of their symptoms within 3 months with or without treatment, the majority of cases resolving in as little as 6 weeks.

Interventional

Interventional procedures such as spinal epidural steroid injections (ESIs) have long been used to treat discogenic LBP. Although no studies support the use of ESIs in the treatment of LBP, their success in selected patients warrants consideration as an alternative to surgical intervention.[7] The use of intradiskal elec-trothermal therapy (IDET) in the treatment of discogenic back pain remains controversial. There are no good long-term studies demonstrating conclusive benefit, and the procedure is not recommended for general use.[8]

Surgical

Surgical intervention for LBP due to DDD that has failed extensive conservative measures can be divided into two broad categories: arthrodesis (fusion) and non-fusion options. Unfortunately, all surgical interventions for discogenic back pain provide inconsistent results and are the subject of significant controversy.

Arthrodesis can be approached in an open or a minimally invasive fashion, and includes posterolateral, posterior lumbar interbody fusion (PLIF), trans-foraminal interbody fusion (TLIF), or anterior lumbar interbody fusion (ALIF). None of these forms of arthrodesis have been demonstrated to be superior to the others in the surgical management of discogenic LBP, and conflicting data exists as to the benefit of arthrodesis compared with nonsurgical management.

A well-established complication of spine fusion surgery is adjacent segment disease.[3] This has led to the development of non-fusion options for the treat-ment of LBP due to DDD, which allow motion to be preserved at the diseased spinal segment, theoretically slowing the degeneration at adjacent segments. The efficacy of this broad class of interventions, including soft-tissue stabiliza-tion procedures, interspinous spacers, and dynamic stabilization systems, has not been validated in the literature for the treatment of LBP.

Finally, total disk arthroplasty (TDA) is being studied as an alternative to fu-sion for the treatment of symptomatic DDD. Much as with other motion-spar-ing non-fusion technologies, the major advantage of TDA is the preservation of motion at the diseased level and prevention of adjacent-level degeneration and disease. TDA has been approved in the United States for the treatment of single-level back pain without instability.[9] TDA has been shown to preserve motion at the surgical level; however, it has not been demonstrated to reduce the in-cidence of adjacent-level disease. Current randomized controlled clinical trials demonstrate that single-level TDA is equivalent to lumbar fusion in reducing back pain.

Summary

LBP due to lumbar DDD is a commonly encountered problem that is challenging to treat. Initial diagnostic imaging should include plain radiographs, and, in the absence of any neurologic findings or "red flags," initial management should be nonoperative. For the select population of patients who fail extensive conser-vative management, available surgical interventions include both fusion and non-fusion options.

References

1. Boden SD, Davis DO, Dina TS, Patronas NJ, Wiesel SW. Abnormal magnetic-resonance scans of the lumbar spine in asymptomatic subjects. A prospective investigation. J Bone Joint Surg Am 1990;72(3):403–408
2. Mroz TE, Steinmetz M. Lumbar degenerative disease and low back pain. In: Lieberman JL. AAOS Comprehensive Orthopaedic Review. Chicago, IL: AAOS; 2009:761–775
3. Madigan L, Vaccaro AR, Spector LR, Milam RA. Management of symptomatic lumbar degenerative disk disease. J Am Acad Orthop Surg 2009;17(2):102–111
4. Modic MT, Masaryk TJ, Ross JS, Carter JR. Imaging of degenerative disk disease. Radiology 1988;168(1):177–186
5. Carragee EJ, Lincoln T, Parmar VS, Alamin T. A gold standard evaluation of the "discogenic pain" diagnosis as determined by provocative discography. Spine 2006;31(18):2115–2123
6. van Tulder MW, Scholten RJ, Koes BW, Deyo RA. Nonsteroidal anti-inflammatory drugs for low back pain: a systematic review within the framework of the Cochrane Collaboration Back Review Group. Spine 2000;25(19):2501–2513
7. DePalma MJ, Slipman CW. Evidence-informed management of chronic low back pain with epidural steroid injections. Spine J 2008;8(1):45–55
8. Freeman BJ, Fraser RD, Cain CM, Hall DJ, Chapple DC. A randomized, double-blind, controlled trial: intradiscal electrothermal therapy versus placebo for the treatment of chronic discogenic low back pain. Spine 2005;30(21):2369–2377, discussion 2378
9. Freeman BJC, Davenport J. Total disc replacement in the lumbar spine: a systematic review of the literature. Eur Spine J 2006;15(Suppl 3):S439–S447

Suggested Readings

Fritzell P, Hägg O, Wessberg P, Nordwall A; Swedish Lumbar Spine Study Group. 2001 Volvo Award Winner in Clinical Studies: Lumbar fusion versus nonsurgical treatment for chronic low back pain: a multicenter randomized controlled trial from the Swedish Lumbar Spine Study Group. Spine 2001;26(23):2521–2532, discussion 2532–2534

This important study found that lumbar fusion in a well-informed and selected group of patients with severe chronic LBP can diminish pain and decrease disability more efficiently than commonly used nonsurgical treatment.

Mirza SK, Deyo RA. Systematic review of randomized trials comparing lumbar fusion surgery to nonoperative care for treatment of chronic back pain. Spine 2007;32(7):816–823

This systematic review determined that surgery may be more efficacious than unstructured nonsurgical care for chronic back pain but may not be more efficacious than structured cognitive-behavior therapy.

Weinstein JN, Lurie JD, Tosteson TD, et al. Surgical vs nonoperative treatment for lumbar disk herniation: the Spine Patient Outcomes Research Trial (SPORT) observational cohort. JAMA 2006;296(20):2451–2459

This important publication of results from the SPORT trial determined that patients with persistent sciatica from lumbar disk herniation improved in both operated and usual care groups. Those who chose operative intervention reported greater improvements than patients who elected nonoperative care. However, the authors were careful to note that nonrandomized comparisons of self-reported outcomes are subject to potential confounding and must be interpreted cautiously.

Madigan L, Vaccaro AR, Spector LR, Milam RA. Management of symptomatic lumbar degenerative disk disease. J Am Acad Orthop Surg 2009;17(2):102–111

This recent summary article provides an excellent outline of the various modalities available for management of symptomatic DDD and the literature supporting each.

Modic MT, Masaryk TJ, Ross JS, Carter JR. Imaging of degenerative disk disease. Radiology 1988;168(1):177–186

> *This classic article describes the imaging modalities available for diagnosing DDD and the benefits of each.*

van Tulder MW, Scholten RJ, Koes BW, Deyo RA. Nonsteroidal anti-inflammatory drugs for low back pain: a systematic review within the framework of the Cochrane Collaboration Back Review Group. Spine 2000;25(19):2501–2513

> *This study provides an excellent systematic review of the utility of NSAIDs for LBP. The authors conclude that the evidence from the 51 trials suggests that NSAIDs are effective for short-term symptomatic relief in patients with acute LBP. Furthermore, there does not seem to be a specific type of NSAID that is clearly more effective than others. Sufficient evidence on chronic LBP still is lacking.*

Kotilainen E, Valtonen S, Carlson CA. Microsurgical treatment of lumbar disc herniation: follow-up of 237 patients. Acta Neurochir (Wien) 1993;120(3-4):143–149

> *Outcomes following a microdiscectomy are reported in 237 consecutive patients. Patients with prolapsed and sequestered disk herniations did better than those with protrusions, and complications included dural tears (4%), diskitis (1.7%), and reoperation for recurrent herniation (4%).*

Lurie JD, Faucett SC, Hanscom B, et al. Lumbar discectomy outcomes vary by herniation level in the Spine Patient Outcomes Research Trial. J Bone Joint Surg Am 2008;90(9):1811–1819

> *An analysis of SPORT for patients treated with discectomy by level versus nonoperative treatment showed greatest improvement at upper lumbar levels L2–L3, L3–L4, intermediate improvement at L4–L5, and smallest improvement at L5–S1.*

Oliphant D. Safety of spinal manipulation in the treatment of lumbar disk herniations: a systematic review and risk assessment. J Manipulative Physiol Ther 2004;27(3):197–210

> *This article discusses the safety of spinal manipulation for lumbar herniated disk and compares its safety to "medically accepted" treatments, including NSAIDs and surgery.*

Olivero WC, Wang H, Hanigan WC, et al. Cauda equina syndrome (CES) from lumbar disc herniations. J Spinal Disord Tech 2009;22(3):202–206

> *A retrospective review of 31 patients with cauda equina syndrome from 1985 to 2004 showed 27 of 28 patients regained bladder continence. Time to surgery did not affect motor and sensory function recovery.*

Parker SL, Xu R, McGirt MJ, Witham TF, Long DM, Bydon A. Long-term back pain after a single-level discectomy for radiculopathy: incidence and health care cost analysis. J Neurosurg Spine 2010;12(2):178–182

> *A retrospective review of 111 patients who underwent primary, single-level lumbar hemilaminotomy and discectomy for radiculopathy. At 37.3 months, 75 patients (68%) had no back pain, 26 patients (23%) had moderate back pain (and were treated conservatively), and 10 patients (9%) had severe back pain requiring additional surgery and fusion.*

Pearson AM, Blood EA, Frymoyer JW, et al. SPORT lumbar intervertebral disk herniation and back pain: does treatment, location, or morphology matter? Spine 2008;33(4):428–435

> *An analysis of 775 of 1191 patients who underwent discectomy showed that leg pain improved more than back pain in both discectomy and nonoperative treatment groups. Additionally, back pain improved more in the discectomy group.*

Toyone T, Tanaka T, Kato D, Kaneyama R. Low-back pain following surgery for lumbar disc herniation. A prospective study. J Bone Joint Surg Am 2004;86-A(5):893–896

> *The authors reported on the relief of low back pain in addition to leg pain following discectomy.*

Türeyen K. One-level one-sided lumbar disc surgery with and without microscopic assistance: 1-year outcome in 114 consecutive patients. J Neurosurg 2003;99(3, Suppl):247–250

> *This article describes excellent outcomes for discectomy with and without use of the microscope.*

Weinstein JN, Lurie JD, Tosteson TD, et al. Surgical versus nonoperative treatment for lumbar disc herniation: four-year results for the Spine Patient Outcomes Research Trial (SPORT). Spine 2008;33(25):2789–2800

> *A prospective randomized and observational cohort study to assess outcomes of surgical and nonsurgical patients with lumbar disk herniation. In an as-treated analysis at 4 years, patients receiving surgery had significantly better outcome scores than those treated nonsurgically.*

Willburger RE, Ehiosun UK, Kuhnen C, Krämer J, Schmid G. Clinical symptoms in lumbar disc herniations and their correlation to the histological composition of the extruded disc material. Spine 2004;29(15):1655–1661

> The authors studied the correlation between the composition of the removed herniated disk material and preoperative pain. More nucleus pulposus was found in the younger patients (<30 years of age), whereas more annulus fibrosus was found in the older patients (>30 years of age).

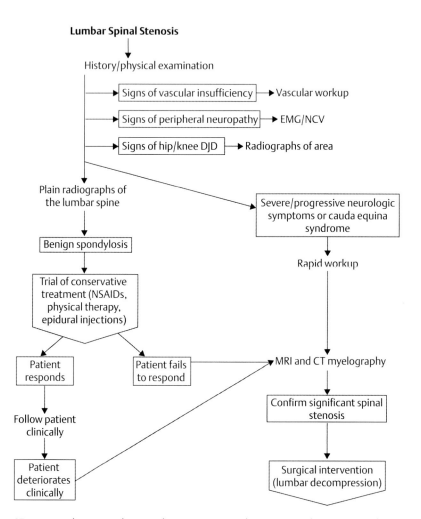

Lumbar Spinal Stenosis

History/physical examination

Signs of vascular insufficiency → Vascular workup

Signs of peripheral neuropathy → EMG/NCV

Signs of hip/knee DJD → Radiographs of area

Plain radiographs of the lumbar spine

Severe/progressive neurologic symptoms or cauda equina syndrome

Benign spondylosis

Rapid workup

Trial of conservative treatment (NSAIDs, physical therapy, epidural injections)

Patient responds

Patient fails to respond

MRI and CT myelography

Follow patient clinically

Confirm significant spinal stenosis

Patient deteriorates clinically

Surgical intervention (lumbar decompression)

CT, computed tomography; DJD, degenerative joint disease; EMG, electromyography; MRI, magnetic resonance imaging; NCV, nerve conduction velocity; NSAIDs, nonsteroidal anti-inflammatory drugs

30

Lumbar Spinal Stenosis

Gregory Gebauer and D. Greg Anderson

Lumbar spinal stenosis involves narrowing of the spinal canal and is a common condition among older adults with spondylosis. Some patients have congenitally smaller spinal canals, and this population is more likely to develop symptoms of stenosis as degenerative changes ensue. The anatomic sites of stenosis within the spine include the central canal, lateral recess (subarticular), and foramen, although a combination of regions is involved in many cases. Clinically, spinal stenosis may be asymptomatic or may involve disabling symptoms. The typical symptoms from spinal stenosis involve crampy buttock and/or leg pain, and subjective weakness with standing or walking. The symptoms are often relieved with spinal flexion or sitting. One third of patients will have unilateral pain more similar to classic radiculopathy.

Pathoanatomy

The causes of stenosis include congenital shortness of the lumbar pedicles, bulging intervertebral disks, infolding/thickening of the ligamentum flavum, and hypertrophy of the facet joints. Spinal canal stenosis is commonly associated with degenerative spondylolisthesis. The narrowing of the spinal canal leads to exclusion of cerebrospinal fluid in the stenotic regions of the spine, which limits the vascular and nutritional supply to the cauda equina. Because the spinal canal and neural foramen are narrowed when the spine is in an extended position, symptoms are generally at their worst with standing and walking. In addition to mechanical compression, vascular effects of stenosis include engorgement of the epidural venous plexus during ambulation, which worsens the compression dynamically.

Workup

History

Stenosis patients classically present with symptoms of neurogenic claudication, causing crampy buttock and/or leg pain brought on by standing and walking. The symptoms may begin in the lumbar region, with more distal migration as the position of spinal extension is maintained. Many patients may also note heaviness or fatigue with prolonged walking, or lower extremity sensory disturbance. The symptoms are generally improved or relieved with sitting or spinal flexion (leaning on shopping cart). A subset of patients present with symptoms of unilateral radiculopathy, with radiating leg pain along a dermatomal distribution. The symptoms can generally be distinguished from vascular claudication, where the crampy leg pain is relieved by rest but not by spinal flexion. In addition to vascular claudication, other items in the differential diagnosis include peripheral neuropathy, nerve entrapment syndromes, hip and knee arthritis, or thromboembolic disease.

Physical Examination

A complete spinal, musculoskeletal, and neurologic examination should be a part of the patient's evaluation, although the findings are often nonspecific. Some typical findings include a flattening of the lumbar lordosis, a slight forward lean during ambulation, and worsening of leg pain with maintained, standing hyperextension. It is rare to find major neurologic abnormalities or positive neural tension signs. It is important to evaluate the distal pulses to rule out vascular insufficiency, and to perform a detailed sensory examination to pick up findings of peripheral neuropathy. Additionally, a careful hip and knee examination should be performed to rule out evidence of symptomatic degenerative joint disease. Some have advocated the use of a "bicycle test," in which the patient rides an exercise bicycle and then walks a fixed distance, with more tolerance of bicycling than of walking.

Spinal Imaging

Standard imaging studies include plain films and an advanced imaging study: magnetic resonance imaging (MRI) or computed tomography (CT)/myelography. The advanced imaging study (typically MRI) will demonstrate narrowing of the spinal canal due to a combination of facet hypertrophy, ligamentum flavum thickening, and annular bulging, causing compression of the neural elements. The axial images can be used to show the dimensions of the spinal canal (**Fig. 30.1**), whereas the parasagittal images are excellent for visualizing the intervertebral foramen. Additionally, MRI can be used to identify associated pathology, such as disk herniations or synovial cyst formation. A subset of patients will also be recognized to have coexistent degenerative spondylolisthesis. It is important to remember that there is a

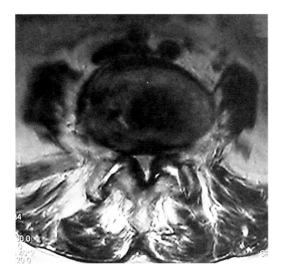

Fig. 30.1 Axial CT demonstrating spinal stenosis.

high occurrence of asymptomatic patients with imaging evidence of spinal canal stenosis and that treatment of asymptomatic stenosis is not currently indicated. CT myelograms can be used for patients who are unable to undergo MRI (**Fig. 30.2A,B**).

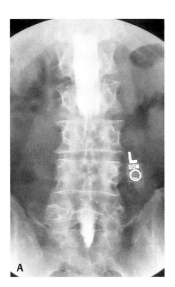
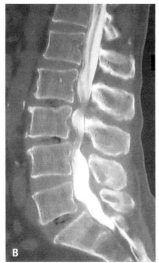

Fig. 30.2 **(A)** Anteroposterior (AP) and **(B)** lateral myelogram demonstrating spinal stenosis. Contrast within the spinal cord and cauda equina is interrupted abruptly at the L4–L5 level by spinal stenosis.

Special Diagnostic Tests

Other tests useful in the workup of patients with symptoms suggestive of spinal stenosis include electromyogram (EMG)/nerve conduction studies to determine whether there are findings supportive of peripheral neuropathy or radiculopathy; vascular studies to rule out vascular occlusive disease; epidural injections/nerve blocks, which may provide temporary symptom relief; and hip or knee radiographs to rule out arthritic involvement in this area.

Treatment

Conservative

Treatment is usually initiated with nonsurgical measures, including nonsteroidal anti-inflammatory drugs (NSAIDs), activity modification, physical therapy, and spinal epidural injections.

Surgical

The mainstay of surgical treatment for stenosis is direct decompression of the neural elements. The classic operation involves a bilateral laminectomy, bilateral medial facetectomy, and bilateral foraminotomy performed through an open surgical approach. This procedure addresses all the sites of neurologic compression and has been studied in a large number of clinical reports. Less invasive techniques using a laminotomy have gained some traction in recent years. Some techniques are being performed with a less invasive surgical approach with the use of a tubular retractor system. When there is associated instability in the form of a degenerative spondylolisthesis, spinal fusion may be added in addition to the decompressive procedure.

Complications

The typical complications with surgical intervention for lumbar stenosis include infection, bleeding, iatrogenic instability, continued low back pain, and recurrence of the neurocompressive disease.

Suggested Readings

Bischoff RJ, Rodriguez RP, Gupta K, Righi A, Dalton JE, Whitecloud TS. A comparison of computed tomography-myelography, magnetic resonance imaging, and myelography in the diagnosis of herniated nucleus pulposus and spinal stenosis. J Spinal Disord 1993;6(4):289–295

> *This study compares the sensitivity, specificity, and accuracy of CT myelography, MRI, and myelography in making the diagnosis of herniated disk and spinal stenosis.*

Boden SD, Wiesel SW. Lumbosacral segmental motion in normal individuals. Have we been measuring instability properly? Spine 1990;15(6):571–576

> *This study reviews dynamic vertebral translation, defined as the change in relative position from flexion to extension, which provides a more accurate assessment of vertebral motion than measurement of static displacement on a flexion or extension view alone.*

Ciol MA, Deyo RA, Howell E, Kreif S. An assessment of surgery for spinal stenosis: time trends, geographic variations, complications, and reoperations. J Am Geriatr Soc 1996;44(3):285–290

> *The authors discuss the temporal trends and geographic variations in the use of surgery for spinal stenosis and in morbidity and mortality of the procedure, and they examine the likelihood of repeat back surgery after surgical repair.*

Dyck P, Doyle JB Jr. "Bicycle test" of van Gelderen in diagnosis of intermittent cauda equina compression syndrome. Case report. J Neurosurg 1977;46(5):667–670

> *A simple clinical adjunct to the routine neurological examination of patients with spinal stenosis syndrome. The "bicycle test" helps exclude intermittent claudication due to vascular insufficiency and frequently confirms the relationship of posture to radicular pain.*

Herno A, Airaksinen O, Saari T. Computed tomography after laminectomy for lumbar spinal stenosis. Patients' pain patterns, walking capacity, and subjective disability had no correlation with computed tomography findings. Spine 1994;19(17):1975–1978

> *This study discuss the relationship between postoperative CT findings and patients' pain patterns, walking capacity, and subjective disability after laminectomy for lumbar spinal stenosis. The authors concluded that the postoperative CT has only limited value because asymptomatic and symptomatic patients yield similar findings after surgery for lumbar spinal stenosis.*

Johnsson KE, Udén A, Rosén I. The effect of decompression on the natural course of spinal stenosis. A comparison of surgically treated and untreated patients. Spine 1991;16(6):615–619

> *The authors studied the natural history of spinal stenosis.*

Katz JN, Lipson SJ, Brick GW, et al. Clinical correlates of patient satisfaction after laminectomy for degenerative lumbar spinal stenosis. Spine 1995;20(10):1155–1160

> *This is a prospective multicenter observational study of the outcome of surgery for degenerative lumbar spinal stenosis in 194 patients. Patients suffering predominantly from back pain preoperatively and those with greater medical comorbidity and functional disability were significantly less satisfied with the results of surgery for degenerative lumbar spinal stenosis than were those with neurogenic symptoms.*

Turner JA, Ersek M, Herron L, Deyo R. Surgery for lumbar spinal stenosis. Attempted meta-analysis of the literature. Spine 1992;17(1):1–8

> *This is a meta-analysis of 74 journal articles to determine the effects of surgery for lumbar spinal stenosis on pain and disability.*

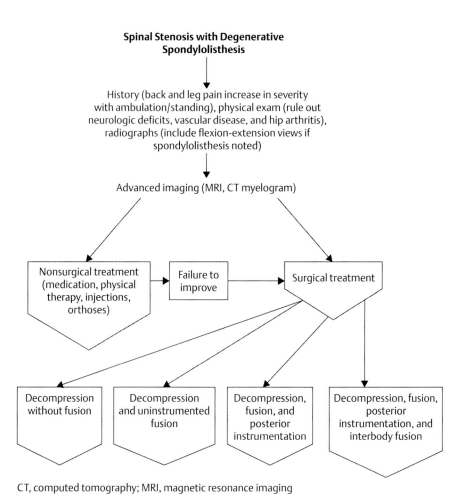

Spinal Stenosis with Degenerative Spondylolisthesis

History (back and leg pain increase in severity with ambulation/standing), physical exam (rule out neurologic deficits, vascular disease, and hip arthritis), radiographs (include flexion-extension views if spondylolisthesis noted)

Advanced imaging (MRI, CT myelogram)

Nonsurgical treatment (medication, physical therapy, injections, orthoses)

Failure to improve

Surgical treatment

Decompression without fusion

Decompression and uninstrumented fusion

Decompression, fusion, and posterior instrumentation

Decompression, fusion, posterior instrumentation, and interbody fusion

CT, computed tomography; MRI, magnetic resonance imaging

31

Lumbar Degenerative Spondylolisthesis

Vincent J. Devlin and Matthew R. Eager

Lumbar degenerative spondylolisthesis is defined as the anterior subluxation of one vertebra relative to the adjacent inferior vertebra in the presence of an intact posterior neural arch. The subluxation results from degenerative changes involving the intervertebral disk and posterior facet joints. As the subluxation increases, secondary hypertrophy of the facet joints and ligamentum flavum contribute to spinal stenosis. The subluxation is usually limited to less than 30% by the intact neural arch and facet joints. Degenerative spondylolisthesis generally occurs in patients greater than 40 years of age. It is more common in females (female-to-male ratio 4:1), blacks (black-to-white ratio 3:1), and diabetic patients. Ninety percent of cases of degenerative spondylolisthesis occur at the L4–L5 level; 10% of cases occur at L3–L4 or L5–S1. Degenerative spondylolisthesis is frequently associated with sacralization of the L5 vertebra.

Classification

Degenerative spondylolisthesis represents a heterogenous process with no universally accepted classification. A variety of factors, including disk space height, segmental motion on flexion-extension radiographs, segmental kyphosis at the level of slip, and the presence/absence of stabilizing osteophytes, have been used to stratify patients into broad treatment groups based on varying definitions of spinal instability.

Workup

History

Presenting symptoms include neurogenic claudication, low back pain, and radicular pain. Neurogenic claudication presents as buttock and thigh pain or cramping pain associated with prolonged standing or walking. Relief of symptoms of neurogenic claudication is achieved by sitting or spinal flexion. Patients may also report numbness, heaviness, or weakness involving the lower extremities.

Physical Examination

Essential components of the physical examination of the patient with suspected lumbar degenerative spondylolisthesis include inspection, palpation, assessment of lumbar range of motion, and a complete neurologic examination, including lower-extremity sensation, motor strength, and reflexes. Physical examination should rule out nonspinal disorders (degenerative hip arthritis, peripheral vascular disease) that may mimic degenerative spondylolisthesis. Hip joint arthrosis may cause buttock and thigh pain that can erroneously be attributed to spinal stenosis. Assessment of hip joint range of motion and the presence of pain at the extremes of motion, especially internal rotation, can determine whether the hip joints are a source of pain and whether hip joint radiographs are indicated. If both hip arthritis and degenerative spondylolisthesis are present, injection of the hip joints under fluoroscopic guidance can aid in sorting out which problem is more symptomatic. Peripheral vascular disease can also cause symptoms of claudication. Assessment of lower-extremity peripheral pulses is an important part of the initial examination of adult patients with spinal disorders. Vascular claudication is associated with increased muscular exertion in the lower extremities independent of trunk position. Symptoms due to vascular claudication typically occur in the distal calf and foot and are not associated with back pain. Generally, these symptoms are exacerbated by walking and are relieved by stopping and standing and not specifically by sitting down or flexing the lumbar spine, as is the case with neurogenic claudication.

Spinal Imaging

Initial imaging studies should include standing anteroposterior (AP) and lateral lumbar radiographs, as well as lateral flexion-extension radiographs. Lumbar magnetic resonance imaging (MRI) is the preferred imaging study for evaluation of the spinal canal for neural compression. In patients who are unable to tolerate MRI (e.g., because of a pacemaker or claustrophobia), a computed tomographic (CT) myelogram is obtained. Parameters to assess on plain radiograph include the degree of subluxation, abnormal mobility at the olisthetic level, segmental kyphosis, and disk space height. In patients who have not undergone prior lumbar spine surgery, degenerative spondylolisthesis presents with a subluxation less than 50% (grade 1 or 2 slippage). Degenerative spondylolisthesis typically results in central spinal stenosis at the level of the subluxation as well as subarticular (zone 1) stenosis with compromise of the traversing nerve root. The exiting nerve root is generally spared from compression unless there is severe loss of disk space height. For example, L4–L5 degenerative spondylolisthesis results in central and subarticular spinal stenosis with compromise of the L5 nerve root (traversing nerve root of the L4–L5 motion segment). The L4 nerve root (exiting nerve root of the L4–L5 motion segment) is generally spared from compression unless severe loss of disk space height results in foraminal narrowing.

Treatment

Nonsurgical

Nonsurgical treatment options include nonsteroidal anti-inflammatory drugs (NSAIDs), physical therapy, orthoses, and injections. Physical therapy should include aerobic conditioning and exercises that emphasize lumbar flexion. Epidural corticosteroid injections are most likely to be effective for patients with significant lower-extremity symptoms rather than for patients whose predominant symptoms are in the low back.

Surgical

Surgical treatment is considered for patients who fail to improve with nonsurgical management or who present with progressive neurologic deficit, persistent or recurrent leg or back pain, neurogenic claudication, and significant reduction in quality of life. Imaging studies should be consistent with the diagnosis of degenerative spondylolisthesis with spinal stenosis, and the patient should be a medically appropriate candidate for spinal surgery. Surgical treatment options that are commonly considered for degenerative spondylolisthesis include (1) decompression; (2) decompression and posterior spinal fusion without spinal instrumentation; (3) decompression and posterior spinal fusion combined with posterior spinal instrumentation; and (4) decompression, posterior spinal fusion, and posterior spinal instrumentation combined with interbody fusion (anterior or posterior).

   Decompression for spinal stenosis associated with L4–L5 degenerative spondylolisthesis typically includes removal of the inferior half of the lamina of L4 and the superior half of the lamina of L5 to decompress central spinal stenosis (**Fig. 31.1**). Subsequently, the L5 nerve roots are decompressed by removing the medial half of the L4–L5 facet joint and accompanying ligamentum flavum. The decompression of the L5 nerve root is continued until mobility of the L5 nerve root is restored and a probe can be passed easily through the neural foramen. The L4 nerve root and neural foramen should also be checked for potential compression.

   Posterolateral fusion is the type of fusion most commonly performed for degenerative spondylolisthesis. After decompression is completed, the transverse processes of L4 and L5 are exposed and soft tissue is removed from their surfaces as well as from the intertransverse membrane. Decortication of the transverse processes is performed with a curette or burr to expose cancellous bone. Bone graft is applied to the intertransverse region to complete the fusion procedure (**Fig. 31.1**). Iliac crest autograft is the traditional gold standard for bone graft material. Some surgeons use only local bone obtained during decompression and increase the graft volume through addition of a bone graft extender (e.g., demineralized bone matrix). Recently, recombinant human bone morphogenetic protein-2 (rhBMP-2) has been utilized in an off-label fashion (per the United States Food and Drug Administration) as the sole graft material

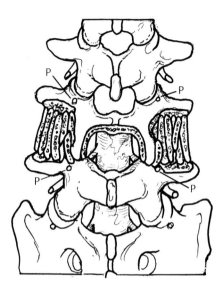

Fig. 31.1 Posterolateral L4–L5 fusion and central canal decompression. P, pedicle.

in the intertransverse region with similar outcomes compared with iliac autograft. If posterior instrumentation is used, a facet fusion may also be performed. However, if no instrumentation is used, facet disruption may increase the risk of postoperative instability.

Posterior spinal instrumentation typically consists of screws placed in the pedicles of the L4 and L5 vertebrae. The entry point to the lumbar pedicle is located at the junction of the pars interarticularis, midpoint of the transverse process, and inferior aspect of the superior articular process (**Fig. 31.2**). The

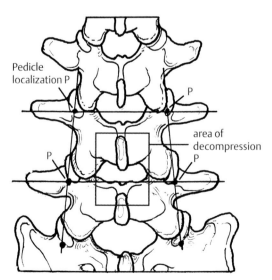

Pedicle
localization P

P

area of
decompression

P

P

Fig. 31.2 Entry points for lumbar pedicle screws and outline of laminectomy.

medial border of the pedicle may be directly visualized to confirm that a medial breach of the pedicle has not occurred. The instrumentation construct is completed by placing rods to connect the L4 and L5 screws. Finally, a cross-link device is placed to connect the rods on each side, thereby increasing the rigidity of the construct. Intraoperative electromyography (EMG) is a valuable technique to aid in the identification of mispositioned pedicle screws.

Interbody fusion is considered in the treatment of an L4–L5 degenerative spondylolisthesis in the following circumstances: (1) when the L4–L5 motion segment has a kyphotic alignment; (2) in the presence of severe L4–L5 disk space narrowing associated with L4 foraminal stenosis, wherein the addition of an interbody fusion will increase the dimensions of the neural foramen between L4 and L5, resulting in indirect decompression of the L4 nerve root; (3) when the required decompression has compromised the available posterior bone surface available for fusion (for example, if the facet joints are completely removed or the pars interarticularis is violated, a posterolateral fusion is less likely to heal because of the decreased surface area available for fusion); and (4) in large-habitus individuals with relatively well-preserved disk space height. An interbody fusion has the potential to improve the fusion success rate and minimize the implant failure rate (**Fig. 31.3**).

Emerging techniques applied to the treatment of degenerative spondylolisthesis include interspinous process distraction devices and dynamic lumbar pedicle screw-rod stabilization. The role of these motion-preserving treatments remains to be clearly defined through future studies.

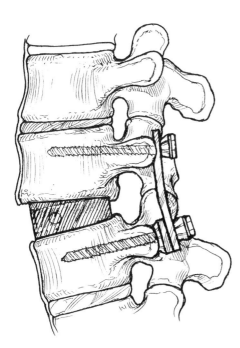

Fig. 31.3 L4–L5 spinal instrumentation consists of pedicle screws at L4 and L5 connected by rods. In select cases, posterior instrumentation and fusion may be performed in combination with interbody fusion. Structural interbody support may be provided by allograft bone or a synthetic cage supplemented with iliac bone graft or bone graft substitutes.

Outcome

Recent outcome studies have shown that degenerative spondylolisthesis patients who undergo surgery improve more than those who are treated nonoperatively with respect to function and pain relief. Outcome studies have shown that the results of decompression combined with posterior fusion are superior to the results of decompression alone. There is lack of consensus regarding routine use of posterior spinal instrumentation and optimal fusion technique as well as the most appropriate source of graft material (autogenous iliac graft, local bone, rhBMP-2, synthetics). Regarding use of posterior spinal instrumentation, short-term studies (2-year follow-up) have shown that although the fusion rate is higher when instrumentation is used, there was no difference in patient outcome. However, longer-term studies (5–8-year follow-up) have shown that patients with solid fusions were significantly improved compared with those who developed a pseudarthrosis. This has led many surgeons to favor the use of posterior spinal instrumentation to increase the chance of successful fusion and to decrease the rate of slip progression. However, others point out that this benefit comes at the cost of a higher rate of surgical and postoperative complications associated with the use of spinal instrumentation. Consensus will be achieved only through performing additional long-term outcome studies.

Complications

Major complications are infrequent, but minor complications are common following surgery for degenerative spondylolisthesis. General perioperative complications associated with surgery include postoperative wound infection as well as general medical problems (acute myocardial infarction, deep vein thrombosis, pulmonary embolism, pneumonia, urinary tract infection). Complications related to decompression include dural tear and neurologic injury as well as persistent back and radicular symptoms. If decompression is performed without fusion, additional complications that may develop include spinal instability with progression of spondylolisthesis and recurrent spinal stenosis. Complications related to posterolateral fusion include pseudarthrosis as well as complications related to harvesting iliac crest bone graft (persistent donor site pain, superior gluteal artery injury, sciatic nerve injury, pelvic fracture). If fusion is performed without the use of posterior spinal instrumentation, additional potential complications include progression of spondylolisthesis and potential for development of a progressive kyphotic deformity. Use of posterior spinal instrumentation is associated with additional potential complications, including implant misplacement, screw fracture, and implant loosening. Other complications associated with the use of posterior spinal instrumentation compared with fusion without instrumentation include longer operative times, greater blood loss, higher reoperation rates, increased incidence of transition syndrome (degeneration and/or stenosis at the level cranial or caudal to the fused segment) and increased procedure cost.

Suggested Readings

Abdu WA, Lurie JD, Spratt KF, et al. Degenerative spondylolisthesis: does fusion method influence outcome? Four-year results of the Spine Patient Outcomes Research Trial. Spine 2009; 34(21):2351–2360

> *No differences were noted in outcomes for degenerative spondylolisthesis patients treated with three different fusion techniques.*

Booth KC, Bridwell KH, Eisenberg BA, Baldus CR, Lenke LG. Minimum 5-year results of degenerative spondylolisthesis treated with decompression and instrumented posterior fusion. Spine 1999;24(16):1721–1727

> *Improved fusion rate and outcome were reported in patients treated with instrumentation and fusion compared to uninstrumented fusion or decompression alone.*

Dimar JR II, Glassman SD, Burkus JK, Pryor PW, Hardacker JW, Carreon LY. Clinical and radiographic analysis of an optimized rhBMP-2 formulation as an autograft replacement in posterolateral lumbar spine arthrodesis. J Bone Joint Surg Am 2009;91(6):1377–1386

> *Use of rhBMP-2 provided similar outcomes to use of iliac autograft and avoided morbidity associated with graft harvest.*

Fischgrund JS, Mackay M, Herkowitz HN, Brower R, Montgomery DM, Kurz LT. 1997 Volvo Award winner in clinical studies. Degenerative lumbar spondylolisthesis with spinal stenosis: a prospective, randomized study comparing decompressive laminectomy and arthrodesis with and without spinal instrumentation. Spine 1997;22(24):2807–2812

> *The authors showed no difference in outcome between groups at 2-year follow-up.*

Glassman SD, Carreon L, Dimar JR. Outcome of lumbar arthrodesis in patients sixty-five years of age or older. Surgical technique. J Bone Joint Surg Am 2010;92(Suppl 1 Pt 1):77–84

> *This is an excellent review of technique for lumbar decompression and instrumented arthrodesis.*

Herkowitz HN, Kurz LT. Degenerative lumbar spondylolisthesis with spinal stenosis. A prospective study comparing decompression with decompression and intertransverse process arthrodesis. J Bone Joint Surg Am 1991;73(6):802–808

> *The authors showed that fusion without instrumentation was superior to decompression alone.*

Kornblum MB, Fischgrund JS, Herkowitz HN, Abraham DA, Berkower DL, Ditkoff JS. Degenerative lumbar spondylolisthesis with spinal stenosis: a prospective long-term study comparing fusion and pseudarthrosis. Spine 2004;29(7):726–733, discussion 733–734

> *Patients with solid arthrodesis have better functional outcomes than patients who develop pseudarthrosis at long-term follow-up (5–14 years).*

Kuntz KM, Snider RK, Weinstein JN, Pope MH, Katz JN. Cost-effectiveness of fusion with and without instrumentation for patients with degenerative spondylolisthesis and spinal stenosis. Spine 2000;25(9):1132–1139

> *The authors document the higher cost and increased complication rate associated with use of spinal instrumentation.*

Majid K, Fischgrund JS. Degenerative lumbar spondylolisthesis: trends in management. J Am Acad Orthop Surg 2008;16(4):208–215

> *This is an excellent review of treatment rationale and contemporary surgical techniques.*

Mardjetko SM, Connolly PJ, Shott S. Degenerative lumbar spondylolisthesis. A meta-analysis of literature 1970-1993. Spine 1994; 19(20, Suppl)2256S–2265S

> *The authors demonstrated that addition of an arthrodesis improved outcome compared to decompression alone. No statistical difference between outcomes or fusion rates was noted when patients with and without posterior spinal instrumentation were compared.*

McNab I. Spondylolisthesis with an intact neural arch. The so-called pseudospondylolisthesis. J Bone Joint Surg Br 1950;32B:325–333

> *This is a classic description of pathology of degenerative spondylolisthesis.*

Weinstein JN, Lurie JD, Tosteson TD, et al. Surgical compared with nonoperative treatment for lumbar degenerative spondylolisthesis. four-year results in the Spine Patient Outcomes Research Trial (SPORT) randomized and observational cohorts. J Bone Joint Surg Am 2009;91(6): 1295–1304

> *The results of this large surgical trial, consisting of randomized and observational cohorts of patients with degenerative spondylolisthesis, show that surgically treated patients improve more than patients treated nonoperatively.*

**Degenerative Scoliosis Patient with Decompensated
Curve with Complaints of Leg and/or Back Pain**

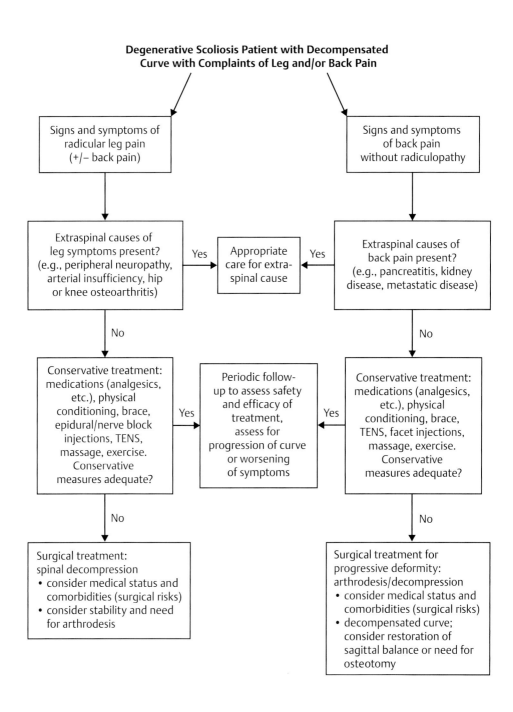

32

Degenerative Scoliosis

Rocco Richard Calderone and Louise E. Toutant

Degenerative or de novo scoliosis presents in adults, in contrast to idiopathic scoliosis of adolescence. Degenerative adult spinal deformity is brought on by asymmetric disk collapse with facet arthropathy and incompetence, leading to unbalancing of the spine into coronal, sagittal, and rotational deformity. Osteo-porotic fractures may contribute to the degenerative deformity. Degenerative scoliosis is present in 6% of the population over 50 years of age, presenting with mechanical back pain from uncompensated sagittal or coronal imbalance and, more commonly, radicular leg pain from stenosis.

Classification

Original classifications of degenerative scoliosis consist of primary or second-ary type. Primary degenerative curves have a predominance of degenerative features. Secondary degenerative curves are those superimposed upon other conditions, such as spondylolysis, congenital anomalies, idiopathic scoliosis, trauma, or infection. A Scoliosis Research Society (SRS) classification system for adult spinal deformity has evolved based upon curve type, degenerative modi-fiers, and global balance. Detailed classification schemes allow comparison of factors that predict need for surgery.

Workup

History

A patient's history of complaints should be carefully defined, distinguishing leg pain from back pain. Degenerative scoliosis patients tend to have a predomi-nance of radicular leg symptoms from stenosis. Adult deformity patients with preexisting adolescent idiopathic deformities tend to have a predominance of mechanical back pain. Patients often complain of asymmetry and loss of the waistline with early satiety. Pelvic obliquity results in one pant leg longer than the other. Pain in the region of the buttocks or gluteal region referred from the lumbar spine is often described by the patient as "hip" pain. Patients relate increased standing and walking intolerance with back pain from sagittal imbalance, which results in muscle fatigue from the attempt to compensate. In contrast to isolated spinal stenosis, radicular complaints associated with degenerative scoliosis tend to be static and unrelieved by sitting, rather than intermittent and relieved by spinal flexion, as seen in classic neurogenic claudication.

Physical Examination

The physical examination begins with observation of the standing spine. Generally, a loss of lumbar lordosis is noted that may be partially compensated for by hip and knee flexion. Observed gait may list to one side of an uncompensated coronal deformity. Coronal imbalance is assessed with a plumb line from the base of the cervical spine to the gluteal crease. Pain on palpation may be present over an inflamed facet joint or along the 12th rib as a result of impingement against the iliac crest. An examination includes evaluation of the lower extremities for leg length discrepancy, pelvic obliquity, contractures, and arthritic deformity of the hips or knees. Pain, numbness, paresthesias, muscle weakness, and atrophy of the lower extremities result from chronic nerve root compression. Anterior thigh pain with femoral stretch testing or lower leg calf pain with straight leg raise may distinguish symptoms emanating from the upper or lower lumbar nerve roots, respectively. Neoplasm and vascular disease are considered in the elderly patient with recent onset of back pain or activity-related leg pain.

Spinal Imaging

Diagnostic testing begins with plain radiographs from thoracic to lumbar regions in the anteroposterior (AP) and lateral plane. Degenerative curves are most commonly in the lumbar spine and centered on L3 (**Fig. 32.1**). Full-length radiographs of the spine assess spinal balance and compensatory thoracic curvatures. Loss of lumbar lordosis is observed on lateral films and presents prior to coronal plane deformities (**Fig. 32.2**). Bending radiographs demonstrate segmental instability in the sagittal plane and curve flexibility in the coronal plane. Magnetic resonance imaging (MRI) provides excellent visualization of the degenerative state of the intervertebral disk and degree of stenosis and nerve impingement. Computed tomography (CT) with 3D reconstructed images or myelography is also useful for assessment of deformity and nerve root foraminal stenosis. Diskography may or may not be helpful. Selective nerve root or facet blocks may be more useful in distinguishing symptomatic levels. Electrodiagnostic studies provide information on the levels of nerve compression or underlying peripheral neuropathy. Bone density tests are an important adjunct for treatment of associated osteoporosis.

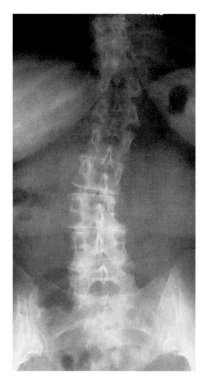

Fig. 32.1 AP radiograph of degenerative lumbar scoliosis with compensatory thoracic curve.

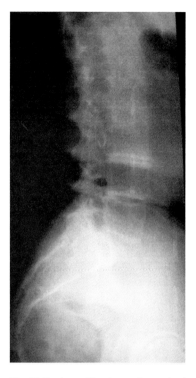

Fig. 32.2 Lateral lumbar radiograph of a degenerative scoliosis patient showing loss of lumbar lordosis.

 Treatment

Treatment is highly individualized depending on the degenerative features and the patient's age and comorbidities. Nonsurgical management is often the initial treatment, although no conservative care option has adequate literature support as the preferred solution. Exercise therapies include aerobic conditioning, trunk stabilization, strengthening exercises, and aquatic exercise. Medical management includes use of analgesics, nonsteroidal anti-inflammatory drugs (NSAIDs), cyclooxygenase-2 (COX-2) inhibitors, narcotics, gabapentin, tricyclic antidepressants (TCAs), and other agents individualized to the patient's circumstances. Rigid braces are rarely tolerated. Soft braces, such as corsets, may provide some degree of symptomatic relief. Adjuncts for short-term symptomatic relief include heat, ice, transcutaneous electrical nerve stimulation (TENS), chiropractic, acupuncture, and massage. Epidural steroids, facet joint injection, and nerve root blocks may play a role in temporary symptomatic relief of radicular or facet pain.

Factors associated with a need for surgical treatment include sagittal and coronal plane decompensation, deformity progression, substantial rotatory subluxations, and spinal stenosis symptoms. Relief of radicular leg symptoms from surgery is more predictable than relief of back pain alone. Surgical candidates require careful selection. Coronal Cobb angle itself is not a primary determinant for surgical intervention. Some risk factors for potential curve progression include a Cobb angle greater than 30 degrees, lateral olisthesis of 6 mm or greater, vertebral rotation of Grade II or greater, and an interiliac crest line that passes through or below the L4–L5 disk space (**Fig. 32.3**). Surgical relief of stenosis requires nerve decompression with laminectomy and foraminotomy. An arthrodesis can be combined with a decompression if there is a risk of further decompensation. The use of segmental pedicle screw fixation allows manipulation, stabilization, and improved spinal balance. Osteoporosis creates challenges to the use of instrumentation and curve correction. Anterior spinal fusion and instrumentation may supplement curve correction and stabilization, particularly when fusing to the sacrum. Minimally invasive surgical approaches involving posterior instrumentation and interbody cage placement now also include lateral access to the disk space. Guidelines for fusion levels in degenerative scoliosis include not ending the fusion at an unstable level with olisthesis, rotatory subluxation, or apex of deformity. Spinal osteotomies are advanced surgical techniques used to correct imbalance that results from deformity.

Outcomes

The SRS Health Related Quality of Life (HRQL) Instrument is responsive to change in assessing adult deformity surgery outcomes. In addition, the Short Form-36 (SF-36) Health Outcomes Assessment has reported worse scores in adult deformity patients treated without surgery compared with general population norms and matched comorbid conditions. The loss of lumbar lordosis with poor standing posture correlated with diminished social function, emotional status, and overall health status. Outcomes indicate sagittal imbalance as the most disabling component. More caudal curve apices and diminished lumbar lordosis are predictors of poorer health than degree of coronal curve. Significant improvements were seen with respect to self-reported health assessment and function among adult spinal deformity patients following corrective surgery. The beneficial results of surgery did not diminish with age or with a more caudal end vertebral level fusion. Regardless of the surgical approach utilized, improved outcomes correlate with solid fusion, sagittal rather than coronal plane balance, and minimized complications.

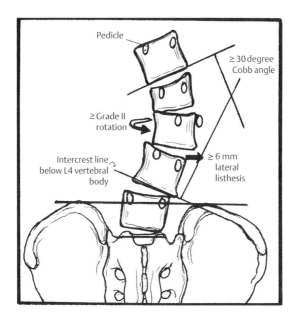

Fig. 32.3 Assessment of sagittal plane balance and risk factors for degenerative curve progression.

Complications

Complications related to the nonsurgical treatment of degenerative scoliosis include medication-specific side effects from long-term use of NSAIDs, opioids, or TCAs. The risks of surgery are increased in the presence of comorbid factors like advanced age, osteoporosis, diabetes, and coronary artery disease.

Surgery-related complications include residual postoperative pain, loss of blood volume, need for transfusion, adjacent-segment degeneration or junctional kyphosis, wound infection, implant failure (especially with osteoporosis), pseudarthrosis (particularly at the lumbosacral junction), direct or indirect neurologic injury, dural injury and spinal fluid leak, and, rarely, retinal artery occlusion with loss of vision. Bone graft donor site morbidity can be complicated by pain, numbness, and dysesthesia. Recent off-label use of recombinant osteoinductive protein has shown promise in avoiding use of donor site harvesting.

Suggested Readings

Everett CR, Patel RK. A systematic literature review of nonsurgical treatment in adult scoliosis. Spine 2007;32(19, Suppl):S130–S134

Conservative care in general may be a helpful option in the care of adult deformity, but no treatment option within conservative care has support within the literature as a preferred solution.

Gill JB, Levin A, Burd T, Longley M. Corrective osteotomies in spine surgery. J Bone Joint Surg Am 2008;90(11):2509–2520

Corrective osteotomies in spinal surgery are reviewed in a current-concepts format.

Glassman SD, Bridwell K, Dimar JR, Horton W, Berven S, Schwab F. The impact of positive sagittal balance in adult spinal deformity. Spine 2005;30(18):2024–2029

Severity of symptoms increases in a linear fashion with progressive sagittal imbalance. Kyphosis is more favorable in the upper thoracic region but very poorly tolerated in the lumbar spine.

Hu SS, Berven SH. Preparing the adult deformity patient for spinal surgery. Spine 2006;31(19, Suppl):S126–S131

A review article of preoperative evaluation. Preoperative risk factor evaluation may help improve patient preparation for surgery with decreased risk of complication.

Li G, Passias P, Kozanek M, et al. Adult scoliosis in patients over sixty-five years of age: outcomes of operative versus nonoperative treatment at a minimum two-year follow-up. Spine 2009;34(20):2165–2170

Adult scoliosis patients over the age of 65 years treated operatively had significantly less pain; had better health-related quality of life, self-image, and mental health; and were more satisfied with their treatment than patients treated conservatively. However, no statistically significant differences in Oswestry Disability Index (ODI) or physical and mental health by Short Form-12 (SF-12) were found. Preoperative radiographic deformity was not a significant factor for predicting an operative or nonoperative treatment course.

Lowe T, Berven SH, Schwab FJ, Bridwell KH. The SRS classification for adult spinal deformity: building on the King/Moe and Lenke classification systems. Spine 2006;31(19, Suppl):S119–S125

A uniform system for classification of adult spinal deformity has significant utility in improving the accuracy of reporting on the outcomes of care for adults with spinal deformity.

Maeda T, Buchowski JM, Kim YJ, Mishiro T, Bridwell KH. Long adult spinal deformity fusion to the sacrum using rhBMP-2 versus autogenous iliac crest bone graft. Spine 2009;34(20):2205–2212

Use of rhBMP-2/collagen in adult spinal deformity fusion demonstrated a pseudarthrosis rate of 4%, as compared to 28% in patients who received iliac crest bone graft.

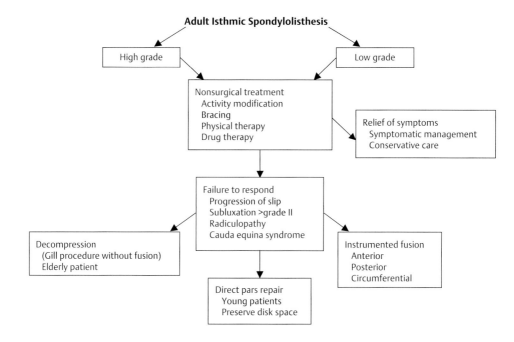

33

Adult Isthmic Spondylolisthesis

Jim A. Youssef, Katie A. Patty, and Douglas G. Orndorff

Adult isthmic spondylolisthesis (ΛIS), a subluxation of a vertebral body (VB) over a subadjacent VB, occurs in 6% of the general population.[1] Although the etiology of AIS is unclear, a genetic basis for isthmic spondylolisthesis is supported by the observation that familial incidence is 25–30%.[2] Acute fatigue-induced spondylolytic lumbosacral stress fractures are also implicated in isthmic spondylolisthesis. Pelvic lordosis correlates with both incidence of AIS and degree of vertebral slip. Regardless of the mechanism, an established defect in the pars interarticularis, or isthmus, progresses to a frank slippage as anatomic and biomechanical forces compromise bone repair. Biomechanical complications arise from forward forces on the spinal axis, and paraspinal muscle strain occurs from prolonged compensation of misaligned sagittal balance. The incidence of slip progression in the asymptomatic adult patient is 5%, with the overall likelihood of progression decreasing with age.[1] Neurologic sequelae arise from changing spinal canal dimensions or compromise of the neural foramina. The most common location of a pars defect is at L5, which accounts for 90% of cases. This results in subluxation at the L5–S1 level.[2] The incidence of spondylolysis in adult high-level athletes (8%) is comparable to that in the general population. Conversely, athletes who participate in throwing sports, gymnastics, rowing, weight lifting, and swimming are found to have higher incidences of spondylolysis.[3]

Classification

Three types of AIS have been described.[2] Subtype A is the classic lytic-fatigue pars lesion. Subtype B is an elongated, but intact isthmus, representing a healed fracture. Subtype C is an acute fracture of the pars. Grading of spondylolisthesis on the lateral radiograph had been proposed by Myerding as follows: grade 1, 1–24% slip; grade II, 25–49% slip; grade III, 50–74% slip; grade IV, 75–99% slip;

grade V, 100% to greater. Angular displacement, expressed as sagittal rotation or slip angle, determines the degree of lumbosacral kyphosis.[2,4]

Workup

History

Isthmic spondylolisthesis is commonly considered a pediatric condition; however, it is becoming more common in adults. Low back pain is typically the initial presenting symptom with adult isthmic spondylolisthesis. Individuals usually remain asymptomatic even with pars defects with or without low-grade spondylolisthesis. It is not until adulthood that some will become symptomatic and seek treatment. Pain may be discogenic or due to the hypermobility at the slip site. As the index disk degenerates and the slip progresses, associated symptoms such as radiculopathy or neurogenic claudication may develop.

Physical Examination

An extensive description of back pain should be captured, particularly the location, chronicity, severity, and quality. Neurogenic claudication or radicular symptoms may be present. Vascular insufficiency and peripheral neuropathy need to be ruled out as alternative causes for symptoms. Subluxation of grade II or greater may result in angular displacement and lumbosacral kyphosis. In such cases, patients present with lumbar hyperextension, pelvic rotation, and hamstring tightness. High-grade slips can also be associated with cauda equina symptoms or radicular complaints. Physical examination may reveal a palpable abnormality over the L4–L5 spinous process junction where the L5 arch is stationary and the L4 arch displaces anteriorly with the L5 VB.

Spinal Imaging

Plain-film radiographs for visualizing isthmic spondylolisthesis include lateral, anteroposterior, and oblique views to reveal pars architecture and the relative positions of vertebral bodies. Dynamic radiographs reveal the amount of translation and angulation. Axial computed tomography (CT) scans are the best for visualizing bony neural arch architecture. They are highly sensitive for spondylolysis and are very useful for assessing healing or chronic pars abnormalities. They can also help assess facet tropism and orientation. Magnetic resonance imaging (MRI) is less useful for identifying the pars defect. However, MRI allows for assessment of central canal and neural foraminal narrowing and is commonly used to determine the need for decompression and fusion. Bone scans are useful in identifying acute pars or acute stress fractures, which are characterized by increased contrast uptake at the affected sites. Single-photon-emission CT has been shown to be more sensitive and superior to MRI and technetium-99m bone scanning. It can be used as a tool to monitor healing during bracing.[1]

Treatment

Nonsurgical options include activity modification, bracing, physical therapy, and the use of nonsteroidal anti-inflammatory drugs (NSAIDs), selective nerve root blocks, or pars injections. Few studies have rigorously analyzed conservative care in the treatment of this population, and treatments generally follow recommendations for nonsurgical management of nonspecific low back pain. Flexible pelvic tilt (PT) has been shown to be superior to extension-based PT in achieving symptomatic relief. After 3–6 months of successful treatment with the use of antilordotic bracing and activity modification, over 75% of adults presenting with symptomatic grade I or grade II spondylolisthesis improve (**Fig. 33.1**).[1]

Surgical intervention criteria, following failure to respond to 6 months of nonsurgical treatment, include progression of slippage of greater than 30%, subluxation greater than grade II, progressive neurologic symptoms, and physical deformity. The goals of surgical intervention via fusion of the affected levels are restoration of disk height; reduction of slip angle and, if possible, forward translation; improvement in sagittal alignment; and improvement of functional outcome. Direct repair of the pars defect to arrest progression of low-grade isthmic spondylolisthesis or spondylolysis in younger patients has been reported.[5]

In the presence of radicular symptoms only, neural decompression and mobilization of exiting nerve roots by removal of the floating posterior elements and cartilaginous tissue (the Gill procedure[6]) has been reported. However, this approach leads to increasing postoperative subluxation in ~27% of cases, though

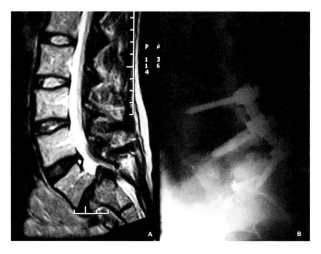

Fig. 33.1   (A) T2-weighted MRI demonstrating grade II spondylolisthesis, degenerative disk disease, and spinal stenosis at L5–S1, and degenerative disk changes, annular tear, and stenosis at L4–L5. **(B)** Postoperative (day of surgery) plain-film lateral radiograph demonstrating anterior lumbar interbody fusion cage at L4–L5, femoral ring allograft at L5–S1, decompressive laminectomy at L5–S1 (Gill procedure), with instrumented posterior fusion at L4–S1, with reduction of spondylolisthesis.

clinical symptoms may not be severe.[7] Decompression alone is now rarely used and is reserved for older patients with stabilizing anterior osteophytes.

Indications for spinal fusion include persistent axial low back pain, progressive slip exceeding 40%, and the presence of a neurologic deficit. Other important risk factors are a slip angle greater than 25 degrees, a trapezoid-shaped VB, rounding of the sacral dome, lumbar hyperlordosis, excess lumbosacral mobility, and evidence of sacral root elongation. The operative approach for bone fusion, commonly combined with decompression, may include the use of interbody constructs and instrumentation to address anterior column failure. The choice of grafting materials has expanded beyond the routine use of autologous iliac crest bone to include structural allograft and intervertebral devices packed with cancellous bone or a variety of bone graft extenders, composites, or substitutes.

Outcome

Most adult isthmic spondylolisthesis patients benefit from nonoperative treatment. Despite the absence of change on the imaging studies, up to 70% of patients with grade I or II disease improve substantially with nonsurgical treatment.[1,2]

Contemporary surgical management generally includes a fusion of the affected segment. The options for fusion include a posterolateral fusion (PLF) with or without a posterior lumbar interbody fusion (PLIF) or transforaminal lumbar interbody fusion (TLIF) or a circumferential fusion with an anterior lumbar interbody fusion (ALIF). The benefits of each approach continue to be debated but do not seem to have a dramatic effect on the clinical outcome in low-grade disease (**Table 33.1**). The role of instrumentation is also still unclear in the literature; however, it is commonly used in most fusion procedures. A meta-analysis compared the outcomes from 35 studies of low-grade AIS and found a statistically significant difference in the fusion rate for circumferential stabilization (98%), as compared with a PLF (83%) or anterior fusion alone (74%).[14] Outcomes of this meta-analysis demonstrated better results for patients who underwent anterior fusion alone (90%) than in patients who underwent circumferential fusion (86%) or PLF (75%).[14]

Complications

Indications for reduction of high-grade isthmic spondylolisthesis are controversial. In situ fusions produce good clinical results in grade I and II disease, which rarely require a reduction. Historically, reduction of high-grade isthmic spondylolisthesis has been associated with a relatively high rate of neurologic sequelae. However, with modern techniques, reduction of high-grade slips appears to be safer and can help to improve or restore abnormalities of sagittal spinal balance. The risks of reduction should be weighed against the risk of spinal decompensation from fusing the spine in the abnormal position in each individual case. Other complications also include infection and nerve root injury/neuropraxia.

Table 33.1 Summary of Results Published in Literature from 2006 to 2010 on Outcomes for Surgical Treatment of AIS

Study	Procedure	Total n	Mean age (yrs)	Mean follow-up (mo)	Mean vertebral slip (%)	Mean slip reduction (%)	Fusion (%)	ODI decrease (%)	VAS decrease (%)	VAS leg decrease (%)
Floman et al.[8]	5 PLIF/7 TLIF	12	47	38	34	95	NR	76/NR	76	88
Kim et al.[9]	Mini-TLIF	46	49.2	29.7	16.7	51	95.7	72	9.3	4.3
Kim et al.[9]	Circumferential fusion	32	51	26.1	17.3	56	100	85	19	41
Kim et al.[10]	Mini-ALIF w/PPF	63	48.5	72	21.8	52	100	50	73	72
Park et al.[11]	MI-TLIF	40 (10 isthmic)	56	35	NR	76	NR	71	71	88
Swan et al.[12]	Combined AP	47	42	24	20.9	53	NR	72	67	NR
Swan et al.[12]	PLF	46	43	24	21.2	8	NR	63	64	NR
Lauber et al.[13]	TLIF	19	NR	50	23	35	94.8	47	NR	NR

Abbreviations: VAS, visual analog scale; ODI, Oswestry disability index; Yrs, years; Mo, months; PLIF, (open) posterior lumbar interbody fusion; TLIF, (minimally invasive) transforaminal interbody fusion; ALIF, anterior lumbar interbody fusion; Combined AP, combined anterior and posterior-lateral instrumented fusion; PLF, posterolateral fusion; NR, not reported; MI, minimally invasive.

References

1. Jones TR, Rao RD. Adult isthmic spondylolisthesis. J Am Acad Orthop Surg 2009;17(10): 609–617
2. Ganju A. Isthmic spondylolisthesis. Neurosurg Focus 2002;13(1):E1
3. Soler T, Calderón C. The prevalence of spondylolysis in the Spanish elite athlete. Am J Sports Med 2000;28(1):57–62
4. Freeman BJC, Debnath UK. The management of spondylosis and spondylolisthesis. In: Szpalski M, et al. Surgery for Low Back Pain. New York, NY: Springer; 2010:Part 4:137–145
5. Agabegi SS, Fischgrund JS. Contemporary management of isthmic spondylolisthesis: pediatric and adult. Spine J 2010;10(6):530–543
6. Gill GG, Manning JG, White HL. Surgical treatment of spondylolisthesis without spine fusion; excision of the loose lamina with decompression of the nerve roots. J Bone Joint Surg Am 1955;37-A(3):493–520
7. Amuso SJ, Neff RS, Coulson DB, Laing PG. The surgical treatment of spondylolisthesis by posterior element resection. J Bone Joint Surg Am 1970;52(3):529–536
8. Floman Y, Millgram MA, Ashkenazi E, Smorgick Y, Rand N. Instrumented slip reduction and fusion for painful unstable isthmic spondylolisthesis in adults. J Spinal Disord Tech 2008;21(7):477–483
9. Kim JS, Kim DH, Lee SH. Comparison between instrumented mini-TLIF and instrumented circumferential fusion in adult low-grade lytic spondylolisthesis : can mini-TLIF with PPF replace circumferential fusion? J Korean Neurosurg Soc 2009;45(2):74–80
10. Kim JS, Choi WG, Lee SH. Minimally invasive anterior lumbar interbody fusion followed by percutaneous pedicle screw fixation for isthmic spondylolisthesis: minimum 5-year follow-up. Spine J 2010;10(5):404–409
11. Park P, Foley KT. Minimally invasive transforaminal lumbar interbody fusion with reduction of spondylolisthesis: technique and outcomes after a minimum of 2 years' follow-up. Neurosurg Focus 2008;25(2):E16
12. Swan J, Hurwitz E, Malek F, et al. Surgical treatment for unstable low-grade isthmic spondylolisthesis in adults: a prospective controlled study of posterior instrumented fusion compared with combined anterior-posterior fusion. Spine J 2006;6(6):606–614
13. Lauber S, Schulte TL, Liljenqvist U, Halm H, Hackenberg L. Clinical and radiologic 2–4-year results of transforaminal lumbar interbody fusion in degenerative and isthmic spondylolisthesis grades 1 and 2. Spine 2006;31(15):1693–1698
14. Kwon BK, Hilibrand AS, Malloy K, et al. A critical analysis of the literature regarding surgical approach and outcome for adult low-grade isthmic spondylolisthesis. J Spinal Disord Tech 2005;18(Suppl):S30–S40

Suggested Readings

Jones TR, Rao RD. Adult isthmic spondylolisthesis. J Am Acad Orthop Surg 2009;17(10): 609–617

This article reviews treatment options for the isthmic spondylolisthesis adult population. Nonsurgical management is generally successful controlling symptoms. Multiple surgical options are available for patients with intractable symptoms despite nonsurgical management. Surgical intervention has shown > 80% success, with low complication rate.

Swan J, Hurwitz E, Malek F, et al. Surgical treatment for unstable low-grade isthmic spondylolisthesis in adults: a prospective controlled study of posterior instrumented fusion compared with combined anterior-posterior fusion. Spine J 2006;6(6):606–614

This prospective controlled study compares single-level posterior-lateral instrumented fusion with combined anterior and posterior-lateral instrumented fusion in matched cohorts. This is a sequential cohort study of two groups, with 50 patients in each treatment arm. At the 2-year follow-up, outcomes showed the combined anterior-posterior operation was superior to the posterior alone surgery.

Weinstein JN, Lurie JD, Tosteson TD, et al. Surgical versus nonsurgical treatment for lumbar degenerative spondylolisthesis. N Engl J Med 2007;356(22):2257–2270

> *This is a randomized or observational cohort study for the treatment of degenerative spondylolisthesis with standard decompressive laminectomy (with or without fusion) or nonsurgical care. Enrollment included 304 patients in the randomized cohort and 303 patients in the observational cohort. Patients with degenerative spondylolisthesis and spinal stenosis treated surgically showed substantially greater improvement in pain and function at 2-year follow-up.*

Wood KB, Fritzell PF, Dettori JR, Hashimoto R, Lund T, Shaffrey C. Effectiveness of spinal fusion versus structured rehabilitation in chronic low back pain patients with and without isthmic spondylolisthesis: a systematic review. Spine 2011;36(21, Suppl):S110–S119

> *A systematic search compared spine fusion versus multidimensional supervised rehabilitation in patients with and without isthmic spondylolisthesis. The concluding argument states that fusion should be considered for patients with low back pain who have failed nonoperative treatment.*

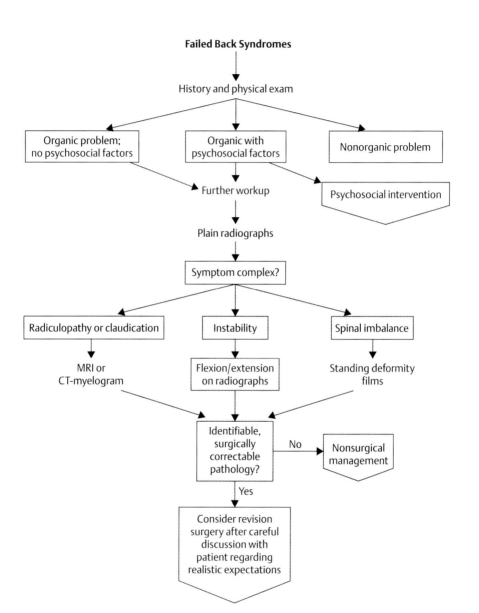

34

Failed Back Syndromes

Gregory Gebauer and D. Greg Anderson

Those with a poor outcome (persistent low back and extremity pain) following lumbosacral spinal surgery are often said to have failed back surgery syndrome (FBSS). Although lumped under this diagnosis, patients with FBSS make up a heterogeneous group with a variety of causes for their persistent symptoms. Treatment for this group is challenging. The workup must consider the possibility of undiagnosed spinal or medical pathology, continued or recurrent spinal pathology, iatrogenic problems related to the prior spinal surgery, psychosocial factors or disorders, and/or secondary gain. By performing a thorough history and physical examination and appropriate studies, it may be possible to identify a specific cause for the ongoing problem. In some cases, patients may be successfully treated with revision surgery. Unfortunately, a leading cause of FBSS is an inappropriate indication for the initial surgical procedure. In this subset, additional surgery is unlikely to resolve the patient's symptoms.

Classification

Although there is no uniformly accepted classification system for FBSS patients, one way to think about this population is to identify the surgical failure in terms of the following:

1. *Wrong patient.* The patient was an inappropriate candidate for the initial surgical procedure. Examples of this type of problem include patients with underlying psychosocial issues contributing to their pain, active litigation, personality disorders, or pathology that is not likely to be helped by surgery. Additional surgery in this group is not indicated.

2. *Wrong diagnosis.* The workup or understanding of the patient's initial clinical problem was incomplete or incorrect, leading to the wrong operative approach. An example of this problem is leg pain due to hip arthritis rather than spinal stenosis, leading to poor results from a lumbar

laminectomy. In some cases, a proper diagnosis may lead to success with further operative intervention.

3. *Wrong surgery.* The pathologic condition was amenable to, but not treated by, an operative approach that was able to correct the problem. The poor outcome could be due to incomplete treatment of the problem (incomplete decompression) or it could be iatrogenic, such as flat back syndrome with the surgical procedure. Some of these patients can be helped by correcting the underlying problem.

4. *Unavoidable complication.* The patient is suffering symptoms from a known complication of the surgical intervention, such as infection, arachnoiditis, or pseudarthrosis.

Workup

History

A thorough history is mandatory when trying to identify the cause of the FBSS patient's continued complaints of pain. The office notes, operative reports, and radiographs from the index procedure should be reviewed whenever possible. The surgeon should seek to understand the initial symptoms and how they responded to surgery. The presence of a pain-free interval after surgery is important and may indicate recurrent or new pathology or a delayed iatrogenic problem, such as iatrogenic instability or pseudarthrosis. Patients without a pain-free interval may have retained pathology, have had improper diagnosis, or simply represent a poor process of patient selection for the index procedure. It is important to thoroughly explore possible psychosocial barriers, pending litigation, and secondary gain from a workers' compensation claim, as these factors would generally be expected to decrease the likelihood of a good outcome from further surgery, regardless of the underlying spinal pathology.

Physical Examination

The physical examination should be complete and focus in particular on identifying musculoskeletal or neurologic abnormalities that may present a clue as to the underlying condition. In addition, the surgeon should search for signs of an exaggeration of pain response or nonorganic symptoms as described by Waddell et al., including a nonanatomic pain distribution, symptoms out of proportion to stimulus, or exaggerated pain behavior.

Spinal Imaging

Imaging studies should be guided by the differential diagnosis generated at the conclusion of the history and physical examination. Plain radiographs may be useful in identifying findings of instability (flexion-extension views) or pseudarthrosis. For patients with symptoms of persistent radiculopathy, magnetic resonance imaging (MRI), with gadolinium to differentiate scar tissue, may be useful, looking for herniated disk material, spinal stenosis, or excessive scar tissue. It is, however, important to remember that degenerative changes in the spine are common and often asymptomatic; thus, any findings must be correlated to the history and physical examination. Fine-cut computed tomography (CT) scans with reconstructed views are helpful in evaluating the status of a prior fusion and in determining the position of spinal implants relative to the neural elements.

 ## Treatment

After compiling the necessary information, the physician should reach a diagnosis when possible. For patients who have an objective that may be corrected with further surgery, it is also important to consider psychosocial factors before proceeding with an operation. Patients without a correctable cause for their pain should be managed nonsurgically, generally with the assistance of other specialists (e.g., pain management team, psychiatry, exercise specialists). The most difficult group of patients are those who have a potentially surgically correctable source of pain but who also have psychosocial barriers impeding an optimal outcome. Treatment in such cases must be highly individualized. When possible, it is beneficial to reduce the barrier through preoperative interventions (e.g., psychological evaluation and counseling) and with frank and open discussions with the patients regarding their problems, the odds of success, and realistic expectations following intervention.

 ## Outcome

The outcome for FBSS patients is less favorable than for patients undergoing primary spinal surgery. The workup and educational process for these patients are demanding. However, there is a subset of patients with an objective and correctable condition who may benefit from additional surgical intervention. With careful patient selection, meticulous preoperative planning, thorough patient education, and good technical execution, some patients (a minority of those with FBSS) can benefit from surgical intervention.

Suggested Readings

Anderson SR. A rationale for the treatment algorithm of failed back surgery syndrome. Curr Rev Pain 2000;4(5):395–406

> *This article identifies the anatomy and pathophysiology of pain and describes an algorithm for treatment.*

Burton CV. Causes of failure of surgery on the lumbar spine: ten-year follow-up. Mt Sinai J Med 1991;58(2):183–187

> *This retrospective review discusses the factors that lead to failures of spinal surgery.*

Finnegan WJ, Fenlin JM, Marvel JP, Nardini RJ, Rothman RH. Results of surgical intervention in the symptomatic multiply-operated back patient. Analysis of sixty-seven cases followed for three to seven years. J Bone Joint Surg Am 1979;61(7):1077–1082

> *In this study of 67 patients who underwent revision lumbar spinal surgery, over 80% had subjective improvement in symptoms. However, perineural fibrosis was predictive of a poor result.*

Frymoyer JW, Rosen JC, Clements J, Pope MH. Psychologic factors in low-back-pain disability. Clin Orthop Relat Res 1985;195(195):178–184

> *In this study, 320 randomly selected males were given a psychological health inventory involving the Minnesota Multiphasic Personality Inventory (MMPI). Patients receiving disability had a significantly higher incidence of psychopathology than patients not on disability.*

Kim SS, Michelsen CB. Revision surgery for failed back surgery syndrome. Spine 1992;17(8): 957–960

> *The authors discuss pseudarthrosis as a potentially treatable cause of FBSS. Thirteen of 16 patients with FBSS secondary to pseudarthrosis improved by surgery to obtain a solid arthrodesis.*

Long DM. Failed back surgery syndrome. Neurosurg Clin N Am 1991;2(4):899–919

> *This is an overview of structural and nonstructural factors that lead to FBSS and the negative incentives for improvement in the current medicolegal system. Emphasis is on prevention through strict surgical indications.*

North RB, Campbell JN, James CS, et al. Failed back surgery syndrome: 5-year follow-up in 102 patients undergoing repeated operation. Neurosurgery 1991;28(5):685–690, discussion 690–691

> *A 5-year follow-up of patients with FBSS who underwent revision surgery found that >50% of patients had a successful outcome.*

Waddell G, McCulloch JA, Kummel E, Venner RM. Nonorganic physical signs in low-back pain. Spine 1980;5(2):117–125

> *This article reviews the nonorganic findings, including clinical tests, to be used to identify patients with nonorganic pathology.*

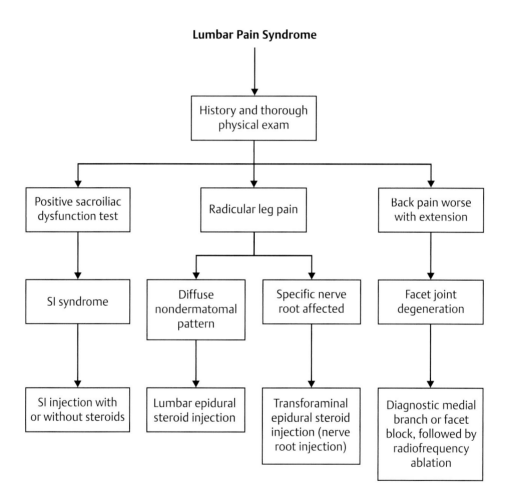

Lumbar Pain Syndrome

History and thorough physical exam

Positive sacroiliac dysfunction test → SI syndrome → SI injection with or without steroids

Radicular leg pain
- Diffuse nondermatomal pattern → Lumbar epidural steroid injection
- Specific nerve root affected → Transforaminal epidural steroid injection (nerve root injection)

Back pain worse with extension → Facet joint degeneration → Diagnostic medial branch or facet block, followed by radiofrequency ablation

35

Lumbar Injections and Procedures

Sapan D. Gandhi and D. Greg Anderson

Because of their high prevalence and debilitating nature, low back pain and radiculopathy have important social, economic, and clinical implications. Although numerous nonsurgical interventions are available for these conditions, lumbar injection therapies have grown to become a popular conservative treatment option because of their dual role as a therapeutic and diagnostic tool. Lumbar injections may serve as a therapeutic tool by temporarily relieving symptoms in some patients, while also serving as a diagnostic tool to confirm pain etiology.

Classification

Lumbar injections can be categorized into one of three groups: those that address neural inflammatory symptoms (epidurals and selective nerve blocks), those that address facet joint pain (facet joint blocks and medial branch blocks), and those directed at sacroiliac (SI) joint dysfunction (SI joint blocks).

Workup

History and Physical Examination

Patients considered for lumbar injections should first give a thorough history and undergo a physical examination.

Spinal Imaging

Spinal imaging is typically performed prior to lumbar injections. Imaging, including radiographs, magnetic resonance imaging (MRI), and computed tomographic (CT) myelography, plays a vital role in determining pain etiology and determining the appropriate course of action. As the treating physician search-es for pain generators in the spine, fluoroscopically guided, contrast-enhanced diagnostic injections may also assume an important role in identifying the pain generators and directing further therapeutic interventions.

Treatment

SI Joint Injections

Pathology in the SI joint can produce pain in the back, buttocks, and thighs. SI pain has been suggested to make up ~15% of low back pain. Because the physi-cal examination is nonspecific, diagnostic injections are crucial to the diagnosis of SI dysfunction. To approach the SI joint, the needle is introduced inferiorly into the diarthrodial portion of the joint (**Fig. 35.1A**).

Epidural Injections

Epidural steroids help decrease the presence of local inflammatory factors and reduce nerve root irritation, leading to some symptomatic relief in some pa-tients. Some patients even temporarily experience complete symptomatic relief if nerve root irritation is the sole etiology of their low back and leg pain. Some authors have hypothesized that the volume of the injectate is important because it may physically dilute the concentration of local inflammatory mediators, al-though there is not strong evidence to support this rationale. In general, these injections are most effective for acute or subacute radicular symptoms. The pro-cedure may be done with or without fluoroscopic guidance, although the accu-racy of the injection is significantly improved with the use of fluoroscopy. Often, epidural injections are done in a series of two to three, performed 2 to 3 weeks apart, tailored to the patient's response. Many different types of injections and approaches have been developed utilizing epidural steroid injections, including:

1. Transforaminal epidural steroid injections (**Fig. 35.1B**), which are per-formed from a lateral approach so that the injectate can be delivered di-rectly into the neural foramen, anterior to the dural sleeve and around the exiting nerve root. This approach is best suited for unilateral leg symptoms in a specific dermatome that can be targeted to a specific symptomatic nerve root.
2. Translaminar epidural steroid injection (**Fig. 35.1C**), which is done through a midline approach. This approach is best suited for symptoms involving multiple dermatomes.

Facet Joints

The term *facet joint syndrome* describes pain in the back that is derived from degeneration of the facet joint. Both the facet joint and the multifidus muscle are innervated by the medial branch of the dorsal ramus. Each nerve supplies

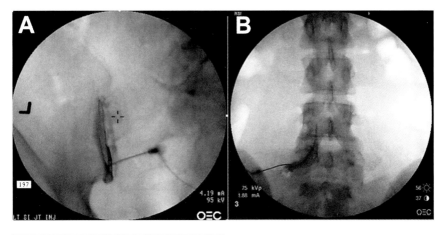

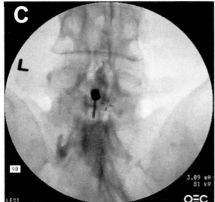

Fig. 35.1 **(A)** SI arthrogram with the needle in the inferior aspect of the left SI joint. **(B)** Anteroposterior view of the left L5–S1 transforaminal (nerve root) injection. Shown here is the contrast spread around the proximal takeoff of the nerve root as well as epidural spread at the corresponding level. **(C)** Translaminar epidural steroid injection with the needle inserted at the L3–L4 interspace. Contrast spread is limited in the caudad direction.

at least two facet joints; therefore, each facet joint may be innervated by more than one nerve. The diagnosis of pain derived from facet joint degeneration depends on a specific clinical presentation and a positive response to diagnostic blocks. Patients whose pain is definitively derived from facet joint degeneration (i.e., consistent positive response to facet or medial branch blocks) may be considered candidates for radiofrequency denervation of medial branches of the dorsal rami. Successful medial branch ablation may prolong the beneficial response to the facet or medial branch blocks.

Diagnostic blocks of medial branches of the dorsal rami involve injecting a small volume of local anesthetic (no more than 0.3 mL) at the junction of the transverse process and the pedicle. Patients with at least 50% pain relief may be considered for denervation of the medial branches.

Outcome

The increasing cost of back pain and the growing socioeconomic implications of the disability have increased the interest in studying the outcomes of care, clinical effectiveness, and cost-effectiveness of interventional techniques in pain management.

The short-term and diagnostic benefit of epidural injections for radicular symptoms is well accepted and plays a vital role in the care of patients with symptomatic lumbar spine pathologies. However, the long-term efficacy of injection procedures and the use of injections to control other symptoms like back pain remain controversial. Patients who stop seeing benefits from procedures like lumbar injections should be considered candidates for surgical intervention.

Complications

Complications discussed with patients undergoing injection procedures include the risk of infection, bleeding, allergic reaction (especially to the contrast agents), pain exacerbation, unintentional intrathecal or intravascular injections, epidural hematomas (especially in anticoagulated patients), temporary anesthesia of the sacral plexus during SI injections, diskitis (diskography), and medical complications. Of particular concern, lumbar transforaminal steroid injections have been linked to very rare complications, with intravascular injections causing neurologic injuries to the cord or brainstem.

To reduce the risk of technical complications, aspiration prior to injection should always be used. Contrast agents are critical for lumbar injection to watch the pattern and spread of contrast and avoid an intravascular injection using real-time fluoroscopy. Prior to a spinal injection, a thorough medical history should be taken, especially concentrating on any history of bleeding disorders, anticoagulants, or allergic reactions to contrast agents (shellfish allergy). Some believe that the use of a water-soluble steroid agent such as betamethasone may be safer in case of inadvertent intravascular injection. Meticulous sterile techniques should always be used to minimize the risk of infection.

Suggested Readings

Benzon H, Rathmell JP, Wu CL, et al. Raj's Practical Management of Pain. Philadelphia, PA: Mosby/Elsevier; 2008

>   *This book provides an overview of pain syndromes and common pain management strategies and techniques.*

Koes BW, Scholten RJPM, Mens JMA, Bouter LM. Efficacy of epidural steroid injections for low-back pain and sciatica: a systematic review of randomized clinical trials. Pain 1995;63(3): 279–288

>   *In this meta-analysis, the authors identified and evaluated 12 randomized clinical trials and concluded that the best studies show inconsistent results. The benefits of steroid injections, if any, seem to be of short duration.*

Rho ME, Tang CT. The efficacy of lumbar epidural steroid injections: transforaminal, interlaminar, and caudal approaches. Phys Med Rehabil Clin N Am 2011;22(1):139–148

> *This is a review of epidural steroid injections for the lumbar spine and an up-to-date summary of studies evaluating its efficacy*

Tsai SP, Gilstrap EL, Cowles SR, Waddell LC Jr, Ross CE. Personal and job characteristics of musculoskeletal injuries in an industrial population. J Occup Med 1992;34(6):606–612

> *In this cross-sectional study, the authors found that estimated relative risks for low-back injuries are significantly higher among smokers, overweight persons, and persons in potentially more physically demanding jobs. They suggest the implementation of an integrated injury prevention program.*

Vlad V, Bhat A, Lutz G, et al. Transformational epidural steroid injections in lumbosacral radiculopathy: a prospective randomized study. Spine 2002;27:11–16

> *In this prospective study randomized by patient choice, the final analysis includes 48 patients with a follow-up period of 16 months. The authors conclude that fluoroscopically guided transforaminal injections serve as an important tool in the nonsurgical management of lumbosacral radiculopathy secondary to a herniated nucleus pulposus.*

Waldman SD. Atlas of Pain Management Injection Techniques. Philadelphia, PA: WB Saunders; 2007

> *This book gives a comprehensive look at injection techniques for pain management.*

VI Scoliosis

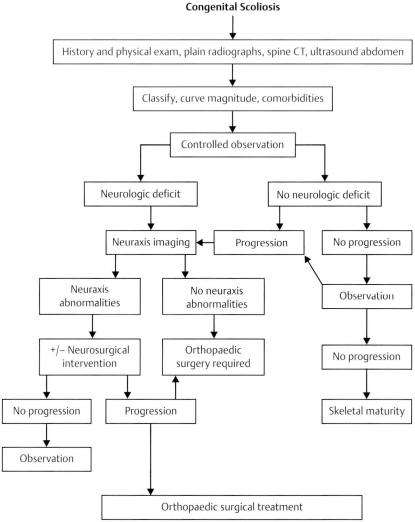

Congenital Scoliosis

History and physical exam, plain radiographs, spine CT, ultrasound abdomen

Classify, curve magnitude, comorbidities

Controlled observation

Neurologic deficit

No neurologic deficit

Neuraxis imaging

Progression

No progression

Neuraxis abnormalities

No neuraxis abnormalities

Observation

+/– Neurosurgical intervention

Orthopaedic surgery required

No progression

No progression

Progression

Skeletal maturity

Observation

Orthopaedic surgical treatment

Primary procedures: in situ posterior spinal fusion (PSF) ± anterior spinal fusion (ASF) ± posterior instrumentation; PSF ± ASF + posterior instrumentation; ASF + anterior instrumentation; hemivertebra excision + ASF/PSF + anterior and/or posterior instrumentation; anterior hemiepiphysiodesis/posterior hemiarthrodesis + instrumentation; vertebral stapling/VEPTR

Salvage procedures: PSF + posterior instrumentation ± ASF; hemivertebra excision + ASF/PSF + instrumentation; spinal osteotomies + ASF/PSF + instrumentation

CT, computed tomography; VEPTR, vertical expandable prosthetic titanium rib

36

Congenital Scoliosis

John P. Lubicky

Congenital scoliosis is a spinal deformity caused by incompletely formed or incompletely segmented vertebrae and has as its essential characteristic *asymmetric growth*. Other associated abnormalities may also be present in patients with congenital scoliosis. Klippel-Feil syndrome is seen in ~25% of these patients, and some form of renal abnormality in 30%. Cardiac abnormalities can be found in ~12% of these patients and some type of dysraphism or other neuraxis abnormalities can be seen in ~15%. It is very important to identify these associated problems because they may have significant impact on the timing and/or the treatment of the spinal abnormality. Knowing the precise anomaly in the case of a congenital spine deformity can help in prognosticating the natural history of the condition. This may help in treatment planning or advising the patient and family with regard to the future and the need for treatment.

Classification

Congenital deformities can be classified as type I: failure of formation (**Fig. 36.1**), type II: failures of segmentation (**Fig. 36.2**), or a combination of both. If healthy growth plates exist on a hemivertebra or between vertebrae connected by a unilateral bar, relentless progression of the deformity can be anticipated. However, the vertebral abnormality (and there can be multiple ones along the entire spinal column) may simply stunt the growth of the spine without causing major coronal or sagittal plane deformities. Therefore, stunting of trunk growth may occur because of the nature of the abnormality and have little or nothing to do with treatment.

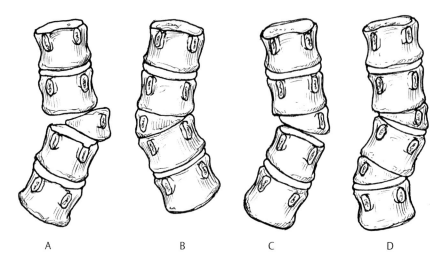

Fig. 36.1 Classification: type I congenital spine deformity, failure of formation. **(A)** Segmented, unincarcerated hemivertebra. **(B)** Nonsegmented hemivertebra. **(C)** Partially segmented hemivertebra. **(D)** Hemimetameric shift.

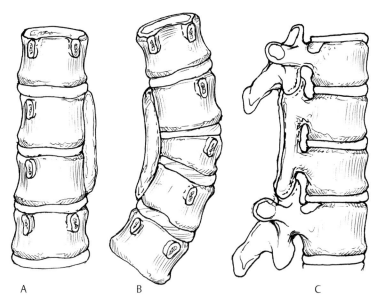

Fig. 36.2 Classification: type II congenital spine deformity, failure of segmentation. **(A)** Unilateral bar with unsegmented adjacent vertebra. **(B)** Unilateral bar with contralateral segmented hemivertebra. **(C)** Posterior bar.

Workup

Physical Examination

The physical examination of a patient with a congenital spine deformity is important and revealing. Even infants with congenital scoliosis can manifest a severe deformity and secondary abnormalities, such as an elevated shoulder or rib hump. The exam may also demonstrate other signs of associated conditions, such as a short stiff neck, a hairy patch on the back, a heart murmur, or even an abdominal mass, which may reflect the presence of hydronephrosis. There also may be a significantly deformed chest and other musculoskeletal abnormalities.

Spinal Imaging

Appropriate spinal imaging techniques should be used to define the skeletal anomaly and also to rule out often-associated neuraxis abnormalities and abnormalities of other organ systems such as the kidneys or heart. Plain radiography in the upright position in the posteroanterior or anteroposterior (PA or AP) and lateral projections helps to define the nature of the deformity and the overall spinal balance and position of the trunk and is the standard image to be used for subsequent radiographic follow-up. Plain radiographs of the neck also can help rule out Klippel-Feil syndrome. Computed tomography (CT) with three-dimensional (3D) reconstruction has become the standard method of demonstrating the pathoanatomy and is extremely valuable in surgical planning. Magnetic resonance imaging (MRI) demonstrates the neuraxis, whose evaluation is absolutely essential in the presence of a recognizable neurologic deficit and/or prior to surgery as a preoperative evaluation. Ultrasound of the abdomen is important to delineate anomalies of the genitourinary tract, and additional workup of cardiac and renal function should be done prior to any surgical treatment.

Treatment

With regard to prognosis and natural history, active growth is the enemy of congenital scoliosis. Winter has noted that 25% of these deformities do not worsen, 50% worsen moderately, and 25% progress a severe amount. To determine which of these three categories a child falls into, a period of "controlled" observation should be instituted as long as there are no impending neurologic problems that may affect the child's prognosis.

Nonoperative measures are ineffective in the treatment of a deformity comprised of congenital vertebral abnormalities. Surgery for congenital scoliosis can be divided into one of two categories: growth-preserving procedures and trunk-shortening procedures. An example of a trunk-shortening procedure is posterior spinal fusion with or without instrumentation. It is important to understand that in a very skeletally immature patient, anterior fusion must generally accompany any posterior fusion to prevent the crankshaft phenomenon, which would tend to negate the improvement seen initially with posterior fusion. Hemivertebra excision is technically a trunk-shortening procedure, but shortening is minimal if only two vertebrae are fused together and good correction is achieved. Growth-preserving techniques include hemiepiphysiodesis/hemiarthrodesis (H/H), growing rods, and vertical expandable prosthetic titanium rib (VEPTR) as well as vertebral body stapling. H/H is used to treat congenital scoliosis secondary to a hemivertebra that does not have an opposite unsegmented bar. The goal of this procedure is to prevent curve progression and, as a secondary benefit, to gain slow spontaneous correction (though somewhat unpredictable), analogous to that seen with physeal stapling of a long bone. Generally only a few levels are involved, thereby limiting the amount of trunk shortening. However, in a situation appropriate for H/H, a hemivertebra excision would often be a better alternative that has the advantage of definitive and acute correction and elimination of the cause of the asymmetric growth (**Fig. 36.3A–D**). Surgery to preserve trunk height should not be performed if it cannot control a deformity that is severe and progressing. Even if a trunk-shortening procedure is chosen, it should not be delayed to the point that a complicated salvage operation is required because of the magnitude of the deformity. Vertebral stapling on the convex side of the curve is a new form of treatment. VEPTR is designed to correct chest deformity caused by fused ribs and to provide some corrective force to the congenital curve without fusing the spine. More experience with spinal correction will be needed to assess its effectiveness fully. However, it is clear that VEPTR can improve the space available for the lung and therefore lung function. Certain forms of treatment, such as H/H and vertebral stapling as well as VEPTR, need to be instituted early, before the deformity is "too big," so that growth can help in the spontaneous correction of the deformity and excessive forces on the bone/implant interface can be avoided. The treatment for this heterogeneous group of spinal anomalies must be individualized for each patient.

Outcome

The outcome is largely dependent on the pattern of congenital deformity and the magnitude of the spinal curve; the nature and severity of associated anomalies of the neurologic, cardiac, and renal systems; and complications of treatment.

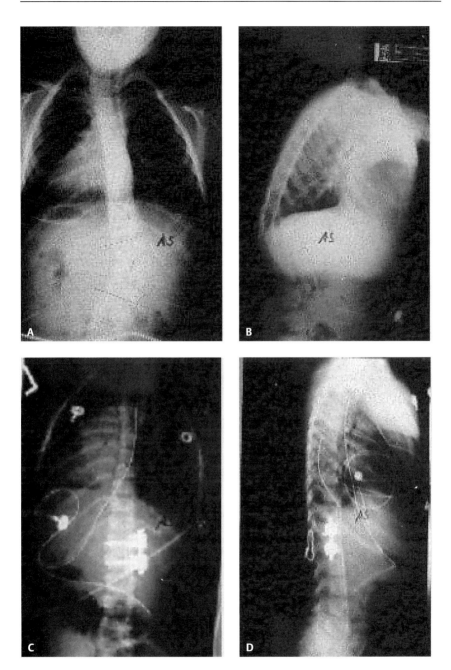

Fig. 36.3 Radiographs of thoracolumbar spine with a hemivertebra causing a scoliosis, treated by hemivertebra resection. **(A)** Preoperative AP. **(B)** Preoperative lateral. **(C)** Postoperative AP. **(D)** Postoperative lateral of the same patient after hemivertebra resection, showing complete correction of the scoliosis and normalization of the sagittal alignment achieved with the fusion of only one motion segment.

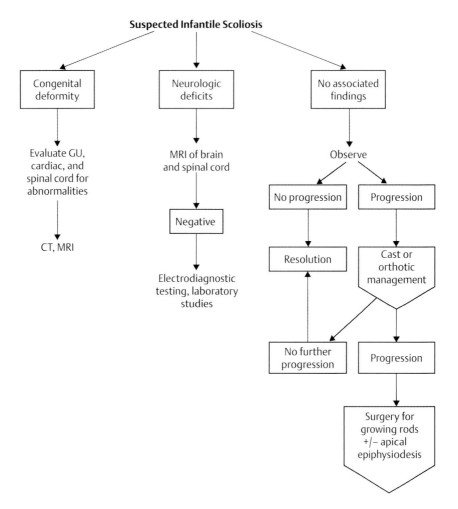

Suspected Infantile Scoliosis

Congenital deformity → Evaluate GU, cardiac, and spinal cord for abnormalities → CT, MRI

Neurologic deficits → MRI of brain and spinal cord → Negative → Electrodiagnostic testing, laboratory studies

No associated findings → Observe
- No progression → Resolution
- Progression → Cast or orthotic management
  - No further progression
  - Progression → Surgery for growing rods +/− apical epiphysiodesis

CT, computed tomography; GU, genitourinary; MRI, magnetic resonance imaging

37

Infantile Scoliosis

Samuel R. Rosenfeld

Infantile idiopathic scoliosis is a coronal plane deformity of the spine exceeding 10 degrees diagnosed prior to the age of 3 years. Weinstein prefers the classification of early-onset idiopathic scoliosis. Infantile scoliosis differs from adolescent scoliosis in that males are more commonly affected than females and the curve patterns are levoconvex (apex toward the left) in 75% of reported cases.

The etiology is unknown, but the main theories include intrauterine molding and postnatal pressure. A segmental radiological study of the spine and rib cage in children with progressive infantile scoliosis determined that the thorax is narrower and the upper chest is funnel-shaped. These findings suggest vertebral rotation is predictive of progressive deformity. By definition, idiopathic infantile scoliosis excludes:

1. Congenital deformities, such as hemivertebrae and spinal dysrhaphism
2. Neuromuscular conditions, such as cerebral palsy, spina bifida, muscular dystrophy, and spinal muscular atrophy
3. Trauma
4. Infection
5. Neoplasm, especially neurofibromatosis and spinal cord tumors (primitive neuroectodermal tumor of infancy)
6. Metabolic bone disease (osteomalacia)
7. Connective tissue diseases (osteogenesis imperfecta, Marfan and Ehlers-Danlos syndromes)

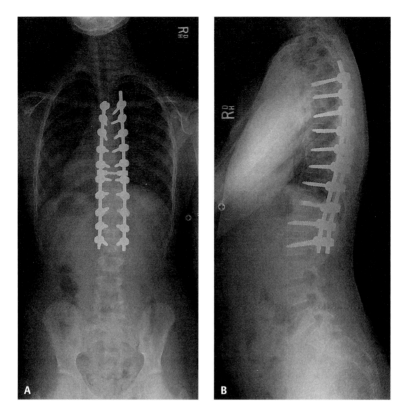

Fig. 38.2 Postoperative standing radiographs after instrumented posterior spinal fusion from T5 to L2 using an all-pedicle screw construct. **(A)** Posteroanterior. **(B)** Lateral.

Outcome

Compared with AIS, JIS is more likely to have underlying neural axis pathology, more likely to progress, and less likely to respond to bracing. Unlike infantile idiopathic scoliosis, JIS is far less likely to undergo spontaneous decrease or resolution. A successful outcome can be achieved by careful neural axis screening, frequent serial clinical and radiographic surveillance, and judicious use of bracing when appropriate. Surgery is required in cases of rapid progression and/or severe curvature (>50 degrees) and should not be delayed in an attempt to achieve some predetermined amount of spinal growth.

References

1. Robinson CM, McMaster MJ. Juvenile idiopathic scoliosis. Curve patterns and prognosis in one hundred and nine patients. J Bone Joint Surg Am 1996;78(8):1140–1148
2. Tolo VT, Gillespie R. The characteristics of juvenile idiopathic scoliosis and results of its treatment. J Bone Joint Surg Br 1978;60-B(2):181–188
3. Gupta P, Lenke LG, Bridwell KH. Incidence of neural axis abnormalities in infantile and juvenile patients with spinal deformity. Is a magnetic resonance image screening necessary? Spine 1998;23(2):206–210
4. Maenza RA. Juvenile and adolescent idiopathic scoliosis: magnetic resonance imaging evaluation and clinical indications. J Pediatr Orthop B 2003;12(5):295–302
5. Masso PD, Meeropol E, Lennon E. Juvenile-onset scoliosis followed up to adulthood: orthopaedic and functional outcomes. J Pediatr Orthop 2002;22(3):279–284
6. Dubousset J, Herring JA, Shufflebarger H. The crankshaft phenomenon. J Pediatr Orthop 1989;9(5):541–550
7. Thompson GH, Akbarnia BA, Kostial P, et al. Comparison of single and dual growing rod techniques followed through definitive surgery: a preliminary study. Spine 2005;30(18):2039–2044
8. Bess S, Akbarnia BA, Thompson GH, et al. Complications of growing-rod treatment for early-onset scoliosis: analysis of one hundred and forty patients. J Bone Joint Surg Am 2010;92(15):2533–2543
9. Shufflebarger HL, Clark CE. Prevention of the crankshaft phenomenon. Spine 1991;16(8,Suppl):S409–S411
10. Newton PO, Marks M, Faro F, et al. Use of video-assisted thoracoscopic surgery to reduce perioperative morbidity in scoliosis surgery. Spine 2003;28(20):S249–S254

Suggested Readings

Bess S, Akbarnia BA, Thompson GH, et al. Complications of growing-rod treatment for early-onset scoliosis: analysis of one hundred and forty patients. J Bone Joint Surg Am 2010;92(15):2533–2543

In a large series of early-onset scoliosis treated with growing rods, 58% of the patients had a minimum of one complication. Complications included implant failures, wound complications, implant prominence, and unplanned spinal procedures. Reduced numbers of overall complications were noted in those patients in whom dual rods were used with submuscular rod placement.

Gupta P, Lenke LG, Bridwell KH. Incidence of neural axis abnormalities in infantile and juvenile patients with spinal deformity. Is a magnetic resonance image screening necessary? Spine 1998;23(2):206–210

This article reported on a prospective and retrospective review of patients from newborn to 10 years of age with idiopathic scoliosis >20 degrees and no neurologic findings, evaluated with total spine MRI. Neural axis abnormalities were found in approximately 20% of patients, leading the authors to recommend MRI evaluation of all patients with juvenile-onset idiopathic scoliosis measuring >20 degrees.

Maenza RA. Juvenile and adolescent idiopathic scoliosis: magnetic resonance imaging evaluation and clinical indications. J Pediatr Orthop B 2003;12(5):295–302

The author reported on a prospective study of 56 patients with JIS and AIS who underwent MRI evaluation of the posterior cerebral fossa (PCF) and spinal cord (SC). Eleven patients (20%) demonstrated abnormalities in both the PCF and SC, 4 patients (7%) demonstrated abnormalities of the SC, and 3 patients (5%) demonstrated anomalies of the osseous spine and abdomen.

Treatment

There are three principal treatment options for AIS: observation, bracing, and surgical arthrodesis. The need for intervention (bracing or surgery) is determined by assessing the likelihood of curve progression, which can be estimated by the magnitude of the Cobb angle and the growth potential. Growth potential is determined by peak growth velocity, menarchal status, and the Risser sign. Because there is a high risk of progression, curves greater than 40 to 50 degrees are generally indications for arthrodesis (surgical fusion) in a growing child.

Observation is warranted for idiopathic curves with a Cobb angle of less than 25 degrees. The SRS currently recommends initiation of brace treatment in skeletally immature patients who present with curves greater than 30 degrees on initial presentation or who progress greater than 10 degrees to a magnitude greater than 25 degrees.[13] Braces are prescribed to be worn 18 to 23 hours a day, although evidence demonstrates the effectiveness of part-time (at least 12 hours per day) brace wear to address patient compliance issues.[14] Brace wear is continued until skeletal growth is complete, as determined by unchanged height measured consecutively 6 months apart, Risser stage 4 (females) or 5 (males), or until 2 years after menarche in females. Generally, one should achieve ~50% curve correction with brace application. Failure to obtain this correction predicts a poor prognosis for successful bracing. Successful bracing will not improve the existing curve and is designed to halt progression of the curve and avoid surgical intervention. An alternative goal for bracing is to allow continued growth in a child with scoliosis who is likely to need surgery but still has significant remaining growth potential.[15] A recent evidence-based review of the literature reported a 23% risk of needing surgery despite best efforts at bracing compared with 22% with observation.[16] There are no level 1 evidence bracing studies currently in the literature, and the efficacy and effectiveness of brace treatment remain unproven and controversial. There is currently an ongoing level 1 study, BrAIST (Bracing in Adolescenet Idiopathic Scoliosis Trial), which will compare full-time and part-time bracing for preventing curve progression.

Of those diagnosed with AIS, only ~10% eventually require surgical treatment. The general indications for surgical treatment in AIS include progressive curves greater than 40 to 45 degrees in skeletally immature patients, curve progression despite bracing, or occasionally an unacceptable cosmetic deformity. The principal goal of surgery is to correct a deformity that is likely to progress and cause functional limitations or cardiopulmonary deterioration. The most critical step in surgical planning is the selection of the approach and the levels to be included in the construct.[15] If a curve is instrumented too short and does not include all levels of the major curve, there is a risk for the development of a progressive junctional deformity or "adding-on" phenomenon cephalad or caudal to the structural curve. When too many levels are included in a construct, this involves additional surgical time, increased instrumentation cost, and a small increased risk of nonunion. Also, overcorrection should be avoided to maintain overall global alignment and balance of the spinal column and prevent postoperative shoulder imbalance.

Surgical approaches may include an anterior, posterior, or circumferential fusion. The choice of surgical approach is based on the type of curve, curve magnitude, curve flexibility, skeletal maturity, and pulmonary function. An anterior-only approach may be considered for single thoracic or thoracolumbar curves of moderate magnitude. The advantages of an anterior-only approach include fusion of fewer levels, reducing postoperative junctional kyphosis, and eliminating paraspinal musculature denervation. A posterior-only approach may be considered in flexible curves with more than 50% correction on bending, traction, push-prone, or fulcrum radiographs.

Historically, severe and rigid curves often require a circumferential (360 degree) approach with an anterior spinal release, followed by posterior spinal fusion with instrumentation. There is good evidence to support a posterior-only procedure with the use of pedicle screws and Ponte-type soft-tissue or bony osteotomies, thereby reducing the need for separate procedures.[17] Relative indications for a circumferential approach include curves more than 100 degrees and curves associated with hyperkyphosis (greater than 70 degrees in the thoracic spine or frank kyphosis in the lumbar spine). Also, patients with open triradiate cartilage are at risk for crankshaft phenomenon, which is progressive rotational deformity that occurs despite a solid posterior fusion, as a result of anterior spinal growth. While the absolute risk of crankshaft phenomenon appears to be less than 50%, curves in young patients may require anterior arthrodesis to prevent progressive deformity, although the three-dimensional control afforded by pedicle screws is thought to decrease this phenomenon.

Outcomes

The natural history of untreated scoliosis, especially in curves >50 degrees, is a slow, continued progression even after the cessation of growth. A recent prospective multicenter study has reported that preoperative bracing negatively impacts postoperative outcome after posterior spine fusion with instrumentation for AIS. Braced patients complained of more pain, were less active, and had lower SRS scores at 2 years after surgical correction.[18] In another recent prospective multicenter study there was significant improvement in SRS scores at 2 years after surgical correction of AIS, with poor outcomes and less satisfaction related to pain and poor function preoperatively, and patients with less spinal appearance issues preoperatively (higher body mass index or Lenke 3 curves).[19] Intermediate-term follow-up after posterior pedicle screw–only constructs for AIS have also reported outcomes with improvement in SRS scores, no neurologic or vascular complications, and maintained radiographic curve correction.[20–22]

Complications

There are various risks associated with the surgical correction of AIS. Although rare, the most concerning is the risk of paralysis or neurologic deficit, with the reported prevalence ranging from 0.3% to 1.4%.[23] Neurophysiologic monitoring, using transcranial electric motor evoked potentials (MEPs) in addition to somatosensory evoked potentials (SSEPs), is recommended for early detection of an evolving or impending spinal cord deficit during surgical correction for AIS.[24] The Stagnara wake-up test is a useful adjunct to neurophysiologic monitoring for the detection of neurologic spinal cord deficits.[24] Pseudarthrosis or fusion failure remains a small risk (1–3% for AIS), but has decreased with the use of modern instrumentation and grafting procedures.[20] The prevalence of nonneurologic postoperative complications following surgery for correction for AIS ranges from 5 to 15%.[25] The factors significantly increasing the rate of complications include increased operative blood loss, prolonged posterior surgery time, and prolonged anesthesia time.[25] Anterior surgery increases the risk of respiratory dysfunction in the postoperative period.

Conclusion

The advances in correctly classifying adolescent idiopathic scoliosis and the development of modern instrumentation allowing advanced correction maneuvers, such as direct vertebral derotation, have changed our approach to the treatment of this condition.[26] There still is controversy, however, in the areas of brace treatment (i.e., whether there are true benefits of being braced), school screening, and the ultimate cause of AIS. Although the knowledge gap has significantly decreased over the past 10 years, there are still strides to make in the understanding and treatment of AIS.

References

1. Kouwenhoven JW, Castelein RM. The pathogenesis of adolescent idiopathic scoliosis: review of the literature. Spine 2008;33(26):2898–2908
2. Heary RF, Madhavan K. Genetics of scoliosis. Neurosurgery 2008;63(3, Suppl):222–227
3. Ogilvie J. Adolescent idiopathic scoliosis and genetic testing. Curr Opin Pediatr 2010; 22(1):67–70
4. Ward K, Ogilvie J, Argyle V, et al. Polygenic inheritance of adolescent idiopathic scoliosis: a study of extended families in Utah. Am J Med Genet A 2010;152A(5):1178–1188
5. King HA, Moe JH, Bradford DS, Winter RB. The selection of fusion levels in thoracic idiopathic scoliosis. J Bone Joint Surg Am 1983;65(9):1302–1313
6. Lenke LG, Betz RR, Clements D, et al. Curve prevalence of a new classification of operative adolescent idiopathic scoliosis: does classification correlate with treatment? Spine 2002; 27(6):604–611
7. Fong DY, Lee CF, Cheung KM, et al. A meta-analysis of the clinical effectiveness of school scoliosis screening. Spine 2010;35(10):1061–1071
8. Richards BS, Vitale M. SRS/AAOS position statement: Screening for idiopathic scoliosis in adolscents. Scoliosis Research Society. Reviewed Aug 2007. http://www.srs.org/professionals/positions/?id=62. Accessed Oct 8, 2010
9. Harrop JS, Birknes J, Shaffrey CI. Noninvasive measurement and screening techniques for spinal deformities. Neurosurgery 2008;63(3, Suppl):46–53
10. Hamzaoglu A, Talu U, Tezer M, Mirzanli C, Domanic U, Goksan SB. Assessment of curve flexibility in adolescent idiopathic scoliosis. Spine 2005;30(14):1637–1642
11. Cheung KM, Natarajan D, Samartzis D, Wong YW, Cheung WY, Luk KD. Predictability of the fulcrum bending radiograph in scoliosis correction with alternate-level pedicle screw fixation. J Bone Joint Surg Am 2010;92(1):169–176

12. Davids JR, Chamberlin E, Blackhurst DW. Indications for magnetic resonance imaging in presumed adolescent idiopathic scoliosis. J Bone Joint Surg Am 2004;86-A(10):2187–2195
13. Schiller JR, Thakur NA, Eberson CP. Brace management in adolescent idiopathic scoliosis. Clin Orthop Relat Res 2010;468(3):670–678
14. Katz DE, Herring JA, Browne RH, Kelly DM, Birch JG. Brace wear control of curve progression in adolescent idiopathic scoliosis. J Bone Joint Surg Am 2010;92(6):1343–1352
15. Angevine PD, Deutsch H. Idiopathic scoliosis. Neurosurgery 2008;63(3, Suppl):86–93
16. Dolan LA, Weinstein SL. Surgical rates after observation and bracing for adolescent idiopathic scoliosis: an evidence-based review. Spine 2007;32(19, Suppl):S91–S100
17. Luhmann SJ, Lenke LG, Kim YJ, Bridwell KH, Schootman M. Thoracic adolescent idiopathic scoliosis curves between 70 degrees and 100 degrees: is anterior release necessary? Spine 2005;30(18):2061–2067
18. Diab M, Sharkey M, Emans J, Lenke L, Oswald T, Sucato D; Spinal Deformity Study Group. Preoperative bracing affects postoperative outcome of posterior spine fusion with instrumentation for adolescent idiopathic scoliosis. Spine 2010;35(20):1876–1879
19. Sanders JO, Carreon LY, Sucato DJ, Sturm PF, Diab M; Spinal Deformity Study Group. Preoperative and perioperative factors effect on adolescent idiopathic scoliosis surgical outcomes. Spine 2010;35(20):1867–1871
20. Lehman RA Jr, Lenke LG, Keeler KA, et al. Operative treatment of adolescent idiopathic scoliosis with posterior pedicle screw-only constructs: minimum three-year follow-up of one hundred fourteen cases. Spine 2008;33(14):1598–1604
21. Cuartas E, Rasouli A, O'Brien M, Shufflebarger HL. Use of all-pedicle-screw constructs in the treatment of adolescent idiopathic scoliosis. J Am Acad Orthop Surg 2009;17(9):550–561
22. Mulpuri K, Perdios A, Reilly CW. Evidence-based medicine analysis of all pedicle screw constructs in adolescent idiopathic scoliosis. Spine 2007;32(19, Suppl):S109–S114
23. Pahys JM, Guille JT, D'Andrea LP, Samdani AF, Beck J, Betz RR. Neurologic injury in the surgical treatment of idiopathic scoliosis: guidelines for assessment and management. J Am Acad Orthop Surg 2009;17(7):426–434
24. Schwartz DM, Auerbach JD, Dormans JP, et al. Neurophysiological detection of impending spinal cord injury during scoliosis surgery. J Bone Joint Surg Am 2007;89(11):2440–2449
25. Carreon LY, Puno RM, Lenke LG, et al. Non-neurologic complications following surgery for adolescent idiopathic scoliosis. J Bone Joint Surg Am 2007;89(11):2427–2432
26. Lee SM, Suk SI, Chung ER. Direct vertebral rotation: a new technique of three-dimensional deformity correction with segmental pedicle screw fixation in adolescent idiopathic scoliosis. Spine 2004;29(3):343–349

Suggested Readings

Carreon LY, Puno RM, Lenke LG, et al. Non-neurologic complications following surgery for adolescent idiopathic scoliosis. J Bone Joint Surg Am 2007;89(11):2427–2432

In this prospective study of patients following surgery for AIS, the prevalence of non-neurologic complications was found to be 15.4%. Risk factors significantly increasing the rate of nonneurologic complications were history of renal disease, increased operative blood loss, prolonged posterior spinal surgery time, and total anesthesia time.

Kim YJ, Lenke LG, Bridwell KH, Cho YS, Riew KD. Free hand pedicle screw placement in the thoracic spine: is it safe? Spine 2004;29(3):333–342, discussion 342

Kim et al. describe the surgical technique for free-hand thoracic pedicle screw placement. The authors found the free-hand technique to be accurate, reliable, and safe after review of 394 patients with over 3204 thoracic pedicle screws placed over 10 years, and found no neurologic, vascular, or visceral complications.

Lehman RA Jr, Lenke LG, Keeler KA, et al. Operative treatment of adolescent idiopathic scoliosis with posterior pedicle screw-only constructs: minimum three-year follow-up of one hundred fourteen cases. Spine 2008;33(14):1598–1604

> *Lehman et al. report the first intermediate-term findings following posterior spinal fusion with pedicle screw–only constructs for surgical correction of AIS. The study included 114 patients having a minimum of 3-year follow-up and found no neurologic, vascular, or visceral complications. The authors reported acceptable radiographic and clinical outcomes using posterior-only deformity correction with pedicle screws for AIS.*

Lenke LG, Betz RR, Harms J, et al. Adolescent idiopathic scoliosis: a new classification to determine extent of spinal arthrodesis. J Bone Joint Surg Am 2001;83-A(8):1169–1181

> *This classic article presents the initial description of the Lenke classification for AIS. In 2001 Lenke et al. developed a new two-dimensional classification for AIS based on coronal and sagittal radiographs, and it was found to be more reliable than the King system.*

Suspected Neuromuscular Scoliosis

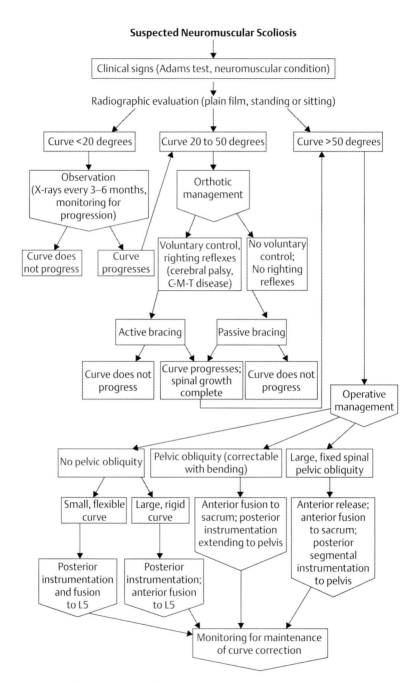

C-M-T, Charcot-Marie-Tooth

40

Neuromuscular Scoliosis

Laura E. Gill, Francis H. Shen, and Vincent Arlet

Neuromuscular disorders are a group of diseases that affect the normal operation of the pathways that allow the brain to communicate with and control the function of the muscles. Neuromuscular scoliosis is a common complication of these diseases, with an incidence of 25–90% depending on the underlying cause.

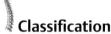

Classification

The accepted classification scheme for neuromuscular disorders has been described by the Scoliosis Research Society (**Table 40.1**). In North America the most frequent diseases contributing to the development of neuromuscular scoliosis are cerebral palsy, myelomeningocele, muscular dystrophies, and post paraplegia. In the developing world, poliomyelitis is still occasionally seen.

Etiology and Natural History

The exact cause of neuromuscular scoliosis is unknown. Contributing factors include paraplegia, mechanical forces, congenital abnormalities, and intraspinal abnormalities, such as tethering of the spinal cord, diastematomyelia, and syringomyelia. Asymmetric tone of the paraspinal muscles may result in increased tone or strength on one side with decreased tone on the other side, resulting in a coronal plane deformity. Mechanical forces causing spinal deformity may result from unilateral hip dislocation or pelvic obliquity with consequential compensatory deformity of the spine.[1] As the spine collapses, pressure builds on the concave side of the vertebral body, increasing the load and decreasing growth on that side (Heuter–Volkmann law). The resultant "wedging" of the vertebral body compounds the curvature and increases the speed of scoliotic progression. In neuromuscular scoliosis, the curves tend to be early-onset, progress after skeletal maturity, and be long sweeping curves that may include the sacrum, with resultant pelvic obliquity. Curves are worse in patients who

Table 40.1 Classification of Neuromuscular Scoliosis Established by the Scoliosis Research Society

Neuropathic	Myopathic

Upper motor neuron
 • Cerebral palsy
 • Spinocerebellar degeneration
   ◦ Friedreich ataxia
   ◦ Charcot-Marie-Tooth disease
   ◦ Roussy-Lévy syndrome
 • Syringomyelia
 • Spinal cord tumor
 • Trauma
 • Spina bifida
	Muscular dystrophy
	 • Duchenne muscular dystrophy
	 • Limb girdle dystrophy
	 • Fascioscapulohumeral dystrophy
	 Arthrogryposis
	 Fiber-type disproportion
	 Congenital hypotonia
	 Myotonia dystrophica

Lower motor neuron
 • Poliomyelitis
 • Other viral myelitides
 • Traumatic
 • Spinal muscular atrophy
   ◦ Werdnig-Hoffmann disease
   ◦ Kugelberg-Welander syndrome
 • Dysautonomia
   ◦ Riley-Day syndrome	

Combined • Myelomeningocele	

are nonambulatory, and the incidence and severity increase with the degree of neurologic involvement, with the severity of mental retardation, and with decreased functional status.[2] Patients with curves greater than 40 degrees before the age of 15 tend to have larger curves in the future, and fusion should be considered in these patients. Spinal deformity, if left untreated, may result in compromise of walking and independent transfers, increased energy consumption in gait, and loss of trunk balance, which may require patients to use their hands for stability, effectively reducing their function because they cannot use their hands for tasks. The deformity may also result in pain and compromise of respiratory function and nutrition as well as pressure sores over the hips and/or ischium. These pressure sores may make sitting difficult and may require surgical correction of the curve even in patients who are nonambulatory.

Workup

History

Because of the early onset and rapid progression of neuromuscular scoliosis, rapid diagnosis and treatment are critical. Central nervous system abnormalities, premature birth, seizure disorders, and hydrocephalus are important to note. A family history of neurologic or muscular disease can provide insight into the likely clinical course. Information about developmental milestones and conditions during the perinatal period, such as maternal diabetes or perinatal anoxia, aids in identifying underlying conditions. For example, nonprogressive neuromuscular disorders like cerebral palsy are apparent early in life, whereas progressive neuromuscular conditions like muscular dystrophies tend to present later with loss of developmental milestones. Finally, a complete review of systems with information about past pulmonary, cardiac, renal, or nutritional disorders as well as symptoms of bladder or bowel dysfunction, weakness, or numbness aids in diagnosis and affects treatment options.

Physical Examination

A complete physical examination is important, as scoliosis may be the first clinical appearance of neuromuscular disease. Examination begins with the inspection of the skin lesions, such as sacral dimpling or hairy patches, which may indicate subtle underlying spinal abnormality. A thorough neurologic examination, including patterns of weakness, reflexes and joint motion, tone, contractures and atrophy, should be performed.

From this one should be able to differentiate spastic-type scoliosis from flaccid neuromuscular. It is not uncommon for patients with myelomeningocele to have a neuromuscular scoliosis that is the consequence of a mixture of spasticity and flaccid paralysis, with possible congenital malformation of the spine as well. The spinal examination should be conducted in a supine position and, if possible, sitting and standing positions to assess overall rigidity of the spine. Sagittal plane abnormalities should also be noted as hyperlordosis of the lumbar spine or kyphosis, as these patients may have a "collapsing spine" secondary to muscular weakness. Other deformities, such as rib prominence, shoulder asymmetry, trunk imbalance, or pelvic tilting, should be identified. Pelvic obliquity is often present in neuromuscular curve, and its cause (suprapelvic/spinal deformity, infrapelvic/hip contracture) can be evaluated with a simple test. The patient is placed prone on the examination table with the hips flexed over the edge of the table. This flexed position of the hips typically eliminates the hips as a cause of pelvic obliquity. It is then possible to visualize whether the pelvis is perpendicular to the trunk and assess whether there is any pelvic obliquity arising from the spine. In the case where the pelvis is oblique to the spine, one can assess the reducibility of the pelvic obliquity by abduction and adduction of the hips. This will determine whether the pelvic obliquity is fixed or not. In this position one will also assess whether there is any pelvic obliquity arising from the hips by looking at the pelvis and extending and abducting and adducting the hips. Functional assessment of the patient is important to help plan treatment choice. The patient's ambulatory status, whether the patient is wheelchair bound, and upper extremity function need to be assessed. If the patient is ambulatory, it is essential to assess gait and see whether the patient is utilizing the lumbosacral junction, as fusion to the sacrum may impede mobility later.

Spinal Imaging

Plain radiographs standing or sitting, including posteroanterior (PA) or lateral views, are most useful for evaluation of curve progression. Supine films or traction films are also useful in assessing curve flexibility. Magnetic resonance imaging (MRI) of the entire spine is performed in cases of neuromuscular scoliosis where one suspects intraspinal lesions, such as syringomyelia, cord tethering, myelomeningocele, or spinal tumor.

Treatment

The goal of treatment in neuromuscular scoliosis is to restore and maintain a spine balanced in the coronal and sagittal planes over a level pelvis, to preserve respiratory function, and to halt progressive loss of functional independence. Management may include observation, orthotic treatment, or surgery.

In general, curves less than 20 degrees can be observed. In nonambulatory patients, seating supports or customized seating systems may help improve trunk support and accommodate spinal or pelvis deformity, especially when curves are smaller or in patients with severe mental retardation and those patients unlikely to gain any functional improvement from surgery.

Bracing should be considered in curves >20 degrees. Although brace management is rarely a definitive measure, it may be used in younger patients to slow curve progression and to delay surgical treatment. Bracing has been shown to be of some benefit in patients with short curves and those <40 degrees with muscle hypotonia or mild spasticity. Types of bracing include the thoracolumbosacral orthosis (TLSO) and the suspension trunk orthosis (STO) for patients who lack voluntary muscle control. The STO attaches to the patient's chair and controls trunk shift and pelvic obliquity without compromising respiratory function or causing pressure ulcers.[3] The Milwaukee brace is rarely used nowadays for ambulatory patients who can maintain trunk control.

Indications for surgery include a progressive deformity, deformity that compromises respiratory or cardiac function, and curve-related pain that is unresponsive to nonoperative measures. Compared with idiopathic curves, neuromuscular curves tend to be more rigid and are often associated with pelvic obliquity (**Fig. 40.1**). Historically, these curves have been treated with posterior or circumferential fusion. The curve severity and rigidity and pelvic obliquity will affect the distal extent of the fusion. Inclusion of the pelvis is usually considered when there is truncal decompensation, when there is fixed pelvic obliquity >15 degrees, and if the sacrum is part of the curve.[2,4] Luque wire segmental instrumentation, often combined with Galveston pelvic fixation and hybrid hook–pedicle screw construct, has been employed (**Fig. 40.2A–D**). Hitesh et al.[5,6] have looked at the posterior approach using all-pedicle screw fixation for neuromuscular scoliosis compared with adolescent idiopathic scoliosis. In their studies they obtained a comparable correction of Cobb angle, pelvic obliquity, and apical derotation without the need for anterior release.

Anterior surgery should be considered for patients with rigid deformities, in skeletal immaturity where there is potential for crankshaft phenomenon,

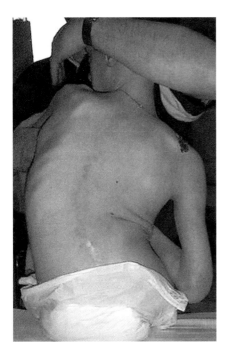

Fig. 40.1 Scoliosis in a patient with spastic quadriparetic cerebral palsy. The curve is long, sweeping and rigid, associated with pelvic obliquity which has affected his sitting balance and function.

or where risk of pseudarthrosis is high (e.g., myelomeningocele). It is usually performed in combination with posterior fusion and instrumentation and has been traditionally shown to have greater correction of scoliosis compared with either procedure alone. However, Basobas et al. and Tokala et al.[7,8] have stated that in select patients, anterior fusion and instrumentation alone may have comparable results while preserving motion segments and, in some cases, avoiding instrumentation of the pelvis or sacrum.

Outcome

Modi et al.[5] retrospectively looked at the outcomes for 52 patients with cerebral palsy who underwent posterior-only instrumentation and fusion at an average of 2 years follow-up. They reported a 63% improvement in Cobb angle and 56% correction in pelvic obliquity. In addition, 42% (21) patients improved their functional ability by grade 1, with 2 patients by grade 2. In an earlier study[6] with 24 patients they also reported improved axial derotation (20.26%) with an all–pedicle screw construct in patients with neuromuscular scoliosis. In a study conducted by Tsirikos and Chang in 2003,[9] 15 patients with neuromuscular scoliosis underwent anterior release followed by posterior fusion and instrumentation. Spinal curve correction averaged 70%, and pelvic obliquity improved by a mean of 80%. Mercado et al.[10] performed a literature review looking at

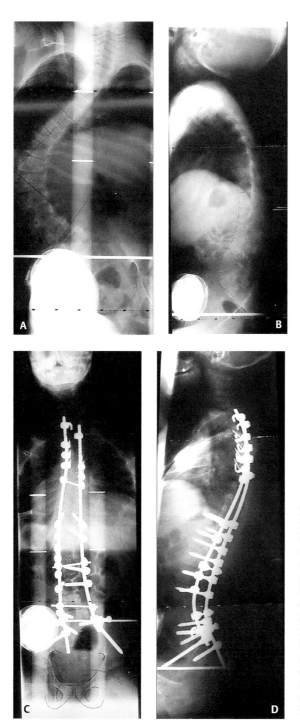

Fig. 40.2 (A,B) Preoperative films showing left-sided, long, sweeping thoracolumbar curve with significant pelvic obliquity. Hypolordosis is evident on the lateral film. **(C,D)** Postoperative film shows excellent correction of this curve and pelvic obliquity and restoration of coronal and sagittal balance using a posterior-only approach with multiple facetectomies and soft-tissue release. Hybrid pedicle screw and hook construct was used for instrumentation.

whether spinal fusion influences the quality of life (QOL) in neuromuscular scoliosis and found that the current literature shows that spinal fusion improves the QOL in patients with cerebral palsy and muscular dystrophy but does not improve the QOL in patients with spina bifida (Grade C recommendations based on level of evidence available). In general, self-reported satisfaction based on parent/caregiver response to questionnaires was high. The expectations, needs, and goals of these patients need to be assessed and weighed against the risk of complications prior to proceeding with surgery.

 Complications

Neuromuscular disorders often involve other bodily systems that affect the risk of complications with surgery. A multidisciplinary approach to correct as many of these risk factors as possible preoperatively is needed to reduce postoperative complications. Often these patients have diminished pulmonary capacity and are prone to perioperative respiratory compromise and pneumonia, requiring prolonged ventilation postoperatively. Poor nutrition is a risk factor for wound breakdown and infection. Hiatal hernia, gastroesophageal reflux disease, and difficulty chewing and swallowing may compound this issue and increase the risk of aspiration. Metabolic bone disease may increase the risk of implant failure. Neuromuscular scoliosis is associated with increased intraoperative blood loss. This may be related to poor nutrition, medications like valproic acid, and underlying connective tissue disorders as well as difficulty and extent of surgery. In the early postoperative period, ileus, urinary tract infections, pancreatitis, and gallbladder disease are also common. Pseudarthrosis is a less common complication and tends to present late as a result of implant failure. In skeletally immature patients undergoing posterior-only surgery, ongoing anterior spinal growth may lead to progressive deformity (crankshaft phenomenon).

References

1. Berven S, Bradford DS. Neuromuscular scoliosis: causes of deformity and principles for evaluation and management. Semin Neurol 2002;22(2):167–178
2. Sarwark J, Sarwahi V. New strategies and decision making in the management of neuromuscular scoliosis. Orthop Clin North Am 2007;38(4):485–496
3. Kotwicki T, Jozwiak M. Conservative management of neuromuscular scoliosis: personal experience and review of literature. Disabil Rehabil 2008;30(10):792–798
4. Broom MJ, Banta JV, Renshaw TS. Spinal fusion augmented by Luque-rod segmental instrumentation for neuromuscular scoliosis. J Bone Joint Surg Am 1989;71(1):32–44
5. Modi HN, Hong JY, Mehta SS, et al. Surgical correction and fusion using posterior-only pedicle screw construct for neuropathic scoliosis in patients with cerebral palsy: a three-year follow-up study. Spine 2009;34(11):1167–1175
6. Modi HN, Suh SW, Song HR, Lee SH, Yang JH. Correction of apical axial rotation with pedicular screws in neuromuscular scoliosis. J Spinal Disord Tech 2008;21(8):606–613
7. Basobas L, Mardjetko S, Hammerberg K, Lubicky J. Selective anterior fusion and instrumentation for the treatment of neuromuscular scoliosis. Spine 2003;28(20):S245–S248
8. Tokala DP, Lam KS, Freeman BJ, Webb JK. Is there a role for selective anterior instrumentation in neuromuscular scoliosis? Eur Spine J 2007;16(1):91–96

9. Tsirikos AI, Chang WN, Dabney KW, Miller F. Comparison of one-stage versus two-stage anteroposterior spinal fusion in pediatric patients with cerebral palsy and neuromuscular scoliosis. Spine 2003;28(12):1300–1305
10. Mercado E, Alman B, Wright JG. Does spinal fusion influence quality of life in neuromuscular scoliosis? Spine 2007;32(19, Suppl):S120–S125

Suggested Readings

Mercado E, Alman B, Wright JG. Does spinal fusion influence quality of life in neuromuscular scoliosis? Spine 2007;32(19, Suppl):S120–S125

> *Authors performed a systematic literature search of articles pertaining to quality of life (QOL) measures for patients with neuromuscular scoliosis. Computer-based databases of literature in English between 1980 and 2006 were reviewed, identifying 198 articles. Based on literature available, authors concluded that spinal fusion improved the QOL in patients with cerebral palsy and muscular dystrophy but not in patients with spina bifida (Grade C Recommendations).*

Modi HN, Hong JY, Mehta SS, et al. Surgical correction and fusion using posterior-only pedicle screw construct for neuropathic scoliosis in patients with cerebral palsy: a three-year follow-up study. Spine 2009;34(11):1167–1175

> *Authors retrospectively reviewed their experience with 52 neuromuscular scoliosis patients with cerebral palsy (CP) who underwent posterior-only pedicle screw constructs. Authors found that at average of 36.1 month follow-up, patients had satisfactory coronal and sagittal correction without higher complication rates.*

Tokala DP, Lam KS, Freeman BJ, Webb JK. Is there a role for selective anterior instrumentation in neuromuscular scoliosis? Eur Spine J 2007;16(1):91–96

> *Retrospective clinical and radiographic study of 148 neuromuscular patients who underwent scoliosis correction, of which 9 patients underwent selective anterior single-rod instrumentation for the management of thoracolumbar and lumbar scoliosis. All patients remained ambulatory. At mean 2-year and 9-month follow-up, the authors concluded that in the short term, selective anterior instrumentation and fusion in the carefully selected patient with neuromuscular scoliosis appears to have satisfactory clinical and radiographic outcome.*

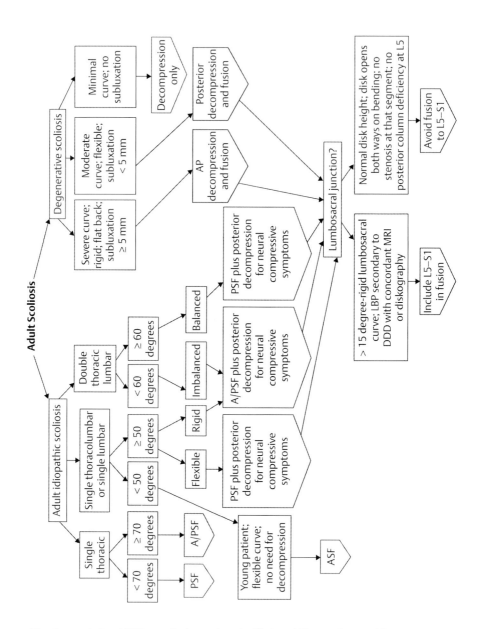

AP, anteroposterior; A/PSF, anterior/posterior spinal fusion; ASF, anterior spinal fusion; DDD, degenerative disk disease; LBP, low back pain; PSF, posterior spinal fusion

41

Adult Scoliosis

Todd J. Albert, Moe R. Lim, Joon Y. Lee, and Conor Regan

Adults with scoliosis often have rigid curves with coexistent degenerative disk disease, spinal stenosis, and osteopenia. As a result, surgical treatment of adult scoliosis tends to be more complex than for adolescent idiopathic scoliosis. The goals of surgical intervention include a fused, stable spine with the head centered over the sacrum, relief of pain, improvement of cosmesis, and prevention of deformity progression.

Classification

Adult scoliosis can be divided into idiopathic and degenerative types. In adult idiopathic scoliosis, the curvature begins prior to skeletal maturity and progresses with age. Patients over the age of 40 with pre-existing idiopathic scoliosis develop degenerative changes that contribute to both the deformity and the clinical symptoms.

In contrast to the well-accepted classification systems for adolescent idiopathic scoliosis, there are no universally accepted radiographic parameters or classification schemes for adult scoliosis. As defined by the Scoliosis Research Society, curves with an apex from T2 to the T11–T12 disk space are classified as thoracic. Curves with an apex from T12 to L1 are classified as thoracolumbar, and curves with an apex from the L1–L2 disk to the L4–L5 disk are considered lumbar (**Fig. 41.1**). The Adult Deformity Classification proposed by Schwab et al. divides the thoracic curve into either upper or lower thoracic and adds sagittal balance, lumbar lordosis, and subluxation modifiers.[1] The Scoliosis Research Society adult scoliosis classification scheme builds upon the Lenke and King/Moe classification systems and includes modifiers for sagittal and coronal balance, olisthesis, and lumbar degenerative disk disease.[2]

In degenerative scoliosis, the deformity typically develops in an elderly patient without preexisting spinal deformity. Degenerative change in the setting of osteopenia is the primary cause of the deformity. Degenerative curves typi-

Treatment

Treatment for most adult patients with scoliosis consists of conservative measures to decrease symptoms. This includes activity modification, physical therapy, nonsteroidal anti-inflammatory drugs (NSAIDs), and occasionally nonstructural bracing. A systematic literature review showed very weak evidence of efficacy for physical therapy, chiropractic treatment, and bracing.[4] Surgery is indicated for patients who continue to have severe pain despite adequate conservative therapy or who demonstrate significant curve progression with coronal or sagittal plane imbalance.

Several key principles should be kept in mind when treating adult scoliosis operatively.[5] The stable and neutral vertebrae should be included in the caudal and cephalad extents of the fusion. In the sagittal plane, the fusion should never end at the apex of the thoracic kyphosis. to avoid progressive junctional kyphosis. Strong consideration should be given to anterior structural grafting when extending a long construct to the sacrum (spanning to above L3), to prevent pseudarthrosis.

Treatment of Adult Idiopathic Scoliosis

Single Thoracic Curves

Patients with curves of less than 70° can usually be treated satisfactorily with posterior instrumentation and fusion. In larger curves with ankylosis or severe facet arthrosis, a combined procedure will likely produce a better correction, solid fusion, and achievement of balance.

Single Thoracolumbar and Single Lumbar Curves

Anterior correction and segmental instrumention can provide optimal fusion rates and outcomes in relatively young patients with mild to moderate thoracolumbar and lumbar curves (<50 degrees) and flexible compensatory curves above and below the deformity. A posterior-only approach is indicated if decompression is required for stenosis or radiculopathy. Combined approaches are indicated in patients with poor bone stock and rigid deformities >50 degrees. Instrumentation should not stop at the thoracolumbar junction or the midthoracic spine due to the possibility of junctional kyphosis.[6]

Double Thoracic and Lumbar Curves

Balanced curves less than 60 degrees can be treated with posterior-only instrumentation and fusion. With larger and more rigid curves, a combined approach should be strongly considered.

Lumbosacral Fractional Curves

In lumbar scoliosis with a significant rigid lumbosacral curve greater than 15 degrees, fusion to S1 is indicated. Correction of more cephalad curves can result in iatrogenic imbalance if a significant lumbosacral curve is not addressed. Iliac screws or an anterior structural graft may be necessary to obtain a biomechanically sound construct. Fusion to S1 can be avoided if the L5–S1 disk height is maintained, there is no stenosis at L5–S1, and the disk space opens both ways on bending films.[7]

Treatment of Degenerative Scoliosis

Treatment of degenerative scoliosis is based on patient symptoms, curve magnitude and flexibility, presence of rotatory subluxation, and the presence of coronal or sagittal imbalance.[8] In keeping with the principles of idiopathic scoliosis treatment, fusions should begin and end with the neutral and stable vertebra and not end at a level with junctional kyphosis or rotatory subluxation.

Typically, adult degenerative scoliosis presents with L3–L4 rotatory subluxation, L4–L5 tilt, and L5–S1 disk degeneration producing lumbar back pain with or without leg pain (**Fig. 41.3**). Operative levels should include the end vertebrae used in determining the Cobb angle and extending to L5 when there is significant listhesis present. Fusion should be extended to S1 in the presence of L5–S1 spondylolisthesis, previous L5–S1 laminectomy, central or foraminal

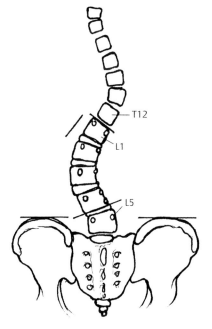

Fig. 41.3 Degenerative scoliosis curves are usually lumbar and have a characteristic lateral tilt at L4–L5, rotatory subluxation at L3–L4, and sequelae of degenerative disk disease.

Pediatric Kyphosis

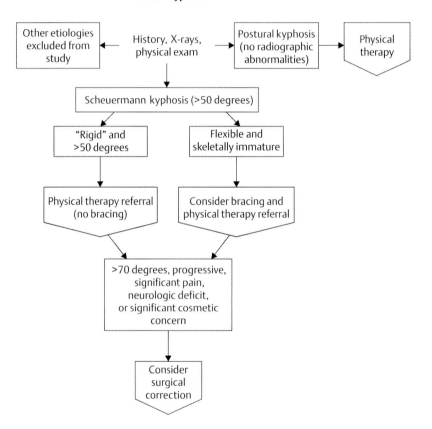

42

Scheuermann Disease

Haim D. Blecher

Kyphotic deformities of the spinal column may result in overall sagittal imbalance and in turn may cause pain, affect gait, and affect neural structures and adjacent segments of the spine. Although there are no absolute measurements of normal lordosis and kyphosis, general ranges are acceptable. Lumbar lordosis of 60 degrees (40–80) and thoracic kyphosis of 35 degrees (20–50) generally constitute normal sagittal contours. The thoracolumbar junction generally has neutral alignment.

Abnormal thoracic kyphosis (over 50 degrees) most commonly is associated with poor posture and has no specific structural pathology. Postural kyphosis carries with it a benign course and responds well to exercises and behavioral modifications.

Structural kyphotic deformities, however, may require a more intensive workup and treatment. Scheuermann disease is the most common structural thoracic kyphotic deformity in the juvenile population.

 ## Classification

Scheuermann described the disease, first reported in 1920, as vertebral wedging with various endplate irregularities seen on radiographs that resulted in the "round back" appearance in the adolescent. Sorensen later described the radiographic pathognomonic findings of the disease to be the anterior wedging of at least 5 degrees in three consecutive thoracic vertebrae.[1] Schmorl described the radiographic appearance of intervertebral disk herniations that are often seen in the anterior vertebral endplates in this disease (Schmorl nodules).

The etiology of the disease is unclear. Aseptic necrosis of the ring apophysis, collagen composition changes, hereditary factors, endocrinologic imbalance, and others have been proposed. Despite the lack of definitive evidence for its pathogenesis, the presentation and treatment of Scheuermann disease are well

Post-Traumatic Kyphosis

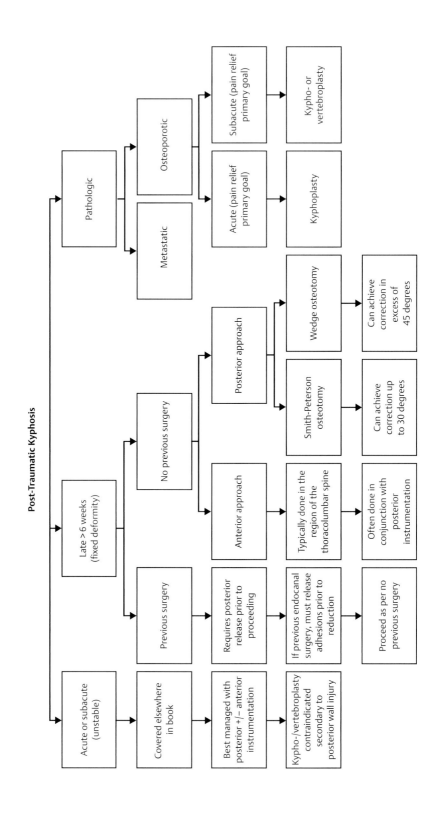

43

Post-Traumatic Thoracolumbar Kyphosis

David M. Neils, Arnima Bhasin, Daniel R. Fassett, and Jeff S. Silber

Trauma to the spinal column, with or without injury to the spinal cord, has life-changing and potentially devastating consequences for patients. With advances in the use of imaging modalities, including radiography, computed tomography (CT), and magnetic resonance imaging (MRI), unstable fractures are often treated with immobilization or surgical stabilization acutely. Despite the advances in the diagnosis and treatment of unstable spinal fractures, delayed complications, including post-traumatic thoracolumbar kyphosis, can develop.

Classification

One likely source for the development of thoracolumbar kyphotic deformities is unrecognized or occult instability with thoracolumbar trauma. Post-traumatic kyphosis typically results from injury to the anterior and posterior columns of the spine. As has been noted in recent classification systems, such as the Thoracolumbar Injury Classification and Severity Score (TLICS), the posterior ligamentous structures play an important role in spinal stability, and disruption of posterior ligaments is likely a key factor in the development of post-traumatic kyphosis. The center of axis for body weight is carried ventral to the spine, and the posterior musculature and ligaments act to hold the spine in an erect posture. Disruption of the posterior tension band allows the body weight to pull the spine ventrally into a kyphotic posture. The posterior ligaments can be evaluated by multiple techniques, including physical examination findings and radiographic studies, but the sensitivity and specificity for detecting ligamentous injuries are questioned with all of these techniques.

Clinical studies of the TLICS classification and other classification systems have found a very poor inter-observer reliability in classifying spinal injuries and, especially, in determining the integrity of the posterior spinal ligaments. As a result, spinal injuries are not treated uniformly, and it can be expected that some unstable fractures do not receive sufficient treatment, resulting in the development of post-traumatic kyphotic deformities.

Aside from underestimating the extent of injury and potential for instability, other causes include pseudarthrosis, instrumentation failure, infections, and inadequate surgical stabilization. Fracture nonunion, with or without evidence of instrumentation fatigue, has been implicated. In cases of suspected nonunion, extensive workup for deep wound infection should be performed, as infections may clinically mimic or even cause chronic nonunions. Implant and instrumentation failure has been reported in as many as 16% of patients requiring reoperation. Causes of implant failure may be related to excessive force on the implants, surgical technical errors, poor implant selection, insufficient number of levels fused, infection, osteoporotic bone, or patient noncompliance with bracing or immobilization devices. Surgical risk factors for delayed formation or progression of kyphotic deformity include laminectomy alone in the setting of an unstable injury or including too few segments in a thoracolumbar fusion procedure. Instrumentation and fusion of five or more spinal segments (two above the injured level and two below) is less likely to result in postoperative deformity. Charcot spine has also been associated with delayed development of thoracolumbar kyphosis.

Presenting Symptoms

Pain

The most common presenting symptom of post-traumatic kyphosis is pain. The pain is usually constant and aching, centered at the apex of the deformity. The pain is typically increased with prolonged standing or activity. The sagittal balance of the kyphotic spine is shifted ventrally with standing, creating a biomechanical disadvantage for the posterior musculature. As a result, the muscles fatigue and pain is produced. The more caudal in the spine the kyphotic deformity, the greater the effect of the deformity on the sagittal balance, and the deformity is subsequently less well tolerated by the patient. Additional factors associated with intolerable pain include the severity of the deformity, disk degeneration, canal compromise, angular deformity, pseudarthrosis/nonunion, and focal instability.

Neurologic Deficit

There is up to a 27% incidence of progressive neurologic deficit in spinal cord injury patients with post-traumatic deformity. Potential causes of neurologic deterioration include spinal cord compression associated with the progressive kyphotic deformity, development of post-traumatic syringomyelia, and possible cystic myelopathy related to arachnoid adhesions at the site of injury. With progressive kyphotic deformity, the spinal cord can become draped over anterior compressive pathology, such as residual bone fragments associated with a burst fracture compromising the ventral spinal canal, and with normal body movements the cord is further damaged as it slides over the anterior pathology. Patients with less than 15 degrees of kyphosis and less than 25%

canal stenosis are less likely to develop hydromelia than are patients with greater deformity.

Evaluation

Radiographic Evaluation

Given the complexity involved in the radiographic evaluation of post-traumatic spinal deformity, multiple imaging modalities are typically necessary. Plain radiographs are crucial in the evaluation of suspected kyphotic deformities. Standing or upright AP and lateral scoliosis films with flexion, extension, and lateral bending are necessary to understand fully the degree of kyphotic deformity and to provide an evaluation of spinal mobility during physiologic range of motion. Likewise, serial plain radiographs are a useful tool for following and documenting changes in the post-traumatic deformity longitudinally.

CT scanning of the affected levels using thin cuts and multiple-planar reconstruction is useful in obtaining detailed bony anatomy as part of preoperative planning. In some instances, such as presence of spinal instrumentation or in the evaluation of intradural pathology like arachnoid adhesions, CT combined with myelography can provide valuable information about neural pathology.

MRI can be helpful in the acute trauma evaluation for ligamentous injury, which may lead to progressive instability in the future. In the setting of a chronic deformity, MRI provides soft-tissue resolution for assessing the spinal cord for compression, myelomalacia, syringomyelia, or arachnoid adhesions.

Treatment

Indications for Surgery

The decision to proceed with surgery is best made after careful discussion with the patient and his or her family about the patient's symptoms and the goals and expectations following surgery to correct the kyphotic deformity. As a general rule of thumb, surgery is indicated when significant pain is combined with altered function in a patient with a sagittal index greater than 20 degrees. The location of the pain is variable and can be associated with the apex of the deformity or in any exaggerations of the normal lordosis or kyphosis of the spine. If the patient has not developed a hyperlordosis of the lumbar spine, there will be a forward listing posture that can be severe enough to limit the patient's line of sight. Additional strong factors in favor of surgical management include pseudarthrosis, disk degeneration, and neurologic deficit caused by neural compression associated with the kyphotic deformity. Cosmetic concerns must also be taken into consideration and must be discussed with the patient. Surgery should be approached with extreme caution in patients with mild deformity and severe pain. There is a percentage of patients who will have persistent pain after spinal trauma, and in some instances this pain is not amenable to surgical intervention.

Surgical Prognosticators

Successful surgical intervention for the treatment of post-traumatic thoraco-lumbar kyphosis is highly dependent upon the surgeon's skill in patient selection, education, and operative techniques. The goal of surgery is always to give reproducible results with low rates of complications. With aggressive surgical correction of deformity, morphological changes in the presenting deformity of greater than 50–70% can be achieved. In assessing patients with pain relief as the primary outcome measure, success rates as high as 60–70% may be achievable. More severe deformities can give the surgeon an increasing confidence in the ability of the surgery to improve pain. Greater patient age, work-related injury, and psychosocial problems are generally regarded to be negative prognosticators for pain relief following surgery.

Surgical Goals

The goals of the surgery must be carefully considered by both the operating surgeon and patient prior to surgery. Typically the goals of surgery are three-fold: (1) Restore sagittal balance of the spine to allow for a normal straight posture. (2) Perform decompression of any neural elements compromised by the deformed level. (3) Cure pain related to pathologic curves by restoring a normal spinal alignment and repairing any spinal instability.

Surgical Procedures

The ultimate decision about the correct and appropriate surgery for a given patient is best made in collaboration with the patient, combining patient symptoms, radiographic studies, and surgeon experience to tailor the treatment plan to each individual case. Thoracolumbar kyphosis can be addressed from either the posterior, anterior, or combined anterior/posterior approach (refer to algorithm at beginning of chapter). There are studies showing efficacy of each approach, but for severe deformities the posterior approach with an osteotomy allows for more radical correction of post-traumatic kyphotic deformities. It is also important to consider the coronal plane balance, and in patients with scoliosis in conjunction with kyphotic deformity, consider asymmetric wedge osteotomies to correct the balance of both the coronal and sagittal planes (**Fig. 43.1**). In situations of progressive neurological deficits, a thorough decompression of the spinal canal is needed in addition to correction of the deformity. For patients with osteopenia or osteoporosis, cement augmentation of the vertebral bodies at the cephalad and caudal extent of the spinal instrumentation may be considered to prevent hardware loosening. There may also be a benefit with the use of cobalt chromium rods over titanium rods for improved strength to reduce the risk of rod breakage in these extensive deformity corrections.

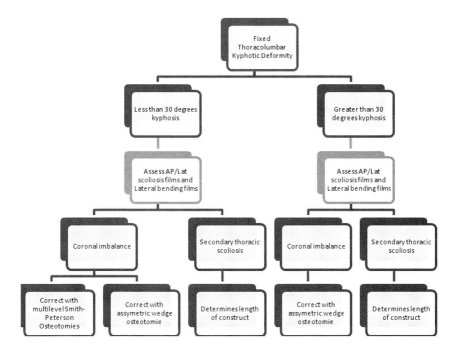

Fig. 43.1   Algorithm for fixed thoracolumbar kyphotic deformity.

Complications

Neurologic Injuries

Patients with kyphotic deformity of the thoracolumbar spine are at increased risk of injury to the neural elements draped over the anterior deformity. The incidence of neural injury in all spinal surgery is 1%; however, this number would intuitively be higher in the setting of aggressive deformity correction. Because of the risk of injury, intraoperative spinal cord monitoring is used by many surgeons to detect any change in neurologic function during each step in the operation.

Dural injury is a potential complication of extensive spinal surgeries and is increased in the setting of previous surgeries due to scarring. Primary dural closure should be considered when possible, and if this is not possible, onlay dural grafting can be substituted. Typically, one or more surgical drains are left in the wound following surgery to prevent seromas as a possible nidus of infection following surgery. The management of these drains becomes complex in the setting of cerebrospinal fluid (CSF) leak at the time of surgery. Typically, patients with durotomies are treated with 24–48 hours of bed rest followed by slow mobilization while monitoring drain output. Upon discontinuation of the drain, the drain site should be over-sewn to prevent CSF leakage.

Infection

Postoperative infection can be a significant problem in the extensive spinal procedures needed to correct these deformities. Infectious complications are typically less than 10%, with deep infections involving a very small subset. These complications can require extensive measures to salvage hardware as maintenance of the deformity correction requires the presence of instrumentation. Preventative measures, such as vigilance with sterile techniques, preoperative antibiotics, double gloving, and washing the wound with antibiotic irrigation, are considerations for these extensive surgeries where an infection can have devastating repercussions.

 Conclusions

Correction of post-traumatic thoracolumbar kyphosis can be highly rewarding for both the surgeon and the patient. Careful patient selection is the key to ensuring good results. If successful, correction of the kyphosis will lead to improved neurologic function, restoration of a more normal spinal biomechanical position and morphology, improvement in patient pain, and improvement in the patient's overall quality of life.

Suggested Readings

Munting E. Surgical treatment of post-traumatic kyphosis in the thoracolumbar spine: indications and technical aspects. Eur Spine J 2010;19(Suppl 1):S69–S73

> *This is a review of indications and techniques to consider for the treatment of post-traumatic kyphosis, with a special emphasis on operative decision making.*

Vaccaro AR, Silber JS. Post-traumatic spinal deformity. Spine 2001;26(24, Suppl):S111–S118

> *This is a review of post-traumatic deformity throughout the spine, emphasizing preoperative evaluation and spinal biomechanics in patient selection for surgery.*

Whang PG, Vaccaro AR, Poelstra KA, et al. The influence of fracture mechanism and morphology on the reliability and validity of two novel thoracolumbar injury classification systems. Spine 2007;32(7):791–795

> *This is a review of the TLICS classification system and an evaluation of the reliability of this fracture classification. It demonstrates the challenges in determining the stability of acute fractures.*

Malcolm BW, Bradford DS, Winter RB, Chou SN. Post-traumatic kyphosis. A review of forty-eight surgically treated patients. J Bone Joint Surg Am 1981;63(6):891–899

> *This review describes a large series of post-traumatic kyphotic deformities treated surgically, with report of results obtained with anterior, posterior, or combined approaches to address these deformities.*

Ikenaga M, Shikata J, Takemoto M, Tanaka C. Clinical outcomes and complications after pedicle subtraction osteotomy for correction of thoracolumbar kyphosis. J Neurosurg Spine 2007; 6(4):330–336

> *This article reports on the clinical outcomes and complications in a series of 67 patients treated with pedicle subtraction osteotomy for correction of thoracolumbar kyphosis. Intraoperative complications decreased with surgical experience.*

Heary RF, Bono CM. Pedicle subtraction osteotomy in the treatment of chronic, posttraumatic kyphotic deformity. J Neurosurg Spine 2006;5(1):1–8

> *The authors describe the pedicle subtraction osteotomy technique in the treatment of post-traumatic kyphotic deformities.*

Osteotomy Type Based on the Character of the Sagittal Deformity

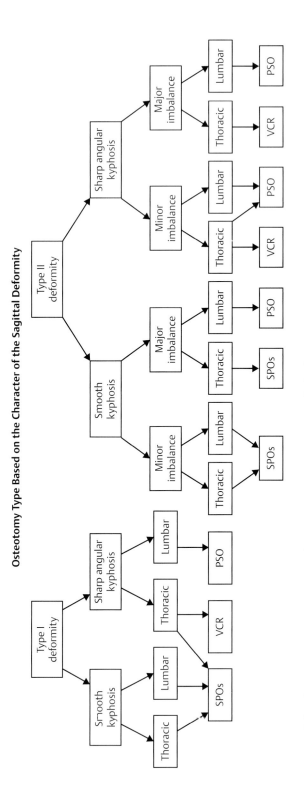

PSO, pedicle subtraction osteotomy; SPO, Smith-Petersen osteotomy; VCR, vertebral column resection

44

Corrective Osteotomies for Kyphosis

Lukas P. Zebala and Keith H. Bridwell

This chapter reviews three techniques for posterior-only correction of kyphotic deformities: Ponte or Smith-Petersen osteotomy (SPO), pedicle subtraction osteotomy (PSO), and vertebral column resection (VCR).

Classification

Kyphosis can be long, smooth, and rounded or short and angular. An example of a smooth kyphosis is Scheuermann kyphosis (see Chapter 42), whereas sharp, angular kyphosis occurs in conditions like congenital kyphosis (see Chapter 36) or post-traumatic kyphosis (see Chapter 43). Another important aspect is the location of the kyphosis: whether the kyphosis occurs in the thoracic or lumbar spine, or in the region of the spinal cord or the cauda equina. Kyphosis may cause sagittal imbalance, which has been classified into Type I and Type II.[1,2] Type I imbalance is segmental, where a portion of the spine is hypolordotic or kyphotic, but overall balance is satisfactory (C7 plumb falls through or within 2 cm anterior to the sacrum) compensated by hyperextension of cranial and caudal segments. A Type II imbalance occurs when the patient cannot compensate because of degenerative changes or the severity of the overall kyphotic deformity.

Workup

A complete history and physical exam are essential when evaluating a patient with kyphosis or sagittal imbalance. Assessing the underlying cause of the kyphosis will help determine whether an osteotomy is appropriate. Certain patients, despite having a structural deformity, are not physically or mentally fit to undergo a major osteotomy procedure. Utilization of a multidisciplinary team to evaluate a patient's overall health is beneficial during preoperative planning.

The patient's coronal and sagittal balance should be assessed both clinically and on standing anteroposterior (AP) and lateral radiographs.[3] For sagittal plane deformity, comparison of standing AP and lateral radiographs to prone and/or supine fulcrum-hyperextension long-cassette radiographs will help assess deformity flexibility. These images help classify the deformity into one of three categories: (1) totally flexible, where deformity autocorrects in a prone position; (2) partially flexible, where some deformity correction occurs through mobile segments; and (3) rigid, where deformity does not correct.[2] Flexion-extension radiographs may also identify areas of pseudarthrosis in prior fusion masses.

Assessment of the spinal canal is an important part of preoperative planning for correction of a kyphotic deformity. If there is a solid fusion, the spinal canal will be patent. However, areas adjacent to a prior fusion are often degenerated, with coexistent spinal stenosis. Magnetic resonance imaging (MRI) may help with this assessment in areas without prior fusion or with uninstrumented fusions, or where titanium implants were used. Stainless steel implants make MRI less useful due to metallic artifact. Computed tomography (CT) or CT myelography may be more helpful.

Treatment

SPOs are commonly used for the treatment of a smooth, gradual fixed kyphosis.[4] An important point to clarify is the often interchangeable nomenclature used in the literature for this osteotomy. As originally described, SPOs were performed through ankylosed segments.[4] Ponte more recently described a technically similar osteotomy that was performed through nonfused regions in patients with Scheuermann kyphosis. While both describe a similar technique, the osteotomy should be called an SPO if done through fused segments and a Ponte osteotomy if performed through unfused segments. For ease, this osteotomy is called an SPO in this chapter.

An SPO involves creating a chevron trough in the posterior elements by removing the posterior bone, ligaments (supraspinous, interspinous, and ligamentum flavum) and facet joints (**Fig. 44.1A–D**). A wide facetectomy is required, as posterior compression closes down the neural foramina and may cause nerve root impingement. An SPO requires a mobile disk space for closure of the posterior and middle columns and opening of the anterior column. In general, the degree of kyphotic correction with a single SPO is 10 degrees/level or 1 degree/mm bone resected.[5,6] A classic example for the use of SPO is Scheuermann kyphosis, where multiple SPOs are performed at the apex of the deformity. Another potential indication for multiple lumbar SPOs would be in a patient with mild sagittal imbalance (6–8 cm), where several lumbar SPOs along with anterior interbody structural support at L4–L5 and L5–S1 would help restore sagittal balance.

When a smooth kyphosis lacks mobile anterior disks, a PSO may be an alternative. More commonly, however, pedicle subtraction procedures are used for sharp, angular kyphosis or sagittal imbalance greater than 10 cm.[7–9] A PSO may

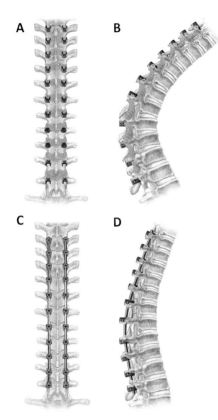

Fig. 44.1   Diagram of a Smith-Petersen (Ponte) osteotomy. **(A)** Placement of pedicle screw fixation prior to starting osteotomies. **(B)** Resection of posterior elements including portion of spinous process, interspinous ligaments, ligamentum flavum, and facets. **(C)** Closure of the osteotomies and placement of rods. Multiple SPOs performed through apex of kyphotic deformity. **(D)** Correction obtained through cantilever and compression techniques on posterior rods, usually obtaining ~10 degrees of kyphosis correction per level.

be performed in the thoracic spine, but more commonly is done in the lumbar spine (at L2 or L3). More distal PSOs carry an increased risk of neurological injury and have fewer distal fixation points.[5] A PSO requires resection of the posterior elements and pedicles and decancellation of the vertebral body in a V-shaped fashion through the transpedicular corridor (**Fig. 44.2A–F**).[8] With osteotomy closure, a large cancellous bone contact area is present as the posterior and middle columns are closed, and the osteotomy hinges on the anterior vertebral body. More aggressive resections include the disk space above the decancellated segment, which may lead to greater kyphotic correction. In addition, asymmetrical pedicle subtraction procedures have been described that can aid in the correction of any concomitant coronal deformity. On average, 30 to 40 degrees of sagittal plane correction can be achieved with a lumbar PSO, and less (~25 degrees) with a thoracic PSO[2,7,9,10] (**Fig. 44.3**).

VCRs are most often used in the thoracic or thoracolumbar spine for the treatment of angular kyphosis or sagittal imbalance associated with coronal malalignment.[11,12] A thoracic VCR necessitates the performance of a costotransversectomy followed by resection of all the posterior elements including the facet joints at the cranial and caudal levels, and the entire vertebral body along

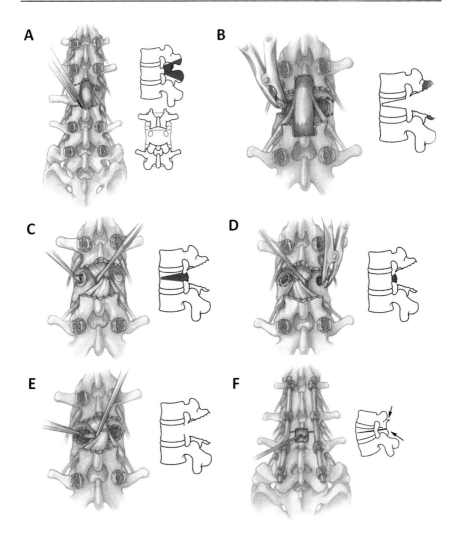

Fig. 44.2 Diagram of a pedicle subtraction osteotomy. **(A)** Wide central decompression is performed from the pars above to the pars below the osteotomy-level pedicle. **(B)** Exiting nerve roots are identified and pedicles are resected down to ventral vertebral body. **(C)** Vertebral body is decancellated through pedicles bilaterally. **(D)** Wedge resection of lateral vertebral body with apex anterior is performed. Vertebral body wedge resection needs to be symmetric to facilitate osteotomy closure and prevent iatrogenic coronal decompensation. **(E)** Dorsal vertebral body is decancellated until thin cortical rim is left. Using a reverse-angled curette or Woodson elevator, the dorsal vertebral body is pushed down ventrally into osteotomy. **(F)** Osteotomy is closed and central decompression is reassessed for residual areas of neural compression.

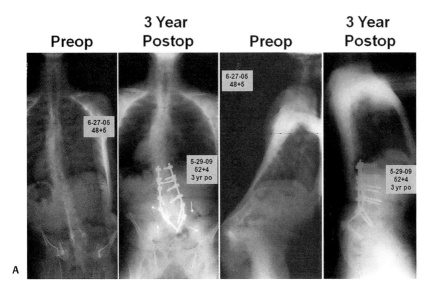

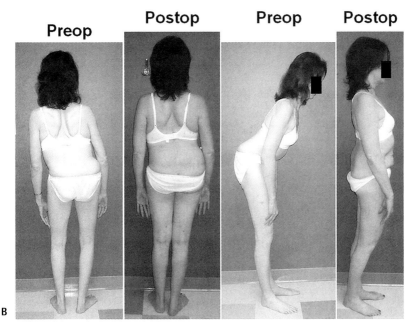

Fig. 44.3 47-year-old female status post a T11–sacrum posterior spinal fusion with Harrington rod instrumentation as a child with subsequent removal of implants. **(A)** Preoperative radiographs show a solid fusion from T11 to sacrum with L5–S1 spondyloptosis and 23 cm of fixed sagittal imbalance with knee extension. Three-year postoperative radiographs after an L3 PSO with correction of sagittal imbalance and reinstrumentation from T11 to sacrum. **(B)** Preoperative clinical photos show dramatic sagittal decompensation and coronal imbalance. Postoperative photos show marked improvement in sagittal balance after L3 PSO.

with the adjacent intervertebral disks (**Fig. 44.4**). The more sharp and angular a thoracic kyphosis, the easier it is to perform a posterior VCR. Key points to remember while performing a VCR are (1) use of temporary rod placement prior to performing the VCR to prevent intraoperative spine subluxation, (2) placement of an anterior structural cage to prevent spinal cord buckling and excessive segment shortening, (3) extensive laminectomy one level above and below the VCR is needed to avoid spinal cord impingement, and (4) rib strut grafts can act as bridge grafts to provide a bony surface for the fusion over the laminectomized region after osteotomy closure. A posterior VCR can offer kyphotic correction in the range of 40 to 50 degrees.[11-13]

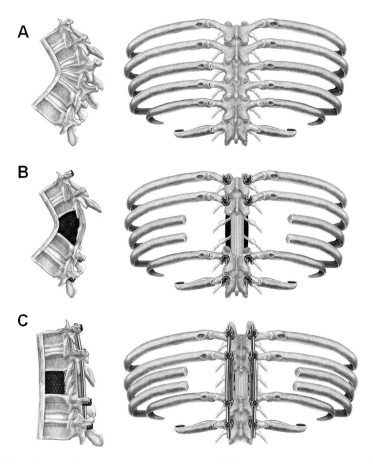

Fig. 44.4 Diagram of a vertebral column resection. **(A)** Bilateral costotransversectomy is performed, removing 4–5 cm of rib. **(B)** Segmental pedicle screws are placed. Laminectomy is widened, and a single thoracic nerve root is usually sacrificed for easier access to vertebral body. Vertebral body and intervertebral disks are resected. **(C)** Osteotomy is closed with placement of anterior cage to act as an anterior hinge for final posterior correction and prevent overshortening of the spinal cord.

There is some overlap between these three techniques, and for a specific indication more than one osteotomy may be used[2] (see the Algorithm). Important points to consider for surgical planning include (1) kyphosis location; (2) the risk of neurologic injury based on the location of surgery; (3) the number of osteotomies necessary to achieve correction; (4) the ideal location of osteotomy; (5) the available fixation points and fusion area; and (6) any areas of prior laminectomy that are present. In addition, the importance of pelvic parameters has recently been emphasized to ensure optimal sagittal correction.[14]

Outcomes

Outcomes after correction of kyphotic deformity depend on several factors, including patient baseline comorbidities, the type of osteotomy employed, and surgeon experience with the osteotomy. In most cases, if the patient's sagittal balance improves and union at all segments is achieved without major complications, a significant improvement in the Oswestry and SRS-22 scores has been reported.[7,12,13]

Kyphosis and sagittal imbalance correction are often greater after PSO and VCR compared with SPOs, but at the expense of greater blood loss, operative time, and a higher risk of complications.[5,9,11,13] Blood loss with a PSO has been reported to be double what it is with three SPOs (for similar 30-degree correction), although similar fusion rate and clinical outcomes were reported.[5] Despite SPO being the least technically challenging of the three osteotomies, complications have been reported and include pseudarthrosis, proximal and distal junctional kyphosis, wound infection, and neurologic deficits (rate ~ 3.3%).[5,6] In addition, if an SPO is performed through an area of residual scoliosis and rotation, there is potential to shift the patient toward the concavity of the scoliotic deformity.[2] This occurs because the posterior elements are on the concavity and the vertebral bodies and disks are on the convexity.

Complications

Patients requiring pedicle subtraction procedures often have multiple comorbidites and have undergone numerous prior spine operations. Early complications after these procedures are often attributable to the patient's underlying comorbidities and vary in severity.[5,7,9] The rate of intraoperative and postoperative neurological deficits has been reported at 11.1%, with a 2.8% rate of permanent deficits.[15] These are usually single-root deficits (L4 or L5) that are identified intraoperatively or in the early perioperative period. The etiology of these injuries is unclear but may be due to one or a combination of spine subluxation, dural buckling, dorsal nerve root compression, or nerve root traction. Despite a large cancellous bed for fusion in a PSO, pseudarthrosis may develop and usually occurs cephalad or caudad to the PSO site.

The potential for a catastrophic neurologic deficit (i.e., paraplegia) is higher with VCR, as this procedure is often performed at the spinal cord level.[11] Blood loss and operative times can be on a similar magnitude as in a PSO. Overall complication rates between 30% and 40% have been reported.[11–13] Rates of neurological deficits have ranged from 10% and 20%, and complete spinal cord injuries have been reported.[11–13,16] Intraoperative neuromonitoring and/or a postoperative wake-up test are important when performing any of these osteotomies.

Lastly, dural deficiencies and tears are risks for any of these procedures. In the event of a dural tear, the preferred treatment is direct repair, if possible. If not possible, then use a material like porcine pericardium, and a fibrin glue product may be utilized. If the osteotomy is closed tightly all the way across, such as in an SPO, then spinal fluid leak is generally less of a concern.

References

1. Booth KC, Bridwell KH, Lenke LG, Baldus CR, Blanke KM. Complications and predictive factors for the successful treatment of flatback deformity (fixed sagittal imbalance). Spine 1999;24(16):1712–1720
2. Bridwell KH. Decision making regarding Smith-Petersen vs. pedicle subtraction osteotomy vs. vertebral column resection for spinal deformity. Spine 2006;31(19, Suppl):S171–S178
3. Bernhardt M, Bridwell KH. Segmental analysis of the sagittal plane alignment of the normal thoracic and lumbar spines and thoracolumbar junction. Spine 1989;14(7):717–721
4. Smith-Petersen MN, Larson CB, Aufranc OE. Osteotomy of the spine for correction of flexion deformity in rheumatoid arthritis. J Bone and Joint Surg 1945;27:1–11
5. Cho KJ, Bridwell KH, Lenke LG, Berra A, Baldus C. Comparison of Smith-Petersen versus pedicle subtraction osteotomy for the correction of fixed sagittal imbalance. Spine 2005; 30(18):2030–2037, discussion 2038
6. Geck MJ, Macagno A, Ponte A, Shufflebarger HL. The Ponte procedure: posterior only treatment of Scheuermann's kyphosis using segmental posterior shortening and pedicle screw instrumentation. J Spinal Disord Tech 2007;20(8):586–593
7. Bridwell KH, Lewis SJ, Lenke LG, Baldus C, Blanke K. Pedicle subtraction osteotomy for the treatment of fixed sagittal imbalance. J Bone Joint Surg Am 2003;85-A(3):454–463
8. Bridwell KH, Lewis SJ, Rinella A, Lenke LG, Baldus C, Blanke K. Pedicle subtraction osteotomy for the treatment of fixed sagittal imbalance. Surgical technique. J Bone Joint Surg Am 2004;86-A(1, Suppl 1):44–50
9. Bridwell KH, Lewis SJ, Edwards C, et al. Complications and outcomes of pedicle subtraction osteotomies for fixed sagittal imbalance. Spine 2003;28(18):2093–2101
10. Yang BP, Ondra SL, Chen LA, Jung HS, Koski TR, Salehi SA. Clinical and radiographic outcomes of thoracic and lumbar pedicle subtraction osteotomy for fixed sagittal imbalance. J Neurosurg Spine 2006;5(1):9–17
11. Suk SI, Kim JH, Kim WJ, Lee SM, Chung ER, Nah KH. Posterior vertebral column resection for severe spinal deformities. Spine 2002;27(21):2374–2382
12. Lenke LG, Sides BA, Koester LA, Hensley M, Blanke KM. Vertebral column resection for the treatment of severe spinal deformity. Clin Orthop Relat Res 2010;468(3):687–699
13. Lenke LG, O'Leary PT, Bridwell KH, Sides BA, Koester LA, Blanke KM. Posterior vertebral column resection for severe pediatric deformity: minimum two-year follow-up of thirty-five consecutive patients. Spine 2009;34(20):2213–2221
14. Rose PS, Bridwell KH, Lenke LG, et al. Role of pelvic incidence, thoracic kyphosis, and patient factors on sagittal plane correction following pedicle subtraction osteotomy. Spine 2009;34(8):785–791
15. Buchowski JM, Bridwell KH, Lenke LG, et al. Neurologic complications of lumbar pedicle subtraction osteotomy: a 10-year assessment. Spine 2007;32(20):2245–2252
16. Wang Y, Zhang Y, Zhang X, et al. A single posterior approach for multilevel modified vertebral column resection in adults with severe rigid congenital kyphoscoliosis: a retrospective study of 13 cases. Eur Spine J 2008;17(3):361–372

Suggested Readings

Bridwell KH, Lewis SJ, Edwards C, et al. Complications and outcomes of pedicle subtraction osteotomies for fixed sagittal imbalance. Spine 2003;28(18):2093–2101

> *Substantial complications associated with PSOs include neurologic deficit, substantial blood loss, and adding on to the sagittal deformity if the entire thoracic and lumbar spine is not fused.*

Bridwell KH, Lewis SJ, Lenke LG, Baldus C, Blanke K. Pedicle subtraction osteotomy for the treatment of fixed sagittal imbalance. J Bone Joint Surg Am 2003;85-A(3):454–463

> *PSOs have a role in patients with fixed sagittal imbalance following idiopathic scoliosis surgery, following distal degenerative lumbar spine surgery, and also for post-traumatic kyphosis and ankylosing spondylitis patients. Most patients receive substantial benefit from the procedures.*

Bridwell KH. Decision making regarding Smith-Petersen vs. pedicle subtraction osteotomy vs. vertebral column resection for spinal deformity. Spine 2006;31(19, Suppl):S171–S178

> *SPOs are most helpful for long, sweeping thoracic kyphotic deformities and mild to moderate sagittal imbalances. Pedicle subtraction osteotomies are most helpful for major sagittal imbalances, sharp angular lumbar kyphosis, and coexistent Type 1 coronal imbalances.*

Buchowski JM, Bridwell KH, Lenke LG, et al. Neurologic complications of lumbar pedicle subtraction osteotomy: a 10-year assessment. Spine 2007;32(20):2245–2252

> *A review of 108 PSOs revealed an intraoperative and postoperative neurological deficit rate of 11.1%, with 2.8% of deficits being permanent.*

Cho KJ, Bridwell KH, Lenke LG, Berra A, Baldus C. Comparison of Smith-Petersen versus pedicle subtraction osteotomy for the correction of fixed sagittal imbalance. Spine 2005;30(18):2030–2037, discussion 2038

> *Three SPOs accomplish approximately what is accomplished with one pedicle subtraction procedure. The blood loss is greater with a pedicle subtraction procedure.*

Rose PS, Bridwell KH, Lenke LG, et al. Role of pelvic incidence, thoracic kyphosis, and patient factors on sagittal plane correction following pedicle subtraction osteotomy. Spine 2009; 34(8):785–791

> *Pelvic incidence and thoracic kyphosis can predict the lumbar lordosis necessary to correct sagittal imbalance with a PSO.*

VIII Spondylolisthesis

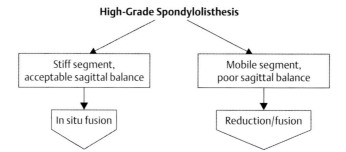

45

High-Grade Spondylolisthesis

Gregory Gebauer, Michael A. Pahl, David T. Anderson, and
D. Greg Anderson

Spondylolisthesis is the forward slippage of one vertebral body on the subadjacent vertebra. A high-grade spondylolisthesis is one in which the upper vertebral body has slipped more than 50% forward on the lower vertebral body. This is most often seen with a spondylolysis or defect in the pars interarticularis. This type of slip is about four times more common in females than in males and most commonly presents during the school years. The L5–S1 disk space is affected ~87% of the time. High-grade spondylolisthesis is more frequent in patients with higher degrees of sacral inclination, meaning that the superior endplate of S1 is oriented more nearly vertically, creating higher shear forces.

Classification

Wiltse et al. classified the different types of spondylolisthesis based on the etiology (**Table 45.1**). Spondylolisthesis can also be classified using Meyerding's system. In this system, the lower vertebral body is divided into quarters. Grade 1 involves a 0–25% slip. Grade 2 is 26–50% slip. Grade 3 is 51–75% slip, and grade 4 is 76–100% slippage. A grade 5 slippage is greater then 100% forward translation of the upper vertebral body and is also called spondyloptosis (**Fig 45.1**).

Workup

Patients with high-grade spondylolisthesis often present with back pain and radiculopathy. The radiculopathy generally affects the exiting nerve root at the level of the slip (i.e., a slip at L5/S1 will likely affect the L5 nerve root). Most patients exhibit hamstring tightness, which may lead to a waddling gait (the *Phalen-Dickson* sign). Physical examination often demonstrates an anterior pel-

Table 45.1   Wiltse and Associates Classification

I – Congenital/Dysplastic	Slippage related to malformation of spinal elements
II – Isthmic	Fracture in pars interarticularis
A – Fatigue fracture of articulating segment	
B – Elongation due to repetitive microfractures without separation	
C – Acute fracture of articulating segment	
III – Degenerative	Degeneration of the intervertebral disk or arthritic facet joints
IV – Traumatic	Acute fracture of the spinal process
V – Pathologic	Underlying bone pathology (i.e., Paget disease, osteoporosis)
IV – Iatrogenic/Postoperative	Excess removal of posterior elements following laminectomy

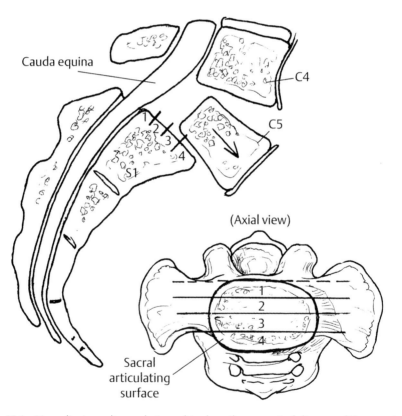

Fig. 45.1   Meyerding's grading scale is used to show the amount of slippage of the superior vertebral body on the inferior vertebral body. If slippage is greater then 100%, it is a grade 5 slippage and termed spondyloptosis. This figure demonstrates a grade 3 slippage.

vic tilt with a protruding abdomen or flattened buttocks. A thorough neurological exam should also be performed.

The lateral plain radiograph is useful in defining the degree of slippage and the slip angle. The amteroposterior (AP) view may show the "Napoleon's hat sign" or an end-on view of L5. Magnetic resonance imaging (MRI) is useful in visualizing the neural elements and generally shows severe stenosis of the exiting nerve root in the foramen.

Treatment

Growing children with a high-grade spondylolisthesis are generally indicated for surgical treatment to prevent further progression. Adults may also require surgery, depending on the degree of slippage (**Fig. 45.2**) and the severity of symptoms as well as the response to conservative treatment. Conservative options include activity modification, strengthening exercises, and anti-inflammatory medications.

The goals of surgical correction include stabilization of the spine through a spinal fusion with or without decompression of the neural elements and resto-

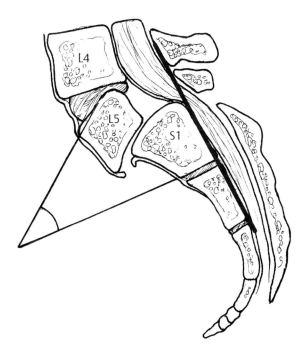

Fig. 45.2 The slip angle is an important measurement in determining treatment options for high-grade spondylolisthesis. As slip angle increases, the risk of further slippage increases. One line of thought is that correction of the kyphotic slip angle with fusion is more important than reduction of the slippage.

ration of the sagittal alignment. Surgical options include an in situ posterolateral fusion with or without instrumentation, interbody fusion, or a reduction of the deformity followed by fusion (**Fig. 45.3A–C**).

Reduction of the deformity increases the risk of a neurologic deficit but may increase the odds of successful healing of the fusion and improves the sagittal alignment.

Outcomes

Patients who achieve successful fusion with normal sagittal alignment generally have favorable clinical outcomes. Of the various factors addressed by surgery, the most important is correction of an abnormal slip angle.

Complications

There are numerous complications associated with treatment of high-grade spondylolisthesis, including major neurologic deficits, loss of fixation, pseudarthrosis, dural laceration, injury to surrounding vital structures, and adjacent segment problems.

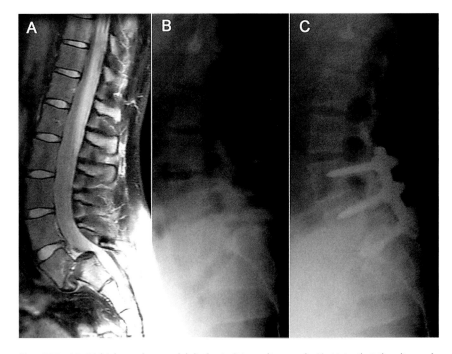

Fig. 45.3 L5–S1 high-grade spondylolisthesis (Meyerding grade 3). Note that the slip angle is neutral. **(A)** Preoperative MRI. **(B)** plain radiograph. Postoperative plain radiograph **(C)** demonstrates reduction with instrumented fusion. Note that the slip angle now is in slight lordosis.

Suggested Readings

Bridwell KH. Surgical treatment of high-grade spondylolisthesis. Neurosurg Clin N Am 2006; 17(3):331–338, vii

> *This is a review of the options, complications, and outcomes for the surgical treatment of high-grade spondylolisthesis.*

Lamberg T, Remes V, Helenius I, Schlenzka D, Seitsalo S, Poussa M. Uninstrumented in situ fusion for high-grade childhood and adolescent isthmic spondylolisthesis: long-term outcome. J Bone Joint Surg Am 2007;89(3):512–518

> *Sixty-nine patients with anterior, posterior, or combined fusion for high-grade spondylolisthesis were followed for an average of 17 years. Increased fusion rates were seen in the anterior-only and combined groups compared to the posterior-only group. Patients who had undergone combined anterior and posterior fusion had significantly better functional outcomes (measured by Oswestry Disability Index) compared with either anterior or posterior alone.*

Lonstein JE. Spondylolisthesis in children. Cause, natural history, and management. Spine 1999;24(24):2640–2648

> *The author gives an excellent overview of the etiology, presentation, and treatment options for spondylolisthesis. He also discusses indications for different surgical options.*

Marchetti PG, Bartolozzi P. Classification of spondylolisthesis as a guide for treatment. In Bridwell KH, DeWald RL, eds: Textbook of Spinal Surgery. Philadelphia, PA: Lippincott-Raven; 1997:1211–1254

> *This chapter classifies spondylolisthesis based on two different etiologies: developmental and acquired.*

Meyerding HW. Spondylolisthesis. Surg Gynecol Obstet (Paris) 1932;54:371–377

> *This article introduces the Meyerding classification system for grading the amount of slippage in spondylolisthesis. This is the most objective and reproducible classification system.*

Moshirfar A, Khanna AJ, Kebaish KM. Treatment of symptomatic spondyloptosis in an adult previously treated with in situ fusion and instrumentation by L5 vertebrectomy and L4–S1 instrumented reduction. Spine J 2007;7(1):100–105

> *The authors present the case of a young woman who had previously had a posterior fusion for her high-grade spondylolisthesis but continued to have significant neurologic deficits and severe back pain. She was treated with an L5 corpectomy, posterior osteotomy, reduction, and revision of the fusion, with full resolution of her symptoms at 2 years.*

Wiltse LL, Newman PH, Macnab I. Classification of spondylolysis and spondylolisthesis. Clin Orthop Relat Res 1976;117(117):23–29

> *This article introduces the Wiltse and associates classification system for spondylolisthesis. It discusses the five (now six) etiologies for spondylolisthesis and the associated anatomy.*

IX Spinal Tumors

Possible Primary Bone Tumor of the Spine

Staging studies: X-rays, CT, MRI, +/– bone scan

```
                                          ┌──────────────────┐     ┌──────────────────┐     ┌──────────────────┐
                                          │ Multiple lesions  │ ──→ │ Determine stage  │ ──→ │ Consider         │
                                          │                   │     │ of disease       │     │ palliative       │
                                          │                   │     │                  │     │ surgery          │
                                          └──────────────────┘     └──────────────────┘     └──────────────────┘
```

Solitary lesion

Progressive neurologic deficit?

Yes → Emergent decompression and biopsy (posterior preferred) → Frozen section analysis

No → Core needle biopsy → Diagnostic?

Diagnostic? No → Open biopsy (posterior preferred)

Yes

Metastatic carcinoma? → Consider radiation therapy or surgery

Benign primary bone tumor?

Osteoid osteoma/osteoblastoma/osteochondroma → Observe or marginal excision

LCH → Observe. Consider intralesional injection of corticosteroids

ABC/GCT → Consider embolization. If it fails, consider intralesional oncologic excision or en bloc excision

Malignant primary bone tumor?

Osteosarcoma/Ewing sarcoma → Neoadjuvant chemotherapy → Consider en bloc excision

Chondrosarcoma/chordoma → En bloc excision

Lymphoma/myeloma → Corticosteroids, chemotherapy +/– radiation therapy (consider percutaneous cementation if mechanical pain persists)

ABC/GCT, aneurysmal bone cyst/giant cell tumor; LCH, Langerhans cell histiocytosis

46

Primary Spinal Tumors

Rex A. W. Marco

Primary bone tumors are those originating in bone (rather than metastasizing to bone). The treatment of benign and malignant primary spinal column tumors is diverse and complex. Most of these tumors present as a solitary lesion. The age, site, clinical presentation, and cell type must be considered prior to initiating treatment.

 ## Classification

There are benign and malignant primary bone tumors. The neoplastic tissue is usually of mesodermal (bone, cartilage, fibrous, vessels, notochord) origin (**Table 46.1**).

Table 46.1 Classification of Benign and Malignant Primary Bone Tumors

Tissue of origin	Benign tumor	Malignant tumor
Fibrous	Fibrous dysplasia Desmoplastic fibroma	Malignant fibrous histiocytoma
Cartilage	Osteochondroma	Chondrosarcoma
Bone	Osteoid osteoma Osteoblastoma	Osteosarcoma
Hematopoietic		Plasmacytoma Lymphoma
Vascular	Hemangioma	
Notochord	Ecchordosis	Chordoma
Unknown	Giant cell tumor Aneurysmal bone cyst Langerhans cell histiocytosis	Ewing sarcoma

Workup

History

The clinical presentation of primary bone tumors varies. A thorough history and physical examination will help direct the most appropriate care. Signs and symptoms of the tumor include persistent back pain, difficulty maintaining balance, wide-based gait, fatigue, bowel or bladder incontinence, paresthesias, and weakness of the extremities.

Physical Examination

A thorough physical examination should be performed in all patients with a solitary spine lesion, because the lesion may represent a metastasic deposit from a palpable organ such as the breast, prostate, rectum, testes, or thyroid. Moreover, sacral chordomas are often palpable on rectal examination.

Spinal Imaging

Conventional radiographs are obtained to evaluate the level of the lesion, the local anatomy, and the overall spinal alignment. A bone scan is helpful to confirm the solitary nature of the tumor. Computed tomography (CT) defines bony architecture and demonstrates characteristic findings of hemangiomas, osteoid osteomas, and osteochondromas. Magnetic resonance imaging (MRI) provides additional information about soft-tissue extension and neural involvement.

Special Diagnostic Tests

The precise diagnosis of the tumor is often dependent on obtaining tissue for pathologic analysis. A biopsy should be performed and thoroughly analyzed prior to proceeding with definitive care unless the patient has a progressive neurologic deficit due to spinal cord compression. However, most patients do not present with a progressive neurologic deficit even in the presence of marked spinal cord compression. Initiation of corticosteroids usually stabilizes the patient's neurologic function and provides some pain control in the short term. However, a biopsy should ideally be obtained prior to initiating steroids because corticosteroids have an oncolytic effect on myeloma and lymphoma, which might impair the diagnostic workup. Suboptimal technique in performing the biopsy may decrease the ability to perform complete excision of the tumor. A core needle biopsy rather than an open biopsy is preferred because a core needle biopsy minimizes contamination of the biopsy tract compared with an open biopsy. Minimizing contamination preserves surgical options, which include en bloc excisions. If the core needle biopsy is not diagnostic, then an open biopsy is indicated.

An emergent decompression with concomitant frozen section analysis is warranted in the rare individual presenting with a severe acute neurological injury or progressive neurological deficit. A posterior biopsy and decompression procedure preserves more surgical options and can function as the first stage of an en bloc excision if deemed necessary. If the pathologist suspects a primary malignant bone tumor, then the thecal sac should be decompressed and an experienced spine tumor surgeon with expertise in en bloc excisions should be consulted as soon as possible. Minimizing local contamination with tumor cells is essential to decrease the likelihood of local recurrence and preserve treatment options. Decompression, tumor removal, and definitive stabilization are considered if carcinoma is identified on the frozen-section analysis.

Treatment

En bloc excisions of benign and malignant primary bone tumors of the spine can prolong survival and decrease the incidence of local recurrence more than intralesional excisions can. Although many symptomatic benign primary bone tumors can be successfully treated with an oncologic intralesional excision (complete removal of pathologic and reactive tissue), an en bloc marginal excision should be considered for patients with benign or malignant tumors isolated to the distal sacrum (below S2), the vertebral body, or the posterior arch of the vertebra. En bloc excisions of benign tumors involving the proximal sacrum or pedicle of the vertebral body may not be warranted because of the morbidity associated with these complex resections. Benign tumors involving the pedicle can be completely removed with an en bloc marginal excision combined with an intralesional excision of the tumor within the pedicle. En bloc excisions of tumors involving the proximal sacrum or vertebral body and pedicle are usually reserved for patients with malignant primary bone tumors.

Maintaining spinal stability by obtaining a solid fusion is especially important when treating patients with aggressive benign (giant cell tumor and osteoblastoma) and low-grade malignant (chordoma and low-grade chondrosarcoma) primary bone tumors, because these tumors have a relatively high incidence of local recurrence. A local recurrence in the setting of a solid fusion is a less challenging situation than a local recurrence in the presence of spinal instability. Appropriate oncologic excisions, combined with meticulous fusion techniques and biomechanically sound reconstructions, improve oncologic and functional outcomes by decreasing the incidence of local recurrence and increasing the likelihood of obtaining a stable spine fusion.

Conventional radiation therapy is not usually advised for the treatment of benign or malignant primary bone tumors. Most benign primary bone tumors are successfully treated with nonoperative measures or an appropriate oncologic excision. The potential benefit of decreasing the incidence of local recurrence thus does not usually outweigh the risk of malignant transformation or damage to the surrounding tissue following radiation therapy. Conversely, radiation therapy is not used for most malignant primary bone tumors because many of these tumors (chondrosarcoma, chordoma, and osteosarcoma) are relatively radioresistant. Ewing sarcoma and osteosarcoma are generally best treated with neoadjuvant chemotherapy followed by an en bloc excision for definitive local control. However, radiation therapy may decrease the incidence of local recurrence in patients with Ewing sarcoma with residual microscopic disease following an oncologic excision with contamination. Additionally, stereotactic radiation therapy has been used to treat primary spinal sarcomas that have been deemed unresectable. Lymphoma is usually treated with chemotherapy alone, but radiation therapy is a useful adjuvant when necessary. Radiation therapy is also useful for patients with plasmacytoma and myeloma.

 ## Complications

Incomplete resection of a lesion is associated with a high rate of recurrence for certain primary bone tumors. Other surgical complications, including infection, bleeding, failed fusion, and neurologic injury, are seen when surgical reconstruction is undertaken.

 ## Outcome

The outcome is dependent on the type of tumor and the adequacy of resection.

Suggested Readings

Bergh P, Kindblom LG, Gunterberg B, Remotti F, Ryd W, Meis-Kindblom JM. Prognostic factors in chordoma of the sacrum and mobile spine: a study of 39 patients. Cancer 2000;88(9): 2122–2134

> *This study reports the improved local control and survival of patients with sacral or mobile spine chordoma treated with en bloc excisions compared to intralesional excisions.*

Boriani S, Bandiera S, Biagini R, et al. Chordoma of the mobile spine: fifty years of experience. Spine 2006;31(4):493–503

> *Forty-eight patients with chordoma involving the mobile spine were evaluated. Fourteen of these patients who received radiation alone, intralesional excision, or a combination had a local recurrence and died. Intralesional, extracapsular excision combined with radiation therapy resulted in local recurrence in 12 of 16 patients (75%), whereas only 6 of 18 patients (33%) who underwent en bloc excision had a local recurrence.*

Boriani S, Biagini R, De Iure F, et al. En bloc resections of bone tumors of the thoracolumbar spine. A preliminary report on 29 patients. Spine 1996;21(16):1927–1931

> *The Weinstein-Boriani-Biagini (WBB) surgical staging system is discussed. This system divides the vertebra into 12 radiating zones in clockwise order from 1 to 12. This system allowed the authors to treat 29 patients with an en bloc resection uniformly. No local recurrences were reported.*

Boriani S, De Iure F, Bandiera S, et al. Chondrosarcoma of the mobile spine: report on 22 cases. Spine 2000;25(7):804–812

> *These authors concluded that en bloc excision, with wide or marginal histologic margins, is the suggested management for chondrosarcoma of the spine. Three local recurrences occurred in 12 patients who had an en bloc excision compared to 10 recurrences in 10 patients treated with an intralesional excision. All patients who had an en bloc excision were alive at last follow-up, while 8 of 10 patients who had an intralesional excision had died.*

Boriani S, De Iure F, Campanacci L, et al. Aneurysmal bone cyst of the mobile spine: report on 41 cases. Spine 2001;26(1):27–35

These authors concluded that selective arterial embolization may be the first treatment option for aneurysmal bone cysts affecting the spinal column because 75% (3/4) of patients were cured with embolization. Moreover, embolization did not affect subsequent surgical treatment options.

Delauche-Cavallier MC, Laredo JD, Wybier M, et al. Solitary plasmacytoma of the spine. Long-term clinical course. Cancer 1988;61(8):1707–1714

Nineteen patients with plasmacytoma of the spine were treated with chemotherapy and radiation therapy. They reported an expected 85% 10-year survival. Dissemination or local recurrence was observed in 13 of 19 patients.

Garg S, Mehta S, Dormans JP. Langerhans cell histiocytosis of the spine in children. Long-term follow-up. J Bone Joint Surg Am 2004;86-A(8):1740–1750

Twenty-six children with biopsy-proven Langerhans cell histiocytosis involving the spine were evaluated. Patients with solitary lesions were treated symptomatically with a spinal orthosis and followed clinically and radiographically. Two (8%) patients required surgical treatment for progressive deformity. These authors concluded that aggressive surgical management is usually not indicated for these patients.

Kawahara N, Tomita K, Murakami H, Demura S, Yoshioka K, Kato S. Total en bloc spondylectomy of the lower lumbar spine: a surgical technique of combined posterior-anterior approach. Spine 2011;36(1):74–82

Ten patients with a spinal tumor of the lower lumbar spine underwent total en bloc spondylectomy (TES) by combined posterior-anterior approach. The authors found that the lumbar nerves were preserved by the combined posterior-anterior approach for spinal tumors of L4 or L5.

Lin PP, Guzel VB, Moura MF, et al. Long-term follow-up of patients with giant cell tumor of the sacrum treated with selective arterial embolization. Cancer 2002;95(6):1317–1325

The authors describe a reasonable alternative to surgical intervention for large giant cell tumors involving the sacrum or spinal column. They conclude that embolization should be considered in the treatment of this difficult disease because the risk-to-benefit ratio of surgical intervention with or without radiation therapy is probably higher than that of embolization.

Mankin HJ, Lange TA, Spanier SS. The hazards of biopsy in patients with malignant primary bone and soft-tissue tumors. J Bone Joint Surg Am 1982;64(8):1121–1127

These authors showed that biopsy-related problems occurred three to five times more often when the biopsy was performed at a referring institution rather than the treating center. The optimal treatment plan was altered in 18% (60/329 patients) of patients, and the prognosis and outcome were adversely affected in 8.5% (28/329) of patients. These authors concluded that the surgeon and the institution should be prepared to perform accurate diagnostic studies and to proceed with the appropriate definitive treatment or refer these patients to a treating center prior to biopsy.

Marco RAW, Gentry JB, Rhines LD, et al. Ewing's sarcoma of the mobile spine. Spine 2005;30(7): 769–773

This study evaluates a homogeneous group of patients with Ewing sarcoma of the mobile spine who were treated with multiagent chemotherapy combined with radiation therapy for definitive local control. These patients demonstrated improved survival rates compared to patients treated with radiation therapy alone. However, these patients had a high risk of local recurrence and postlaminectomy kyphosis. The authors concluded that current spinal resection and reconstruction techniques may lead to improved oncologic and clinical outcomes.

Marco RA, An HS. Complications of surgical and medical care: anticipation and management. In: McLain RF, Benzel E, eds. Cancer in the Spine (Handbook of Comprehensive Care): Complications, Anticipation and Management. Totowa, NJ: Humana Press; 2006:169–197

This is an excellent comprehensive review of the potential pitfalls involved with spine tumor surgery of the cervical, thoracic, lumbar, and sacral spine.

Rao G, Ha CS, Chakrabarti I, Feiz-Erfan I, Mendel E, Rhines LD. Multiple myeloma of the cervical spine: treatment strategies for pain and spinal instability. J Neurosurg Spine 2006;5(2): 140–145

The authors report the results of radiotherapy and surgical treatment of patients with myeloma involving the cervical spine. The authors suggest that external-beam radiation can effectively treat most patients with clinical or radiographically documented instability.

Schoenfeld AJ, Hornicek FJ, Pedlow FX, et al. Osteosarcoma of the spine: experience in 26 patients treated at the Massachusetts General Hospital. Spine J 2010;10(8):708–714

The authors confirm a poor prognosis for patients with osteosarcoma of the spine. They find that a combination of therapies, including surgery, chemotherapy, and high-dose radiation, achieve adequate short-term survival, but the 5-year mortality rate remains high.

Sundaresan N, Schmidek H, Schiller A, Rosenthal D, Eds. Tumors of the Spine: Diagnosis and Clinical Management. Philadelphia, PA: WB Saunders; 1990

This is an excellent review of the evaluation and treatment of benign and malignant primary bone tumors.

Tomita K, Kawahara N, Baba H, Tsuchiya H, Fujita T, Toribatake Y. Total en bloc spondylectomy. A new surgical technique for primary malignant vertebral tumors. Spine 1997;22(3): 324–333

These authors provide a step-by-step description of their en bloc spondylectomy technique.

Metastatic Tumor

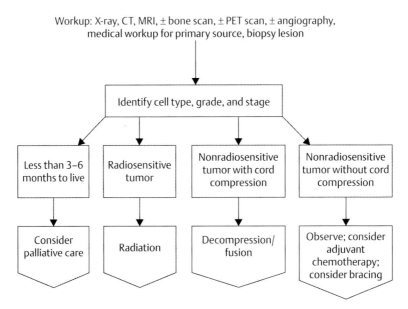

Workup: X-ray, CT, MRI, ± bone scan, ± PET scan, ± angiography, medical workup for primary source, biopsy lesion

Identify cell type, grade, and stage

Less than 3–6 months to live

Radiosensitive tumor

Nonradiosensitive tumor with cord compression

Nonradiosensitive tumor without cord compression

Consider palliative care

Radiation

Decompression/ fusion

Observe; consider adjuvant chemotherapy; consider bracing

CT, computed tomography; MRI, magnetic resonance imaging; PET, positron emission tomography

47

Metastatic Spinal Tumors

Paul Kraemer and Rick C. Sasso

The spine is the most common site of skeletal metastatic disease. Spinal metastases account for the majority of spinal tumors encountered by spine surgeons. Breast carcinoma is the most common primary in women (**Fig. 47.1A,B**), while lung and prostate carcinoma are the most common primary sources in men. Renal, thyroid, and gastrointestinal tumors are also commonly seen, but in lesser frequency then the former mentioned tumors. Breast, prostate, and renal metastases are more likely to be seen by spine surgeons because of the longer relative survival compared with lung and gastrointestinal carcinoma.

Workup

The most common first symptom of spinal metastasis is mechanical pain, often well localized, insidious in onset, positional, and severe enough to disturb sleep. Patients may also present with various neurologic symptoms ranging from mild sensory or motor radiculopathy to complete paralysis due to neurologic compression, either directly from excessive tumor load or through instability of a pathologic fracture. Spinal metastasis may be the presenting complaint in a patient previously unaware of having a malignancy. The history should also address constitutional symptoms, such as fever, chills, malaise, and weight loss, as well as malignancy in the patient history and family history.

Radiographic evaluation begins with plain films looking for tumor location, bony destruction, soft-tissue extension, and pathologic fracture. Classic radiographic signs such as the "winking owl" (missing pedicle) or vertebra plana are present only after significant bony destruction. Magnetic resonance imaging (MRI) allows excellent evaluation of the neurologic elements and soft-tissue tumor involvement. Key tumor characteristics, such as density and vascularity, are also readily seen on MRI. Computerized tomography (CT) scans are helpful in evaluating bony lesions, determining stability, and preoperative planning.

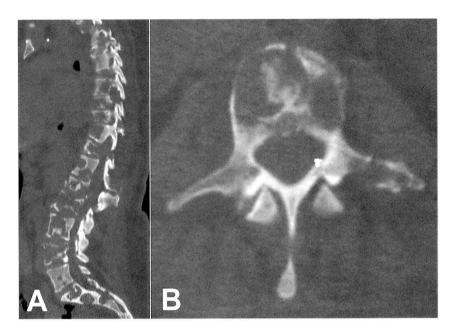

Fig. 47.1 CT of metastatic breast carcinoma of the vertebral column. **(A)** Sagittal. **(B)** Axial.

Pathologic diagnosis should be obtained by biopsy, either CT-guided or open. Bone scans may be used as screening tools to identify other sites of metastasis, both in the spine and in the apical skeleton. Areas of metastasis identified outside of the spine, especially if they occur around the hips, should be imaged to evaluate for potential impending pathologic fracture.

For patients who present with metastatic lesions in the spine and who have not previously been diagnosed with cancer, a thorough examination should be performed. This often includes blood work, including complete blood count (CBC), erythrocyte sedimentation rate (ESR), C-reactive protein (CRP), ionized calcium level, and serum and urine electrophoresis (SPEP and UPEP). Prostate-specific antigen (PSA) levels should be checked in men. CT scans of the chest, abdomen and pelvis should be obtained. Biopsy of either the spinal lesion or another lesion identified on imaging studies is necessary to make a definitive diagnosis.

Treatment

Goals of any intervention are improved quality of life via palliation of pain and prevention of neurologic worsening. The patient's overall health and prognosis must be taken into account when considering surgery or radiation, and close consultation with the medical oncologist, patient, and family should be the first step. Surgery should not be considered in patients who are hopelessly bedridden with an expected survival of less than six weeks.

Bracing is generally not considered except in terminal cases where no other options are reasonable, as there is no defined endpoint other than death. Surgical options should provide definitive stability without the need for adjunct bracing.

Vertebroplasty or kyphoplasty is useful for palliative treatment of select tumors wholly contained within a vertebral body. Indications for use are refractory pain without neurologic deficit. The posterior vertebral body wall must be intact to prevent extravasation of cement into the spinal canal.

Radiation therapy may be extremely useful for pain and tumor control in select pathologies, particularly germ cell and hematopoietic lines. Close coordination with the radiation oncologist is mandatory, as protocols change often, and variability in the direction of external beam may avoid irradiating a potential surgical approach.

Indications for surgical management include an isolated spinal lesion, pathologic fracture or deformity causing a neurologic deficit, or refractory pain and radioresistant tumors. The mainstay of treatment is intralesional excision and spinal reconstruction. Strong consideration should be given to "overfixing" with instrumentation, as immediate unbraced activity is necessary to maintain constitutional fitness, and solid osseous union may never be achieved in the face of an immunocompromised cancer patient. Anterior, posterior, and combined approaches all have a place in reconstructive efforts, largely depending on level, degree of instability, and surgeon preference. Multiple noncontiguous lesions may create a very difficult situation.

Patchels et al. in 2005 presented the only level I evidence comparing radiation to surgery. Exquisitely radiosensitive tumors were not studied and should be treated with radiation. Patients randomized to surgery had statistically better return of neurologic function, preservation of bowel and bladder function, relief of lower pain, and improved ambulation. Those who crossed over from radiation to surgery did not improve as much as those who were randomized to surgery, and the complication rate was higher. The study was stopped early by the review board because the results so heavily favored surgery over radiation. Though these results strongly favor surgical treatment of carcinoma and adenocarcinomas, a thorough discussion of the risks and benefits of all options must be undertaken.

Outcome

Outcomes and prognosis for spinal metastasis vary based on several interrelated factors: primary tumor site, general health of the patient, number of extraspinal metastases, number of spinal metastases, metastatic involvement of internal organs, and severity of neurologic deficit on presentation.

Complications

Wound healing in cancer patients is often challenging. If radiotherapy is used as an adjunct to definite surgical stabilization, serious consideration should be given to deferring radiotherapy until after surgery to minimize complications of operating in an irradiated bed. Discussing the approach and incision with the radiation oncologist may help avoid unnecessary radiation to the incision.

Patients with diffuse metastatic disease may be systemically ill, cachectic, and malnourished. Aggressive nutritional support should be considered mandatory preoperatively as well as postoperatively and can help avoid or limit wound healing problems.

Suggested Readings

Abe E, Kobayashi T, Murai H, Suzuki T, Chiba M, Okuyama K. Total spondylectomy for primary malignant, aggressive benign, and solitary metastatic bone tumors of the thoracolumbar spine. J Spinal Disord 2001;14(3):237–246

> *Total spondylectomy was used to treat 14 patients with malignant or aggressive benign vertebral tumors. All patients had good pain relief and there were no serious complications. There were three local recurrences at 3.2 years.*

Dudeney S, Lieberman IH, Reinhardt MK, Hussein M. Kyphoplasty in the treatment of osteolytic vertebral compression fractures as a result of multiple myeloma. J Clin Oncol 2002;20(9):2382–2387

> *This article reports prospective evaluation of 55 kyphoplasties in 18 patients. Mean follow-up was 7.4 months. SF36 scores for bodily pain, physical function, vitality, and social function all significantly improved.*

Fourney DR, Schomer DF, Nader R, et al. Percutaneous vertebroplasty and kyphoplasty for painful vertebral body fractures in cancer patients. J Neurosurg 2003;98(1, Suppl):21–30

> *Sixty-five vertebroplasties and 32 kyphoplasties were done in 56 patients with myeloma and primary malignant tumors. Median follow-up was 4.5 months with 84% complete pain relief.*

Patchell RA, Tibbs PA, Regine WF, et al. Direct decompressive surgical resection in the treatment of spinal cord compression caused by metastatic cancer: a randomised trial. Lancet 2005;366(9486):643–648

> *This landmark randomized controlled trial compared surgery to radiotherapy for metastatic lesions to the spine; it was ended early because significant benefits were seen for surgical patients.*

Ryu S, Fang Yin F, Rock J, et al. Image-guided and intensity-modulated radiosurgery for patients with spinal metastasis. Cancer 2003;97(8):2013–2018

> *In this evaluation of 10 patients, most had significant pain relief within 2 to 4 weeks after treatment.*

Sundaresan N, Rothman A, Manhart K, Kelliher K. Surgery for solitary metastases of the spine: rationale and results of treatment. Spine 2002;27(16):1802–1806

> *This is a retrospective review of 80 patients with solitary spinal metastasis from solid tumors. Median survival after surgery was 30 months. Surgical excision is recommended before radiotherapy to increase the chances of palliation and cure.*

Wai EK, Finkelstein JA, Tangente RP, et al. Quality of life in surgical treatment of metastatic spine disease. Spine 2003;28(5):508–512

> *In this prospective evaluation of 25 patients undergoing surgery for spinal metastasis, the greatest improvement was with pain; however, improvements in constitutional symptoms were also seen.*

Whyne CM, Hu SS, Lotz JC. Burst fracture in the metastatically involved spine: development, validation, and parametric analysis of a three-dimensional poroelastic finite-element model. Spine 2003;28(7):652–660

> *A finite-element study was undertaken to investigate features that contribute to burst fracture risk. The primary factors affecting fracture initiation were tumor size, magnitude of spinal loading, and bone density.*

X Spinal Infections and Inflammatory Disease

Pyogenic Spinal Infection

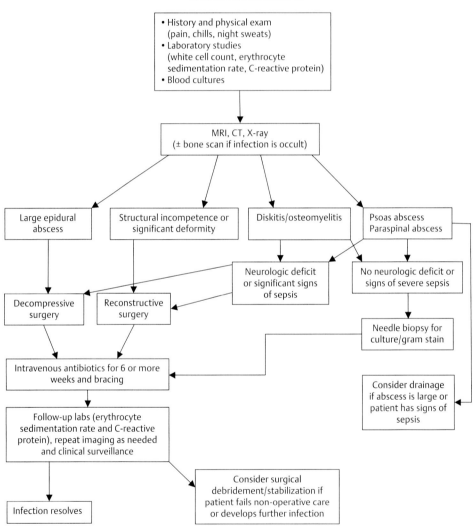

49

Pyogenic Infections of the Spine

Olga A. Perlmutter and D. Greg Anderson

Purulent infections of the spinal column are relatively rare. Risk factors for a purulent spinal infection include diabetes, rheumatoid arthritis, alcoholism, human immunodeficiency virus (HIV), chronic steroid usage, the presence of an extraspinal infection, malignancy, prior surgery, and intravenous (IV) drug abuse. Most pyogenic infections are hematogenous in origin (i.e., spread to the spine via the vascular system). In some cases, direct extension of a local infection (e.g., empyema) can involve the spinal column. Purulent spinal infections are serious, with a mortality rate approaching 20% if not treated promptly and aggressively. The most frequent causative organisms include gram-positive aerobic cocci (80%), such as *Staphylococcus aureus* (60%), *Streptococcus* (10–20%), and coagulase-negative *Staphylococcus* (10%). Gram-negative aerobic cocci are found in 15–20% of cases, including *Escherichia coli*, *Pseudomonas aeruginosa*, and *Proteus* species. A significant number of infections may be polymicrobial, especially in diabetic and immunosupressed patients or those with a history of IV drug abuse.

Classification

Infections of the spinal column are most commonly classified on the basis of anatomical location. The most common locations for the infection include the vertebral bodies and disk space, facet joints, spinal canal, and perispinal soft tissues (e.g., psoas muscle). Infections of the spinal canal are often subclassified into epidural, subdural, and intramedullary, depending on the location of the abscess. Another related area of infection includes the sacroiliac joint.

Workup

History

Patients with a pyogenic infection most commonly present with pain at the site of the infection and generalized symptoms, such as fevers, chills, or night sweats. The pain is often "nonmechanical" and is severe even at rest. Fever may not be present, depending on the location of the infection and the status of the patient's immune system. Neurologic symptoms may be present for infections involving the spinal canal and may include anything from minor deficits to complete paralysis.

Physical Examination

Patients with spinal infections often appear grossly ill, but this is not always the case. Vital signs may show an elevated temperature. Patients with severe sepsis may exhibit findings of tachycardia and hypotension. There may be local tenderness around the site of the infection. A thorough neurologic examination is mandatory in cases where infection is suspected. The examination should be repeated frequently during treatment, as changes may occur.

Special Diagnostic Tests

Laboratory Studies

Serum laboratory studies, including white cell count with differential, erythrocyte sedimentation rate (ESR), and C-reactive protein level (CRP), are commonly ordered. Blood cultures are useful and may identify the organism in some patients. In patients with related medical conditions, such as diabetes or HIV, additional laboratory work may help to define the severity of the condition.

Imaging Studies

Plain radiographs are often taken and may show destructive changes with chronic vertebral osteomyelitis; however, radiographic signs lag behind clinical ones, and radiographs may be negative for the first 3 weeks of a bony infection. Computed tomography (CT) is useful to visualize chronic destructive changes of the spinal column as well and may show an air/fluid level within the site of an abscess. However, in early spinal infections, plain radiographs and CT may be negative. Magnetic resonance imaging (MRI) is thus the imaging modality of choice in most cases of pyogenic infection (**Fig. 49.1**). It is highly sensitive for spinal canal abscesses, diskitis, psoas abscess, and even early vertebral osteomyelitis. Gadolinium enhancement may be useful, especially in cases where the infection involves the spinal cord. MRI can be used to define the location and extent of the infection. Bone scans are helpful in cases of multifocal osteomyelitis and in subtle cases where the site of the infection is not evident. Gallium

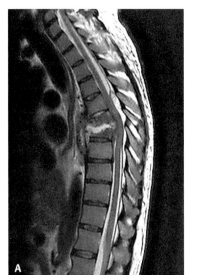
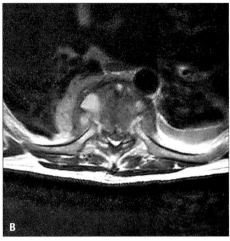
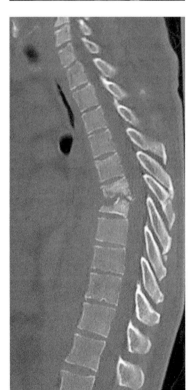
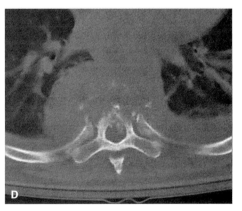

Fig. 49.1 A patient with a significant spinal infection. Notice that there is evidence of bone and disk destruction and a large dorsal epidural abscess. **(A,B)** Sagittal and axial MRI. **(C,D)** Sagittal and axial CT scans.

scanning has been described as useful in cases of chronic postsurgical infections in the setting of spinal hardware. Indium scanning is neither sensitive nor specific in the setting of spinal infections.

Biopsy and Culture

If no organism is identified on blood cultures, a biopsy sample of the infectious material should be obtained. Depending on the location and size of the infection, this may be done with fluoroscopic guidance, with CT guidance, or as an open surgical procedure. An adequate sample should include any abscess material and surrounding soft tissue from the focus of infection. The material should be evaluated with gram stain, aerobic, anaerobic, acid-fast, and fungal cultures. A biopsy for histology is also useful, as tumors may occasionally present with findings similar to infection.

 ## Treatment

Nonsurgical Treatment

Nonsurgical treatment is indicated as the initial therapy for patients with infections involving the vertebral body, disk space, and perispinal tissues as long as there is no finding of significant involvement of the spinal canal and the neurologic examination is normal. After biopsy to identify the organism, treatment consists of targeted antimicrobial drugs and bracing/immobilization of the spinal column. Antimicrobial therapy generally involves intravenous dosing, which continues for at least 6 weeks. Serum laboratory test results including CRP level and ESR are followed during the course of treatment and should be returning to normal by the point that treatment is discontinued. Some authors have recommended oral antibiotics following the discontinuation of intravenous antibiotics. Patients with major immune dysfunction (e.g., patients with HIV or patients on chemotherapy for malignancy) are much more likely to fail nonsurgical treatment and, in some cases, are better served with early surgery. Patients with significant destruction of the spinal column leading to a kyphotic spinal deformity are also better served with surgical reconstruction.

Surgical Treatment

Surgical treatment involves an adequate débridement of the site of the infection, followed by reconstruction of any structurally significant bony defects. Rigid internal fixation is used to maintain stability at the site of the infection, and this facilitates resolution of the infection and bony fusion across the area (**Fig. 49.2**). Autogenous bone graft is preferred over allograft or other synthetic materials in the face of a serious pyogenic infection. When possible, the spinal instrumentation should be placed in a region of the spine that is not involved with the infection (e.g., posterior instrumentation following anterior

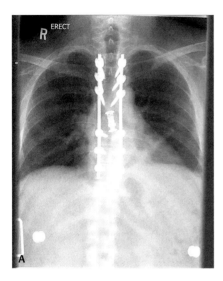
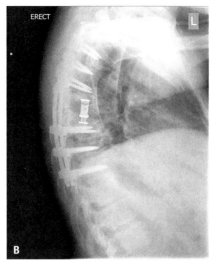

Fig. 49.2   **(A,B)** Postoperative images following reconstruction. The patient was treated with a decompressive laminectomy with evacuation of the epidural abscess followed by stabilization of the infected section using a pedicle screw and rod construct. The anterior column débridement and reconstruction were achieved from an extracavitary approach with resection of the infected bone in the vertebral bodies and reconstruction with an expandable titanium cage filled with autologous bone graft. Postoperatively, cultures grew out methicillin-resistant *Staphylococcus aureus,* which was treated with intravenous vancomycin for 6 weeks, resulting in resolution of the infection.

débridement and grafting of diskitis/osteomyelitis. Postoperative antimicrobial therapy

Outcome

The outcome for most patients with appropriate treatment for pyogenic infection is favorable. Control of the infection and reconstitution of the spinal segment can generally be obtained with medical and/or surgical therapy. Delay in diagnosis or inadequate therapy is associated with a significant decline in rate of success and may lead to mortality.

Complications

Complications following pyogenic infections include generalized sepsis, death, spinal instability, neurologic deterioration, or late recurrence.

Suggested Readings

Baker AS, Ojemann RG, Swartz MN, Richardson EP Jr. Spinal epidural abscess. N Engl J Med 1975; 293(10):463–468

Thirty-nine patients with spinal epidural abscess were evaluated at Massachusetts General Hospital. Progression from spinal ache to root pain to weakness followed by paralysis continues to be characteristic of spinal epidural abscess.

Carragee E, Iezza A. Does acute placement of instrumentation in the treatment of vertebral osteomyelitis predispose to recurrent infection: long-term follow-up in immune-suppressed patients. Spine 2008;33(19):2089–2093

The authors followed 32 immunocompromised patients who were treated with dé-bridement and instrumentation for acute spinal infections for 10 years. One patient was treated for recurrent infection and was treated with débridement and retention of the hardware. The authors conclude that the use of hardware in the setting of infection even in immunocompromised patients resulted in a low risk of recurrent infection.

Danner RL, Hartman BJ. Update on spinal epidural abscess: 35 cases and review of the literature. Rev Infect Dis 1987;9(2):265–274

Thirty-five cases of spinal epidural abscess were evaluated retrospectively and com-pared with 153 cases reported in the literature. Early diagnosis and treatment led to a significant improvement in outcome. The combination of antibiotics and surgical drainage remains the treatment of choice.

Del Curling O Jr, Gower DJ, McWhorter JM. Changing concepts in spinal epidural abscess: a re-port of 29 cases. Neurosurgery 1990;27(2):185–192

Authors state that the spectrum of organisms causing epidural abscess has broad-ened over the past 50 years, and distinction between acute and chronic spinal epi-dural abscesses has minimal clinical significance.

Hlavin ML, Kaminski HJ, Ross JS, Ganz E. Spinal epidural abscess: a ten-year perspective. Neuro-surgery 1990;27(2):177–184

A retrospective study of spinal epidural abscess spanning 10 years and encompass-ing 40 patients was done. Preoperative paralysis and neurologic deterioration from normal were identified as poor prognostic features.

Korovessis P, Repantis T, Iliopoulos P, Hadjipavlou A. Beneficial influence of titanium mesh cage on infection healing and spinal reconstruction in hematogenous septic spondylitis: a retro-spective analysis of surgical outcome of twenty-five consecutive cases and review of literature. Spine 2008;33(21):E759–E767

The authors report the successful treatment of 25 cases of spondylodiskitis with anterior débridement and stabilization with titanium mesh cages packed with autograft and supported with posterior pedicle screw instrumentation. They sug-gested that minimally invasive insertion of the posterior pedicle screws may help to minimize soft-tissue trauma, resulted in shorter operating room times and fewer complications, and did not adversely affect healing.

Leys D, Lesoin F, Viaud C, et al. Decreased morbidity from acute bacterial spinal epidural ab-scesses using computed tomography and nonsurgical treatment in selected patients. Ann Neu-rol 1985;17(4):350–355

Authors describe antibiotic treatment parenterally for a minimum of 8 weeks, fol-lowed by oral antibiotic therapy in patients with epidural abscess.

Post MJD, Quencer RM, Montalvo BM, Katz BH, Eismont FJ, Green BA. Spinal infection: evalua-tion with MR imaging and intraoperative US. Radiology 1988;169(3):765–771

Twenty-four patients with spinal infections were reviewed, and the clinical and pathological data were correlated to MRI images of the spine or intraoperative ul-trasound. MRI is recommended as the initial screening procedure in spinal infection.

Russell NA, Vaughan R, Morley TP. Spinal epidural infection. Can J Neurol Sci 1979;6(3): 325–328

> *Thirty cases of spinal epidural abscess were reviewed, focusing on presentation and results of treatment. Study points out that late diagnosis can lead to severe or complete paralysis before surgical treatment can be carried out.*

Thelander U, Larsson S. Quantitation of C-reactive protein levels and erythrocyte sedimentation rate after spinal surgery. Spine 1992;17(4):400–404

> *CRP and ESR were prospectively measured after four types of uncomplicated spinal operations. CRP is presumably a better test than ESR for early detection of postoperative infection.*

Wang Z, Lenehan B, Itshayek E, et al. Primary pyogenic infection of the spine in intravenous drug users: a prospective observational study. Spine 2011

> *A prospective analysis in which 51 patients with osteodiskitis and a history of IV drug abuse (IVDA) were compared to 51 patients with osteodiskits and no history of IVDA. The patients with a history of IVDA more commonly presented with cervical involvement and paralysis, while non-IVDA patients were more likely to have involvement of the thoracolumbar spine. Of the IVDA patients, 37 were caught at least once using illegal drugs while in the hospital. IVDA patients were more likely to have surgical site infections and early hardware failure. Given these factors and the unreliable nature of drug-abusing patients, the authors advocate for halo immobilization in addition to surgical stabilization.*

of prednisone).[19] Current recommendations state that aspirin should be discontinued ~7–10 days prior to surgery, and the cyclooxygenase-2 (COX-2) inhibitors should be discontinued 5 half lives before surgical intervention, with a reported range between 9 hours and 1 week.[9]

Recent recommendations regarding the perioperative management of methotrexate have suggested continuing the usual dose perioperatively unless the patient has poorly controlled diabetes, liver, kidney, or lung disease or is elderly. Of note, a recent prospective randomized study revealed no increase in wound infections or other surgical complications with continued methotrexate use. It is recommended that both sulfasalazine and hydroxychloroquine be continued for all procedures, with care to look for any possible drug interactions or side effects. The perioperative management of biologic modifiers such as the TNF antagonists (etanercept, infliximab, and adalimumab) has not been formally studied. It has been recommended that these agents be withheld for 2–4 weeks before surgery and restarted 1–2 weeks after surgery.[20,21] The effect of these medications on postoperative complications of wound infection and cervical pseudarthrosis remain unknown. Ultimately, decisions regarding medication management should be made on a case-by-case basis and often require the involvement of the treating rheumatologist.[22]

Surgical Management

Initial teaching suggested surgical stabilization of the cervical spine in RA patients with progressive neurologic changes or intractable pain.[23] Ultimately, a subset of patients with radiographic changes of the cervical spine without neurologic or pain symptoms was identified who would benefit from surgical arthrodesis to prevent neurologic injury.[12] Absolute indications for surgery do not exist; care should be individualized to the patient. Nonetheless, general recommendations can be made (**Table 51.1**).

When AAS is reducible, posterior fusion can be performed with wiring, transarticular screws or C1–C2 lateral mass fixation. With irreducible subluxation, laminectomy must be considered to provide more room for the spinal cord. There remains some controversy as to the optimal surgical approach for AAS. A study of 15 consecutive patients treated with transoral decompression via odontoid resection with anterior plating and posterior fusion showed reliable improvements in pain control, neurologic status, and subjective evaluation of function.[24] However, MRI studies have shown significant pannus resorption after surgical stabilization, suggesting that odontoid resection may be unnecessary in patients without significant anterior impingement of the cord.[25] The morbidity and complications from the transoral approach can, therefore, be avoided with a posterior arthrodesis. Sublaminar wire fixation is best avoided in patients with irreducible AAS because of the risk of neurologic injury.

AAI requires both decompression and stabilization. Decompression can be performed via preoperative skeletal traction. However, if traction fails to reduce the cranial settling, a posterior decompression (C1 laminectomy, suboccipital decompression) or odontoid resection must be performed along with the posterior fusion to decompress the ventral compression adequately.[26] Stabilization

Table 51.1   Relative Indications for Operative Intervention in RA

Progressive neurologic deficit

Intractable neck pain with radiographic changes

Radiographic risk factors of impending neurologic injury:

 PADI < 14 mm in presence of AAS

 Odontoid migration > 5 mm rostral to McGregor's line in presence of AAI

 Sagittal canal diameter < 14 mm in patients with SAS

 Cord compression or cervicomedullary angle > 135 degrees on MRI evaluation

is usually obtained with posterior occipitocervical fusion, with segmental fixation from the occiput to the C2 or C3 level.

SAS can be treated with either an anterior or a posterior arthrodesis. Preoperative skeletal traction is a useful adjunct to allow gradual, protected reduction of the subluxations. Additionally, traction provides insight into the degree of reducibility of the cervical spine. Posterior procedures allow direct decompression of dorsal compressive structures (ligamentum flavum, cervical lamina). Posterior stand-alone procedures are contraindicated in the setting of cervical kyphosis and fixed subluxation with significant ventral cord compression. In these settings, the optimal treatment is anterior decompression and arthrodesis. The extent of the arthrodesis remains uncertain because of the progressive nature of the disease. Because of the potentially high risk of adjacent-segment degeneration, some authors have recommended including all involved levels rather than only the levels with the worst stenosis.[27] Other authors have suggested including the entire cervical spine in their fusion construct because of the risk of adjacent level disease.[11] This approach may be aggressive given the 20–25% complication rate associated with a multilevel instrumented arthrodesis.[28]

The chronic subluxations associated with rheumatoid disease may recur after stand-alone anterior or posterior fusions, resulting in recurrent stenosis.[29,30] Furthermore, the risk of pseudarthrosis increases with a greater number of surgical levels. To mitigate these risks, combined anterior and posterior procedures can be performed.

Outcomes

With our increased understanding of the rheumatoid cervical spine, patient outcomes continue to improve. This progression is likely multifactorial, with earlier diagnosis of myelopathy, earlier surgical referral, and more aggressive medical management. In general, outcomes studies have shown surgical treatment to be superior to medical management for patients with neurologic deficits, and postoperative neurologic function is most closely related to preoperative neurologic status. These findings have supported a more aggressive surgical environment in the treatment of patients with RA, including recommendations for surgery in patients with radiographic indices shown to predict functional decline.

In AAS, a PADI of < 14 mm has been shown to predict neurologic deterioration. Further, it has been shown to be an excellent predictor of neurologic recovery, with all surgically treated patients with measurements > 14 mm having a complete neurologic recovery and no recovery seen in patients with a PADI < 10 mm.[8] The rate of postoperative neurologic deterioration is not known, but has been reported in 4–8% of patients.[12] The rate of pseudarthrosis formation has been reported as high as 50% after fusion for AAS, with 12% of patients requiring revision operations.[31]

Casey et al. prospectively studied 116 patients with AAI treated with posterior decompression with instrumented fusion. Transoral odontoid resection was performed only in those patients with anterior cord compression. The authors reported neurologic recovery in 50% and significant pain relief in 97% of patients. A higher revision rate was seen in patients without inclusion of the occiput in the fusion construct, and adjacent-level degeneration was a common complication. They also reported a perioperative mortality rate of 10%.

Surgical treatment of SAS has been shown to improve neck pain reliably, with less consistent results in relieving upper extremity symptoms. Patients with myelopathy have been shown to have significantly worse surgical outcomes, prompting authors to suggest early stabilization of SAS before the onset of myelopathic symptoms.[32]

A recent meta-analysis compared the neurologic outcomes of patients with RA and cervical spine subluxations treated surgically and nonsurgically.[33] Comparing 23 studies of surgical treatment with 7 studies of patients treated nonsurgically, the authors concluded that surgical neurologic outcomes were superior to conservative treatment in all patients with neurologic symptoms (Ranawat Grade II, IIIA and IIIB). No difference in the outcomes of patients without neurologic deficits (Ranawat I) was identified.

It has been suggested that patients with severe neurologic deficits have higher risk of morbidity from surgical intervention and less potential for neurologic improvement.[34] Not surprisingly, patients with a higher Ranawat classification have a poorer overall prognosis, although most patients still improve at least one Ranawat class after surgical intervention.[35] However, in patients with severe mutilating-type seropositive RA, surgical stabilization has been shown to prolong life, improve neurologic function, and improve ability to perform activities of daily life.[36]

Conclusion

Cervical spine surgery in patients with RA is complicated by medical comorbidities, increased infection rates, and, often, poor bone quality. Despite these challenges, surgical stabilization of AAS, AAI, and SAS reliably improve neurologic and functional status in a well-chosen patient population.

References

1. Reiter MF, Boden SD. Inflammatory disorders of the cervical spine. Spine 1998;23(24): 2755–2766
2. Arnett FC, Edworthy SM, Bloch DA, et al. The American Rheumatism Association 1987 revised criteria for the classification of rheumatoid arthritis. Arthritis Rheum 1988;31(3): 315–324
3. Yelin E, Henke C, Epstein W. The work dynamics of the person with rheumatoid arthritis. Arthritis Rheum 1987;30(5):507–512
4. Geborek P, Crnkic M, Petersson IF, Saxne T; South Swedish Arthritis Treatment Group. Etanercept, infliximab, and leflunomide in established rheumatoid arthritis: clinical experience using a structured follow up programme in southern Sweden. Ann Rheum Dis 2002;61(9):793–798
5. Oda T, Fujiwara K, Yonenobu K, Azuma B, Ochi T. Natural course of cervical spine lesions in rheumatoid arthritis. Spine 1995;20(10):1128–1135
6. Nguyen HV, Ludwig SC, Silber J, et al. Rheumatoid arthritis of the cervical spine. Spine J 2004;4(3):329–334
7. Casey AT, Crockard HA, Pringle J, O'Brien MF, Stevens JM. Rheumatoid arthritis of the cervical spine: current techniques for management. Orthop Clin North Am 2002;33(2): 291–309
8. Dreyer SJ, Boden SD. Natural history of rheumatoid arthritis of the cervical spine. Clin Orthop Relat Res 1999;(366):98–106
9. Krauss WE, Bledsoe JM, Clarke MJ, Nottmeier EW, Pichelmann MA. Rheumatoid arthritis of the craniovertebral junction. Neurosurgery 2010;66(3, Suppl):83–95
10. Sherk HH. Atlantoaxial instability and acquired basilar invagination in rheumatoid arthritis. Orthop Clin North Am 1978;9(4):1053–1063
11. Kraus DR, Peppelman WC, Agarwal AK, DeLeeuw HW, Donaldson WF III. Incidence of subaxial subluxation in patients with generalized rheumatoid arthritis who have had previous occipital cervical fusions. Spine 1991;16(10, Suppl):S486–S489
12. Boden SD, Dodge LD, Bohlman HH, Rechtine GR. Rheumatoid arthritis of the cervical spine. A long-term analysis with predictors of paralysis and recovery. J Bone Joint Surg Am 1993;75(9):1282–1297
13. Pellicci PM, Ranawat CS, Tsairis P, Bryan WJ. A prospective study of the progression of rheumatoid arthritis of the cervical spine. J Bone Joint Surg Am 1981;63(3):342–350
14. Mikulowski P, Wollheim FA, Rotmil P, Olsen I. Sudden death in rheumatoid arthritis with atlanto-axial dislocation. Acta Med Scand 1975;198(6):445–451
15. Weissman BN, Aliabadi P, Weinfeld MS, Thomas WH, Sosman JL. Prognostic features of atlanto-axial subluxation in rheumatoid arthritis patients. Radiology 1982;144(4):745–751
16. Riew KD, Hilibrand AS, Palumbo MA, Sethi N, Bohlman HH. Diagnosing basilar invagination in the rheumatoid patient. The reliability of radiographic criteria. J Bone Joint Surg Am 2001;83-A(2):194–200
17. Takahashi M, Yamashita Y, Sakamoto Y, Kojima R. Chronic cervical cord compression: clinical significance of increased signal intensity on MR images. Radiology 1989;173(1):219–224
18. Bundschuh C, Modic MT, Kearney F, Morris R, Deal C. Rheumatoid arthritis of the cervical spine: surface-coil MR imaging. AJR Am J Roentgenol 1988;151(1):181–187
19. Howe CR, Gardner GC, Kadel NJ. Perioperative medication management for the patient with rheumatoid arthritis. J Am Acad Orthop Surg 2006;14(9):544–551
20. Rosandich PA, Kelley JT III, Conn DL. Perioperative management of patients with rheumatoid arthritis in the era of biologic response modifiers. Curr Opin Rheumatol 2004;16(3): 192–198
21. Pieringer H, Stuby U, Biesenbach G. Patients with rheumatoid arthritis undergoing surgery: how should we deal with antirheumatic treatment? Semin Arthritis Rheum 2007; 36(5):278–286
22. Grennan DM, Gray J, Loudon J, Fear S. Methotrexate and early postoperative complications in patients with rheumatoid arthritis undergoing elective orthopaedic surgery. Ann Rheum Dis 2001;60(3):214–217
23. Ferlic DC, Clayton ML, Leidholt JD, Gamble WE. Surgical treatment of the symptomatic unstable cervical spine in rheumatoid arthritis. J Bone Joint Surg Am 1975;57(3):349–354

24. Kim DH, Hilibrand AS. Rheumatoid arthritis in the cervical spine. J Am Acad Orthop Surg 2005;13(7):463–474
25. Kerschbaumer F, Kandziora F, Klein C, Mittlmeier T, Starker M. Transoral decompression, anterior plate fixation, and posterior wire fusion for irreducible atlantoaxial kyphosis in rheumatoid arthritis. Spine 2000;25(20):2708–2715
26. Crockard HA. Surgical management of cervical rheumatoid problems. Spine 1995; 20(23):2584–2590
27. Grob D, Würsch R, Grauer W, Sturzenegger J, Dvorak J. Atlantoaxial fusion and retrodental pannus in rheumatoid arthritis. Spine 1997;22(14):1580–1583, discussion 1584
28. Cloyd JM, Acosta FL Jr, Ames CP. Effect of age on the perioperative and radiographic complications of multilevel cervicothoracic spinal fusions. Spine 2008;33(26):E977–E982
29. Christensson D, Säveland H, Rydholm U. Cervical spine surgery in rheumatoid arthritis. A Swedish nation-wide registration of 83 patients. Scand J Rheumatol 2000;29(5):314–319
30. Olerud C, Larsson BE, Rodriguez M. Subaxial cervical spine subluxation in rheumatoid arthritis. A retrospective analysis of 16 operated patients after 1-5 years. Acta Orthop Scand 1997;68(2):109–115
31. Papadopoulos SM, Dickman CA, Sonntag VK. Atlantoaxial stabilization in rheumatoid arthritis. J Neurosurg 1991;74(1):1–7
32. Olerud C, Larsson BE, Rodriguez M. Subaxial cervical spine subluxation in rheumatoid arthritis. A retrospective analysis of 16 operated patients after 1–5 years. Acta Orthop Scand 1997;68(2):109–115
33. Wolfs JF, Kloppenburg M, Fehlings MG, van Tulder MW, Boers M, Peul WC. Neurologic outcome of surgical and conservative treatment of rheumatoid cervical spine subluxation: a systematic review. Arthritis Rheum 2009;61(12):1743–1752
34. Nguyen HV, Ludwig SC, Silber J, et al. Rheumatoid arthritis of the cervical spine. Spine J 2004;4(3):329–334
35. Casey AT, Crockard HA, Stevens J. Vertical translocation. Part II. Outcomes after surgical treatment of rheumatoid cervical myelopathy. J Neurosurg 1997;87(6):863–869
36. Mori K, Imai S, Omura K, Saruhashi Y, Matsusue Y, Hukuda S. Clinical output of the rheumatoid cervical spine in patients with mutilating-type joint involvement: for better activities of daily living and longer survival. Spine 2010;35(13):1279–1284

Suggested Readings

Boden SD, Dodge LD, Bohlman HH, Rechtine GR. Rheumatoid arthritis of the cervical spine. A long-term analysis with predictors of paralysis and recovery. J Bone Joint Surg Am 1993; 75(9):1282–1297

This article reported on the radiographic and clinical progression of 73 patients followed for over 7 years and found that 58% of patients developed paralysis. All paralyzed patients treated nonoperatively died within 4 years, while 71% of patients treated operatively improved at least one neurologic class.

Dreyer SJ, Boden SD. Natural history of rheumatoid arthritis of the cervical spine. Clin Orthop Relat Res 1999;(366):98–106

This article is an excellent review of the natural history of the cervical spine manifestations of rheumatoid arthritis. The authors focus on the risk of neurologic injury with disease progression and the role of prophylactic surgical stabilization.

Howe CR, Gardner GC, Kadel NJ. Perioperative medication management for the patient with rheumatoid arthritis. J Am Acad Orthop Surg 2006;14(9):544–551

With the recent major advances in the medical treatment of rheumatoid arthritis, this article provides a much-needed review of medical treatment options for rheumatoid arthritis. It outlines the risks and benefits associated with common medication regimens as well as guidelines for managing medications to optimize surgical outcomes.

Krauss WE, Bledsoe JM, Clarke MJ, Nottmeier EW, Pichelmann MA. Rheumatoid arthritis of the craniovertebral junction. Neurosurgery 2010;66(3, Suppl):83–95

> *This article provides a thorough review of the surgical management of rheumatoid arthritis of the cervical spine. The article outlines the surgical indications and the surgical techniques used in the treatment of basilar invagination, atlanto-axial instability, and SAS.*

Mori K, Imai S, Omura K, Saruhashi Y, Matsusue Y, Hukuda S. Clinical output of the rheumatoid cervical spine in patients with mutilating-type joint involvement: for better activities of daily living and longer survival. Spine 2010;35(13):1279–1284

> *This recent study found that in patients with severe mutilating-type seropositive RA, surgical stabilization was associated with longer life expectancy, improved neurologic function, and improved ability to perform activities of daily life.*

XI Osteoporosis

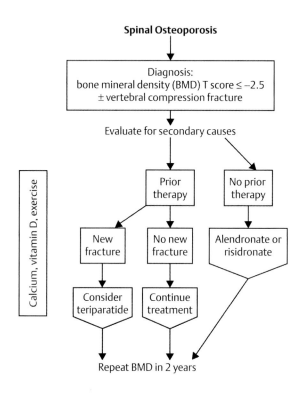

52

Medical Management of Spinal Osteoporosis

Daniel Mazanec and Tagreed M. Khalaf

Osteoporosis is a skeletal disorder characterized by compromised bone strength that predisposes to fractures. Bone mineral density (BMD) accounts for ~70% of the strength of a bone and is the strongest predictor of fragility fracture. BMD can be directly measured in the spine or hip using dual-energy X-ray absorptiometry (DEXA). The magnitude of BMD is quantified by a T score, which is defined as the number of standard deviations (SDs) above or below the mean BMD for a healthy, young white woman. Osteoporosis has been defined as a T score of less than –2.5, whereas osteopenia is defined as a T score of between –1.5 and –2.5.

The consequence of spinal osteoporosis is vertebral compression fractures (VCFs). Only one third of VCFs are acutely symptomatic. Long-term consequences of VCFs include kyphosis, mechanical back pain, gastrointestinal symptoms, and restrictive pulmonary disease. A 23% increase in age-adjusted mortality is seen in older women with a VCF.

 ## Workup

History

Spinal osteoporosis should be suspected in patients with nontraumatic vertebral body fractures. Multiple risk factors may contribute to osteoporosis (**Table 52.1**), but in up to one-third of women and 50% of men with osteoporosis, a secondary cause can be identified (**Table 52.2**). A detailed history, including risk factor assessment, and screening laboratory studies are appropriate in all patients (**Table 52.3**).

Table 52.1 Risk Factors for Osteoporosis

Female sex

Increased age

Estrogen deficiency

White race

Low weight and body mass index

Family history of osteoporosis

Cigarette smoking

History of prior fracture

Table 52.2 Secondary Causes of Osteoporosis

Endocrine: hyperthyroidism, hyperparathyroidism, hypogonadism, Cushing disease

Medication: glucocorticoids, heparin, excess thyroid hormone replacement, anticonvulsants, omeprazole

Nutritional: malabsorption, alcoholism, liver disease

Malignancy: multiple myeloma

Table 52.3 Laboratory Evaluation of Osteoporosis

Complete blood count

Serum calcium, phosphorus, alkaline phosphatase, creatinine

Serum albumin and total protein

24-hour urine calcium

Thyroid-stimulating hormone (if indicated by history)

Parathyroid hormone (if indicated by screening laboratory)

Serum free testosterone (men)

25-hydroxyvitamin D

Special Diagnostic Tests

In asymptomatic populations, BMD measurements have been recommended for all women over 65 and for women over 60 with risk factors for osteoporosis. Measurement of BMD in the spine most accurately reflects spinal bone mass. However, persons with significant lumbar spondylosis may have artificially elevated spinal BMD values with DEXA scanning, making hip BMD values more predictive of true bone mass in this patient population.

Treatment and Outcome

All persons meeting BMD criteria for osteoporosis, with or without fractures, should be treated. In addition, treatment is recommended for individuals with a T score less than –2.0 or less than –1.5 with risk factors. While bone mineral density is an excellent predictor of fracture risk, density combined with clinical risk factors for fracture is a better predictor than density or clinical risk factors alone. The World Health Organization Fracture Risk Assessment Tool, FRAX, is a clinical software tool developed to calculate fracture risk on the basis of bone mineral density of the femoral neck as well as multiple clinical risk factors, including patient's age, sex, height, weight, personal history of previous fracture, history of parental hip fracture, current smoking, history of long-term glucocorticoid use, rheumatoid arthritis, and daily alcohol consumption. The tool also incorporates the presence or absence of other secondary causes of osteoporosis. It estimates the 10 year probability of a major osteoporotic fracture. FRAX is available to clinicians online (www.shef.ac.uk/FRAX).

Ensuring adequate calcium and vitamin D intake is fundamental to osteoporosis therapy. Postmenopausal women not receiving estrogen should ingest 1500 mg of calcium daily from all sources. The optimal dose of vitamin D should be based on titration to normal serum 25-hydroxyvitamin D levels. Weight-bearing exercise such as walking should be encouraged. Back extensor strengthening exercises have been shown to decrease the risk of vertebral fracture as well as falls.

The antiresorptive bisphosphonates (diphosphonates) alendronate and risedronate are the first-choice agents for spinal osteoporosis, reducing vertebral fracture risk by ~50% in postmenopausal women with osteoporosis. Both drugs reduce risk of nonvertebral fractures to a similar extent. Another bisphosphonate, ibandronate, approved for the treatment of osteoporosis has also been shown to reduce the incidence of vertebral fracture by ~50%, but reduction in hip fracture risk remains unproven. An intravenous bisphosphonate, zolendronic acid, is administered once yearly and may be more effective than oral agents in vertebral fracture reduction (70% versus 50%). There is currently no consensus on how long to continue bisphosphonate therapy. However, stopping therapy after 5 years for some women may be reasonable, as there appears to be residual benefit on BMD and fractures for at least 5 years.

A newly available, novel antiresorptive agent, denosumab, is a human monoclonal antibody administered subcutaneously twice yearly for 36 months. Denosumab has been shown to decrease risk of vertebral, nonvertebral, and hip fractures in women with osteoporosis comparably to zolendronic acid. Unlike bisphosphonates, which interfere with osteoclast function, denosumab inhibits development of osteoclasts by inhibition of receptor activator of nuclear factor kappa-B ligand (RANKL).

The alternative antiresorptive agents raloxifene and calcitonin are probably less effective in bone preservation and fracture reduction. Raloxifene, acting as an estrogen receptor agonist in bone, reduces vertebral fracture risk by 30% to 50% but has not been shown to reduce nonvertebral fractures. Hormone replacement therapy with estrogen is no longer recommended as primary treatment for osteoporosis since the Women's Health Initiative Study, which found that the combination of estrogen plus progesterone reduces fracture risk but increases the risk of breast cancer and cardiovascular events. Limited data suggest that salmon calcitonin nasal spray may reduce vertebral fracture risk by one-third in women with osteoporosis, but reduction of nonvertebral fractures has not been demonstrated.

Teriparatide (human parathyroid hormone 1–34) is the only currently available anabolic agent for treatment of osteoporosis, increasing bone density by ~10% and reducing vertebral fracture risk by 70% and nonvertebral fracture risk by at least 50%. Teriparatide is administered daily by subcutaneous injection and is considerably more expensive than oral bisphosphonates. Indications for teriparatide are evolving, but the drug should be considered in patients who sustain fractures or continue to lose bone mass on antiresorptive therapy. Antiresorptive therapy should be discontinued when teriparatide therapy is initiated.

 Complications

Complications include intolerance to medications or rarely osteonecrosis of the jaw, mainly in cancer patients receiving high-dose intravenous bisphosphonates. Recent reports have suggested increased risk of atypical subtrochanteric femoral shaft fractures in women treated with bisphophonates, but retrospective secondary analyses of large randomized bisphophonate trials failed to substantiate an increased risk.

Suggested Readings

Black DM, Kelly MP, Genant HK, et al; Fracture Intervention Trial Steering Committee; HORIZON Pivotal Fracture Trial Steering Committee. Bisphosphonates and fractures of the subtrochanteric or diaphyseal femur. N Engl J Med 2010;362(19):1761–1771

> *A secondary analysis completed on three large randomized trials demonstrated no significant risk associated with bisphosphonate use and atypical femur fractures.*

Cummings SR, San Martin J, McClung MR, et al; FREEDOM Trial. Denosumab for prevention of fractures in postmenopausal women with osteoporosis. N Engl J Med 2009;361(8):756–765

> *A randomized controlled trial demonstrated reduction in the risk of vertebral, nonvertebral, and hip fractures in women with osteoporosis given denosumab subcutaneously twice yearly for 36 months.*

Kanis JA, Johnell O, Oden A, Johansson H, McCloskey E. FRAX and the assessment of fracture probability in men and women from the UK. Osteoporos Int 2008;19(4):385–397

> *This paper reviews the FRAX model and process of development.*

Kennel KA, Drake MT, Hurley DL. Vitamin D deficiency in adults: when to test and how to treat. Mayo Clin Proc 2010;85(8):752–757, quiz 757–758

> *This general review article provides an overview on vitamin D deficiency and supplementation.*

National Osteoporosis Foundation. Clinician's Guideline to Prevention and Treatment of Osteoporosis. Washington, DC: National Osteoporosis Foundation; 2008

This is an overview on osteoporosis treatment.

Nelson HD, Haney EM, Dana T, Bougatsos C, Chou R. Screening for osteoporosis: an update for the U.S. Preventive Services Task Force. Ann Intern Med 2010;153(2):99–111

This article gives current recommendations for osteoporosis screening.

Osteopenic Patient Requiring Surgery

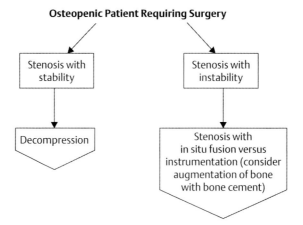

53

Surgical Treatment of the Osteopenic Patient

Safdar N. Khan and Frank M. Phillips

Within the next decade, spine surgeons will encounter an increasing number of patients with osteopenia/osteoporosis requiring surgical intervention for spinal disorders as the longevity of the general population increases. The patient with osteoporosis poses a considerable challenge for spine surgeons, with issues including frequent preoperative medical comorbidities and suboptimal nutrition to intraoperative and postoperative concerns regarding poor bone quality leading to hardware cutout and failure. Similarly, postoperative adherence to rigorous physical therapy protocols is unlikely in this patient population.

 ## Surgical Indications

As in a younger cohort of surgical spine patients, indications for surgery in the elderly continue to be neurogenic claudication, radiculopathy, myelopathy, mechanical back pain, progressive spinal deformity with or without vertebral fractures, or any combination of these findings. That said, a serious discussion with the patient and caregiver must be undertaken when a reasonable course of nonoperative care is feasible prior to surgical intervention in this high-risk population.

 ## Treatment

Once nonoperative management has been exhausted and the patient has been medically cleared for the physiologic challenge of spine surgery, direct decompression of the involved neural elements remains the mainstay of treatment for spinal stenosis that gives rise to claudication and/or myeloradiculopathy. When diffuse multilevel spinal degenerative changes are present, it is helpful if the symptoms can be isolated to a particular spinal level or nerve root, thus allowing for a limited decompressive procedure and obviating the need for large, multilevel procedures. If indicated, a concomitant arthrodesis may be considered in the presence of deformity or preexisting instability or when surgical decompression creates instability as a result of excessive bony resection, as in a complete facetectomy or pars resection. Limited in situ fusion for instability or deformity may be effective without instrumentation when the risk of progressive deformity is minimal.

Often, segmental instrumentation is necessary to correct deformity and to stabilize the destabilized spine. Such a construct must be able to withstand the three-dimensional forces across the area of fixation until fusion is complete. Pedicle screw instrumentation enables segmental control of all three columns of the spine from a posterior approach alone. The implant–bone interface remains the weak link in the instrumentation construct in the osteoporotic spine. The majority of instrumentation failures involve screw loosening and pullout, which may lead to failure of fusion or the development of recurrent or de novo deformity. Inserting larger-diameter pedicle screws and undertapping may enhance screw stability. Triangulating the screws in the axial plane to increase posterior pullout strength and diverging the screws in the sagittal plane to increase axial load-bearing capacity are important. Increasing screw length and diameter does increase screw pullout strength, although this effect may be less pronounced in osteoporotic bone. Precoating pedicle screws with hydroxyapatite has been shown to reduce the incidence of screw cutout significantly in preclinical and clinical series. At the sacrum, medially directed, triangulated bicortical purchase aiming toward the promontory may protect against distal construct failure. In certain instances, purchase within the ilium may be necessary, especially in long fusion constructs for deformity. Another strategy to improve construct rigidity in osteoporotic bone is to increase the number of levels instrumented. This approach must be weighed against the morbidity of the additional level surgery as well as the potential for junctional breakdown in the future.

Several studies have indicated that the bone–screw interface may be improved by injecting bone cement (polymethylmethacrylate, PMMA) into the pedicle at the time of screw insertion. A two- to threefold increase in screw pullout resistance has been demonstrated with the use of bone cement injected into the vertebral body through a specially designed fenestrated-cannulated pedicle. Bioactive cements such as calcium phosphate and carbonated apatite have also been shown to contribute to the screw–bone interface and increase pedicle screw pullout strength. The surgeon may also augment the pedicle screw construct with offset sublaminar hooks or wires that are well suited for use in the osteoporotic spine by relying on the relatively spared cortical laminar bone for fixation.

Another approach in reconstruction for the patient with osteopenic deformity is to utilize both the anterior and posterior column for support at a given level. Anterior devices may function to share load that would otherwise be concentrated on posterior pedicle screw or hook constructs. In general, anteriorly placed metallic interbody devices have a modulus mismatch with bone and tend to subside in osteopenic bone. Since the cortical rim is the strongest part of the vertebral body in axial loading, the graft or implant should have a wide footprint and engage as much of the rim circumference as possible. The potential benefit to use of interbody load-sharing devices must be carefully weighed against increased surgical time, risk, and morbidity associated with their use. Consideration may be given to staging such patients for an anterior release/ reconstruction prior to tackling the posterior fusion construct.

Segmental deformity correction with the use of posterior-based osteotomies may correct sagittal balance and indirectly minimize the stresses borne by instrumentation. Modest correction can be obtained using the Smith-Petersen osteotomy, and a greater correction can be obtained with the pedicle subtraction osteotomy. Accepting a lesser degree of deformity correction when full spinal balance cannot be achieved is an alternative to avoid implant overload and subsequent instrumentation failure. Such procedures severely stress the physiologic baseline of these patients and must be approached with caution.

Outcomes

Outcomes in these patients can be optimized with a careful, well-thought-out surgical plan with appropriate decompression and judicious use of fusion with or without instrumentation to achieve the goals of surgery, including pain relief, improved physical function, and restoration of spinal alignment. Perioperative complications have been shown to occur with significantly greater frequency in patients older than 60, prolonging the postoperative recovery time to 6 months or longer in this population.

Complications

Intraoperative and early postoperative surgical complications include neurologic injury, durotomy, infection, wound breakdown, and failure of fixation. Coexistent medical comorbidities, leading to prolonged intubation and intensive care unit (ICU) stay, are not uncommon in these patients. Complications for which patients with osteoporosis are specifically at risk include instrumentation failure, progression of deformity, and adjacent-level compression fracture. These complications are best avoided by meticulous surgical planning and an understanding of the capabilities of the instrumentation as well as of the biomechanical environment across which the instrumentation is applied.

Suggested Readings

Albert TJ, Purtill J, Mesa J, McIntosh T, Balderston RA. Health outcome assessment before and after adult deformity surgery. A prospective study. Spine 1995;20(18):2002–2004, discussion 2005

   This excellent article details health outcome analysis before and after adult deformity surgery.

Bridwell KH. Spine osteotomy and resection. In: DeWald RL, ed. Spinal Deformities: The Comprehensive Text. New York, NY: Thieme; 2003:551–561

This chapter discusses the indications and techniques of kyphotic deformity correction using the pedicle subtraction and Smith-Petersen osteotomies. It also considers the complications and results of these osteotomies.

Cho W, Cho SK, Wu C. The biomechanics of pedicle screw-based instrumentation. J Bone Joint Surg Br 2010;92(8):1061–1065

This excellent recent review focuses on the biomechanics of pedicle screw instrumentation and cross-connectors in challenging clinical scenarios.

Chao EY, Inoue N, Koo TK, Kim YH. Biomechanical considerations of fracture treatment and bone quality maintenance in elderly patients and patients with osteoporosis. Clin Orthop Relat Res 2004;(425):12–25

An excellent overview of nonsurgical management of osteoporosis and the biomechanics of fixation in the osteoporotic spine.

Andersson GBJ, Weinstein JN. Focus issue on osteoporosis. Spine 1997;22(24 Supplement)

This issue presents an excellent compendium of articles on the medical management of osteoporosis and provides a framework for surgical management of the osteoporotic spine.

Hu SS. Internal fixation in the osteoporotic spine. Spine 1997;22(24, Suppl):43S–48S

This article provides a thorough discussion of biomechanical and patient factors to be considered along with surgical techniques and principles to improve fixation in the osteoporotic spine, including bailout and revision strategies.

Manson NA, Phillips FM. Minimally invasive techniques for the treatment of osteoporotic vertebral fractures. J Bone Joint Surg Am 2006;88(8):1862–1872

Review of the current minimally invasive modalities for the treatment of osteoporotic vertebral compression fractures.

Vertebral Compression Fracture (Wedge or Biconcave Configuration)

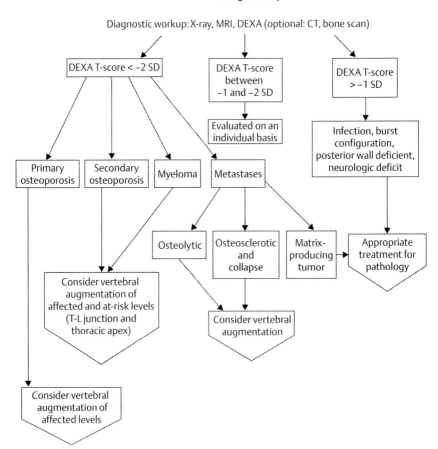

Diagnostic workup: X-ray, MRI, DEXA (optional: CT, bone scan)

CT, computed tomography; DEXA, dual-energy X-ray absorptiometry; MRI, magnetic resonance imaging; SD, standard deviation; T-L, thoracocolumbar

54

Vertebroplasty and Kyphoplasty

D. Greg Anderson

There are over 700,000 osteoporotic vertebral compression fractures (VCFs) each year in the United States, making this a major health concern. Although many patients respond to bracing, there is a subpopulation of those with VCFs who are not adequately treated with nonoperative care and for whom traditional open surgery is overly invasive. These patients may be helped by a percutaneous vertebral augmentation procedure. These procedures are able to achieve rapid pain relief in most patients, with a relatively low overall complication rate. Both vertebroplasty and kyphoplasty involve the injection of polymethylmethacrylate (PMMA) into the compressed vertebral body. In contrast to vertebroplasty, kyphoplasty first utilizes an inflatable bone tamp to make a space for the cement, and in some cases, it can help to restore vertebral body height (**Fig. 54.1**).

Classification

Vertebroplasty and kyphoplasty are both indicated for the treatment of patients with VCFs who are experiencing severe, unmanageable pain or progressive deformity. These procedures have also been shown to have a role in the management of certain painful, osteolytic VCFs. Contraindications include any systemic pathology, such as sepsis or an anticoagulated state. Relative contraindications include non-osteolytic infiltrative spinal metastases, vertebral bodies with deficient posterior cortices (burst fractures), or patients presenting with a neurologic deficit.

Workup

History

The onset, duration, location, and character of the patient's pain/injury should be clearly understood. Pain related to other spinal issues, such as spondylolisthe-

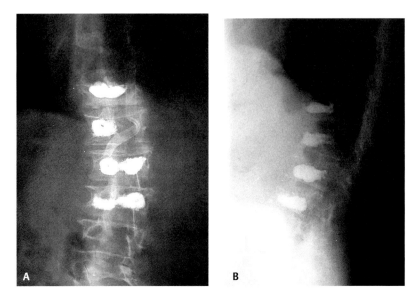

Fig. 54.1 Plain radiographs demonstrating vertebral compression fractures after correction with kyphoplasty. **(A)** Anteroposterior. **(B)** Lateral.

sis, will not benefit from cement augmentation, and an attempt should be made to exclude patients with other painful processes. It is also important for the physician to ensure that the underlying osteoporosis is diagnosed and treated.

Physical Examination

In addition to a complete neurologic exam, the spine should be palpated or percussed over the fracture site to confirm direct tenderness. Symptoms may be shown to increase with upright positioning (as opposed to recumbency) or worsen with gentle range of motion.

Spinal Imaging

Radiographs and magnetic resonance imaging (MRI) are generally used to diagnose the fracture. The MRI can help to determine the acuity of the fracture by showing edema at the fracture site. The MRI should be carefully studied to rule out any findings of metastatic disease or burst component to the fracture. In cases where the diagnosis or fracture pattern is unclear, nuclear bone scans or computed tomography (CT) scans can be useful.

Special Diagnostic Tests

Bone densitometry (dual-energy X-ray absorptiometry [DEXA]) is used to assess the degree of osteoporosis. A T-score of –2.5 or lower is diagnostic of osteoporosis, which should be treated in addition to the fracture. In cases that suggest tumors or metabolic bone diseases, serum markers for these conditions can be ordered.

Treatment

Patients deemed to be appropriate candidates for vertebral augmentation can be treated under either local anesthesia with sedation or general anesthesia. Under sterile conditions, Jamshidi needles are introduced into the vertebral body using either a transpedicular or extrapedicular approach. Biplanar fluoroscopy is used throughout the procedure to document the accuracy of needle and cement placement. With vertebroplasty, the PMMA is generally injected in a less viscous form under live fluoroscopy. With kyphoplasty, an inflatable bone tamp is utilized to create a void in the vertebral body and the PMMA is introduced in a more viscous form under live fluoroscopy. After curing, the needles are withdrawn and the wounds are dressed.

Outcome

Pain reduction is expected in 70% to 90% of patients. Additionally, physical function scores have been shown to increase in responsive patients. Although there have been no reports of cement failure, refracture or adjacent-level fracture remains a problem for some patients.

Complications

The most frequently reported complication with vertebral augmentation is cement extravasation. PMMA can leak through the fracture clefts or be introduced into the draining vertebral venous plexus. In most cases, there are no clinical consequences of minor cement extravasation, but there have been case reports of either death (related to cement pulmonary emboli) or paralysis (related to cement extravasation into the spinal canal). Some studies suggest that cement extravasation is less likely with kyphoplasty, because of the void creation and increased viscosity at the time of cement introduction. Infection and bleeding are rarely a problem with cement augmentation procedures.

Suggested Readings

Barr JD, Barr MS, Lemley TJ, McCann RM. Percutaneous vertebroplasty for pain relief and spinal stabilization. Spine 2000;25(8):923–928

> *A retrospective review of 47 patients treated by vertebroplasty found pain relief in a high percentage of patients with osteoporotic fractures. Only 50% of patients with osteolytic metastases had improvment.*

Spinal Imaging

Plain radiographs and an advanced imaging study, either magnetic resonance imaging (MRI) or computed tomography (CT) myelography, should be evaluated for findings of neural element compression. On plain films, it is important to ensure that the patient has no findings of kyphosis, which would contraindicate the foraminotomy approach. The advanced imaging study should show compression of the exiting nerve root that correlates to the pain on history and physical examination. It is important that the compression be in the region of the lateral spinal canal and foramen and not in the central canal. Patients with significant compression in the central spinal canal should be managed by an alternative means. Also, a patient with findings requiring surgery at more than two levels should also be managed by an alternative approach.

Treatment

The initial management for cervical radiculopathy should be nonsurgical and may include rest, nonsteroidal anti-inflammatory drugs (NSAIDs), physical therapy, traction, and spinal injections. In cases that are recalcitrant to this approach for at least 6 weeks, surgical intervention may be considered. For those with lateral compression and no evidence of deformity, an anterior foraminotomy may be considered.

The approach to the cervical spine is achieved in similar fashion to the standard Smith-Robinson approach. After radiographic confirmation that the correct level has been exposed, the longus colli muscle is dissected and retracted laterally to expose the lateral portion of the disk in the region of the uncovertebral joint. A small retractor is placed between the uncovertebral joint and the vertebral artery and is used to protect the vertebral artery during the procedure. Next, using microscopic magnification, the uncovertebral joint is drilled away until the nerve root is identified and decompressed. Soft disk material can be swept away from the nerve root with a small nerve hook. The nerve hook can also be used to confirm the adequacy of the decompression. Closure of the wound is similar to that in other anterior cervical procedures.

Outcome

For properly selected patients, the anterior foraminotomy should yield good or excellent outcomes in 85% to 98% of patients. This procedure is more technical than the traditional discectomy and fusion approach and should be learned in an appropriate setting.

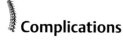 **Complications**

It is important to protect the vertebral artery during this procedure, and injury may ensue if the artery is not well protected. Excessive drilling of the segment may lead to segmental instability with recurrent pain symptoms, requiring a spinal fusion. All other complications inherent to the anterior approach, such as swallowing problems and vocal cord paralysis, are also possible with the anterior foraminotomy approach.

Suggested Readings

Jho HD, Kim WK, Kim MH. Cervical microforaminotomy for spondylitic cervical myelopathy. Neurosurgery 2002;51(5):S2-54–59

> *This article describes the technique for anterior microforaminotomy.*

Narayan P, Haid RW. Treatment of degenerative cervical disc disease. Neurol Clin 2001;19(1): 217–229

> *This article details the evaluation process and decision-making for patients with cervical disk disease.*

Thongtrangan I, Le H, Park J, Kim DH. Minimally invasive spinal surgery: a historical perspective. Neurosurg Focus 2004;16(1):E13

> *This article reviews the development of minimally invasive surgical techniques.*

Anterior Thoracic Spinal Pathology

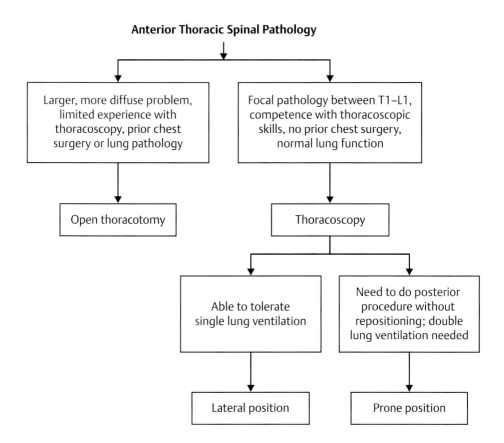

57

Thoracoscopy

Dominick A. Tuason and Daniel J. Sucato

Thoracoscopy is the endoscopic technique of gaining access to the intrathoracic cavity using small (~1–2 cm) incisions to enable surgical procedures on structures within the chest. Although thoracoscopy was first utilized in the treatment of lung conditions, applications for treatment of the spine have become common and effective.[1] Visualization of the structures within the chest is accomplished using a fiberoptic camera. This thoracoscope is usually 10 mm in diameter, has a 30- or 45-degree angled lens, and is long enough to reach significant depths within the chest, thus providing the surgeon the ability to look around corners and allowing improved visualization as compared with open techniques. The remaining working portals allow for long rongeurs, electrocautery, curettes, osteotomes, suction devices, and suturing instruments to be placed into the chest (**Fig. 57.1**). These instruments allow the surgeon to perform many types of surgical procedures for anterior thoracic spinal pathology. The goal of the thoracoscopic approach is to provide excellent visualization and the ability to duplicate the safety and efficacy of performing anterior thoracic surgery achieved through an open thoracotomy approach.[2,3]

Indications and Contraindications for Thoracoscopy

The indications for thoracoscopy in the treatment of spinal conditions are essentially the same as those for an open thoracotomy approach. Candidates for thoracoscopy include patients with severe spine deformity requiring anterior release, skeletally immature patients requiring anterior fusion to avoid the crankshaft phenomenon, and patients requiring anterior instrumentation and fusion (**Fig. 57.2A–D** and **Fig. 57.3A–D**).[4] Thoracoscopy can be used in the setting of spinal infection or vertebral column or spinal cord tumors to obtain cultures/biopsy or for débridement/resection and placement of anterior structural support. Often these anterior surgeries can be supplemented with a posterior approach.[5-7] Thoracoscopy can also be used to treat herniated thoracic disks

437

ter decompression of the canal. Anterior instrumentation, such as plates and cages, can be placed with possibly less radiation exposure than with posterior pedicle screw fixation. Newer reduction plates are available that offer the capability of applying lordotic forces through swivel heads at both ends of the plate. After the plate is fixed to the bridging vertebral bodies, the angulation of the cranial and caudal swivel heads can be changed to provide the appropriate amount of lordosis.[14] Finally, thoracoscopic-assisted stabilization of burst fractures may be associated with less postoperative pain and improved restoration of spinal alignment.[15,16]

References

1. Han PP, Kenny K, Dickman CA. Thoracoscopic approaches to the thoracic spine: experience with 241 surgical procedures. Neurosurgery 2002;51(5, Suppl):S88–S95
2. Huntington CF, Murrell WD, Betz RR, Cole BA, Clements DH III, Balsara RK. Comparison of thoracoscopic and open thoracic discectomy in a live ovine model for anterior spinal fusion. Spine 1998;23(15):1699–1702
3. Wall EJ, Bylski-Austrow DI, Shelton FS, Crawford AH, Kolata RJ, Baum DS. Endoscopic discectomy increases thoracic spine flexibility as effectively as open discectomy. A mechanical study in a porcine model. Spine 1998;23(1):9–15, discussion 15–16
4. Reddi V, Clarke DV Jr, Arlet V. Anterior thoracoscopic instrumentation in adolescent idiopathic scoliosis: a systematic review. Spine 2008;33(18):1986–1994
5. Mazel Ch, Grunenwald D, Laudrin P, Marmorat JL. Radical excision in the management of thoracic and cervicothoracic tumors involving the spine: results in a series of 36 cases. Spine 2003;28(8):782–792, discussion 792
6. Kan P, Schmidt MH. Minimally invasive thoracoscopic approach for anterior decompression and stabilization of metastatic spine disease. Neurosurg Focus 2008;25(2):E8
7. Mückley T, Schütz T, Schmidt MH, Potulski M, Bühren V, Beisse R. The role of thoracoscopic spinal surgery in the management of pyogenic vertebral osteomyelitis. Spine 2004;29(11):E227–E233
8. Burke TG, Caputy AJ. Treatment of thoracic disc herniation: evolution toward the minimally invasive thoracoscopic technique. Neurosurg Focus 2000;9(4):e9
9. Sucato DJ, Newton PO, Betz R, et al. Defining the learning curve for performing a thoracoscopic anterior spinal fusion and instrumentation for AIS: A multi-center study. 39th Annual Meeting of the Scoliosis Research Society. Buenos Aires, Argentina, 2004
10. Sucato DJ, Erken YH, Davis S, Gist T, McClung A, Rathjen KE. Prone thoracoscopic release does not adversely affect pulmonary function when added to a posterior spinal fusion for severe spine deformity. Spine 2009;34(8):771–778
11. Sucato DJ, Elerson E. A comparison between the prone and lateral position for performing a thoracoscopic anterior release and fusion for pediatric spinal deformity. Spine 2003;28(18):2176–2180
12. Patel AA, Vaccaro AR. Thoracolumbar spine trauma classification. J Am Acad Orthop Surg 2010;18(2):63–71
13. Kocis J, Wendsche P, Muzík V, Bilik A, Veselý R, Cernohousová I. [Minimally invasive thoracoscopic transdiaphragmatic approach to thoracolumbar junction fractures]. Acta Chir Orthop Traumatol Cech 2009;76(3):232–238
14. Schnake KJ, Scholz M, Marx A, Hoffmann R, Kandziora F. Anterior, thoracoscopic-assisted reduction and stabilization of a thoracic burst fracture (T8) in a pregnant woman. Eur Spine J 2011;20(8):1217–1221
15. Khoo LT, Beisse R, Potulski M. Thoracoscopic-assisted treatment of thoracic and lumbar fractures: a series of 371 consecutive cases. Neurosurgery 2002;51(5, Suppl):S104–S117
16. Ringel F, Stoffel M, Stüer C, Totzek S, Meyer B. Endoscopy-assisted approaches for anterior column reconstruction after pedicle screw fixation of acute traumatic thoracic and lumbar fractures. Neurosurgery 2008;62(5, Suppl 2):ONS445–ONS452, discussion ONS452–ONS453

Suggested Readings

Burke TG, Caputy AJ. Treatment of thoracic disc herniation: evolution toward the minimally invasive thoracoscopic technique. Neurosurg Focus 2000;9(4):e9

> *Detailed technique of thoracoscopic discectomy is presented along with the historical progression of treatment methods for thoracic disk herniation.*

Han PP, Kenny K, Dickman CA. Thoracoscopic approaches to the thoracic spine: experience with 241 surgical procedures. Neurosurgery 2002;51(5, Suppl):S88–S95

> *This article reports on 241 thoracoscopic procedures. Over all, there was excellent outcome in these patients, and the authors conclude that thoracoscopic techniques can be very effective for many conditions and the complications of an open thoracotomy are avoided.*

Huntington CF, Murrell WD, Betz RR, Cole BA, Clements DH III, Balsara RK. Comparison of thoracoscopic and open thoracic discectomy in a live ovine model for anterior spinal fusion. Spine 1998;23(15):1699–1702

> *This animal study compared the open and thoracoscopic anterior thoracic release, demonstrating similar disk removal (76% open vs 68% thoracoscopic), which was not statistically significant. When the disk areas were analyzed with respect to the number in which greater than 50% of the disk was removed, there were 29 of 30 (97%) in the open group, 27 of 30 (90%) in the thoracoscopic approach.*

Kan P, Schmidt MH. Minimally invasive thoracoscopic approach for anterior decompression and stabilization of metastatic spine disease. Neurosurg Focus 2008;25(2):E8

> *A small series of five patients treated with thoracoscopic approach for treatment of thoracic and thoracolumbar metastatic spinal cord compression demonstrated improvement in preoperative symptoms and neurologic deficit and no reported complications.*

Khoo LT, Beisse R, Potulski M. Thoracoscopic-assisted treatment of thoracic and lumbar fractures: a series of 371 consecutive cases. Neurosurgery 2002;51(5, Suppl):S104–S117

> *This article presents a retrospective review of 371 patients who had a thoracic or thoracolumbar fracture treated with thoracoscopic techniques for fixation of the spine. Anterior surgery alone was done in 35%, with the rest supplemented with posterior surgery. Operative time was long in the early cases but improved with surgeon experience. Complications included one aortic injury, one splenic contusion, one neurologic deterioration, one cerebrospinal fluid (CSF) leak, and one wound infection. A comparison to patients who had treatment with an open technique demonstrated less use of narcotics postoperatively.*

Kocis J, Wendsche P, Muzík V, Bilik A, Veselý R, Cernohousová I. [Minimally invasive thoracoscopic transdiaphragmatic approach to thoracolumbar junction fractures]. Acta Chir Orthop Traumatol Cech 2009;76(3):232–238

> *This is a retrospective study of 127 patients with thoracolumbar junction fractures treated with reconstruction of the anterior spinal column via a thoracoscopic procedure with minithoracotomy. Bony fusion occurred within a year of surgery, with average loss of correction of 2 degrees. Improvement of neurologic status by at least one Frankel grade occurred in 10 of the 19 patients with neurologic deficit.*

Mazel Ch, Grunenwald D, Laudrin P, Marmorat JL. Radical excision in the management of thoracic and cervicothoracic tumors involving the spine: results in a series of 36 cases. Spine 2003;28(8):782–792, discussion 792

> *The authors describe a combined posterior and thoracoscopic anterior approach to remove tumors en bloc for the small and medium-size thoracic tumors. Thirty-six cases were reported that had the combined technique, with complete vertebrectomy in 7 cases and partial in 29 cases. The authors describe the learning curve but state that selective preoperative screening of patients is essential.*

Mückley T, Schütz T, Schmidt MH, Potulski M, Bühren V, Beisse R. The role of thoracoscopic spinal surgery in the management of pyogenic vertebral osteomyelitis. Spine 2004;29(11): E227–E233

> Three patients who had endoscopic treatment of vertebral osteomyelitis without conversion to an open procedure or posterior procedure. The surgery included radical débridement with anterior reconstruction with good results.

Newton PO, Upasani VV, Lhamby J, Ugrinow VL, Pawelek JB, Bastrom TP. Surgical treatment of main thoracic scoliosis with thoracoscopic anterior instrumentation. Surgical technique. J Bone Joint Surg Am 2009;91(Suppl 2):233–248

> This article provides a review of surgical technique and examines 5-year results of 25 patients treated at one center with anterior thoracoscopic spinal instrumentation for thoracic scoliosis. Five-year results show that outcomes are comparable with those reported for open anterior and posterior techniques in terms of percent correction of Cobb angle, average total Scoliosis Research Society (SRS) scores, and average total lung capacity as a percent of predicted value. However, there was hardware failure and need for surgical revision in 12% of the patients in this report.

Patel AA, Vaccaro AR. Thoracolumbar spine trauma classification. J Am Acad Orthop Surg 2010; 18(2):63–71

> This review article discusses the TLICS, which was developed to address the inadequacies of previous classification systems in terms of prognostic information and guiding surgical management. This scoring system defines injury based on three clinical characteristics: injury morphology, integrity of the posterior ligamentous complex, and neurologic status of the patient. The severity score offers prognostic information and is helpful in medical decision making.

Reddi V, Clarke DV Jr, Arlet V. Anterior thoracoscopic instrumentation in adolescent idiopathic scoliosis: a systematic review. Spine 2008;33(18):1986–1994

> This review of patients with adolescent idiopathic scoliosis treated with anterior thoracoscopic instrumentation compared with open anterior and posterior procedures was based on eight included articles from multiple literature search databases. It concluded that curve correction was similar between techniques, and two studies showed increased patient satisfaction with thoracoscopy, but there was slightly greater operative and ICU time compared to open procedures.

Ringel F, Stoffel M, Stüer C, Totzek S, Meyer B. Endoscopy-assisted approaches for anterior column reconstruction after pedicle screw fixation of acute traumatic thoracic and lumbar fractures. Neurosurgery 2008;62(5, Suppl 2):ONS445–ONS452, discussion ONS452–ONS453

> This is a prospective study of 83 patients with 100 acute thoracic or lumbar vertebral fractures treated with posterior pedicle screw instrumentation followed by thoracoscopic or endoscopic anterior approach for anterior column reconstruction. Conversion to an open approach was needed in five cases. Complications included: need for repositioning of ventral graft, L1 nerve root injury, posterior wound infection, pleural empyema in one case each, and two cases of transient neurologic worsening.

Schnake KJ, Scholz M, Marx A, Hoffmann R, Kandziora F. Anterior, thoracoscopic-assisted reduction and stabilization of a thoracic burst fracture (T8) in a pregnant woman. Eur Spine J 2011;20(8):1217–1221

> This is a case report of a pregnant 24-year-old woman whose burst fracture was treated using an anterior thoracoscopic-assisted reduction and stabilization. The body of T8 was removed and a titanium plate was placed from T7 to T9 to stabilize the fracture. Correction of kyphosis was achieved with distraction through the plate. Tricortical iliac bone graft was then press-fitted into the defect.

Sucato DJ. Thoracoscopic anterior instrumentation and fusion for idiopathic scoliosis. J Am Acad Orthop Surg 2003;11(4):221–227

> *This review article discusses thoracoscopically assisted surgery along with indications for this procedure, anesthesia considerations, surgical technique (including instrumentation and correction maneuvers), early results, and complications associated with this technique. It highlights the advantages of improved cosmesis and limitation of chest wall compromise compared to open anterior procedures, and preservation of motion segments compared to posterior surgery. In addition, the article emphasizes that great attention must be paid to proper patient selection, anesthesia considerations, and potential complications.*

Sucato DJ, Newton PO, Betz R, et al. Defining the learning curve for performing a thoracoscopic anterior spinal fusion and instrumentation for AIS: A multi-center study. 39th Annual Meeting of the Scoliosis Research Society. Buenos Aires, Argentina, 2004

> *This retrospective study from 9 institutions evaluated 147 patients, demonstrating a significant improvement in the surgical time and the incidence of complications. A probability analysis demonstrated that surgeons will have a 95% chance of no complications once they have done 35 thoracoscopic anterior instrumentations and fusions.*

Sucato DJ, Erken YH, Davis S, Gist T, McClung A, Rathjen KE. Prone thoracoscopic release does not adversely affect pulmonary function when added to a posterior spinal fusion for severe spine deformity. Spine 2009;34(8):771–778

> *This prospective clinical study compared patients who had prone thoracoscopic release with double lung ventilation followed by posterior spinal fusion and instrumentation (PSFI) to patients who had only PSFI for severe idiopathic scoliosis. Excellent coronal correction was achieved without detrimental effect on pulmonary function. Thoracoplasty had a negative effect on pulmonary function.*

Sucato DJ, Elerson E. A comparison between the prone and lateral position for performing a thoracoscopic anterior release and fusion for pediatric spinal deformity. Spine 2003;28(18): 2176–2180

> *This retrospective study demonstrated that patients who had a thoracoscopic release followed by a PSFI in the prone position had similar postoperative curve corrections as those who had the anterior release performed in the lateral position. However, because of the same position for the anterior and posterior surgeries with a regular endotracheal tube, the surgical times were less, patients had less postoperative respiratory difficulties, and the need for postoperative oxygen was less.*

Wall EJ, Bylski-Austrow DI, Shelton FS, Crawford AH, Kolata RJ, Baum DS. Endoscopic discectomy increases thoracic spine flexibility as effectively as open discectomy. A mechanical study in a porcine model. Spine 1998;23(1):9–15, discussion 15–16

> *This animal model studied the flexibility of the thoracic spine following anterior thoracic discectomy comparing the open and thoracoscopic techniques. There was no difference in the flexibility of the spines when the two techniques were compared.*

Degenerative Disk Disease

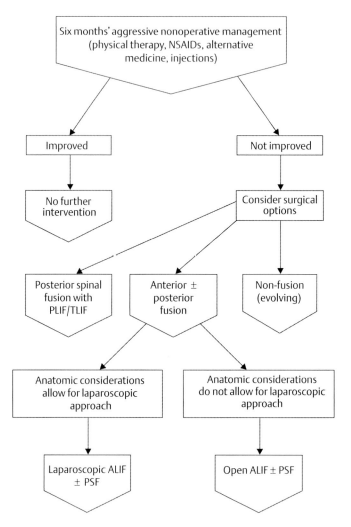

NSAIDs, nonsteroidal anti-inflammatory drugs; PLIF, posterior lumbar interbody fusion; PSF, posterior spinal fusion; TLIF, transforaminal lumbar interbody fusion

58

Lumbar Laparoscopy

Haim D. Blecher

Anterior lumbar interbody fusion (ALIF) has traditionally been a technique widely utilized by spine surgeons for the treatment of many disorders. Given the ability to visualize the anterior lumbar spine directly, ALIF has been used to treat spondylolisthesis, degenerative disk disease (DDD), spinal deformities, spinal infections, trauma, and tumors. When used to treat DDD, ALIF may be performed as a stand-alone procedure or in combination with a posterior surgery. Traditionally, open retroperitoneal approaches have been the mainstay of treatment. Limited-access approaches have been developed over the years, including laparoscopic techniques. Over the past decade, laparoscopic approaches for DDD have lost popularity to other techniques that may accomplish similar goals. With the increased use of transforaminal lumbar interbody fusion (TLIF) and a variety of direct lateral techniques, laparoscopic techniques are not commonly used today for the treatment of DDD.

Classification

There are no current classifications that direct toward a specific ALIF or interbody technique for DDD. Generally, ALIF may be performed as a stand-alone procedure or in combination with posterior fusion and instrumentation. ALIF can be performed through an open, mini-open, or laparoscopic approach.

Workup

History

ALIF, regardless of the technique, should be considered for DDD only when the patient has been carefully selected. Surgical candidates for lumbar fusion should have an anatomically identifiable pain generator that corresponds to

447

their symptoms and have failed at least 6 months of extensive nonoperative treatment for their condition. As it pertains to laparoscopy, the patient's previous peritoneal or retroperitoneal surgical history is of utmost importance when considering an anterior approach.

Physical Examination

Laparoscopic approach or not, the patient's physical examination should be consistent with the location and nature of symptoms. There are many non-specific sources of back pain that are not amenable to spinal surgery and that should be kept closely in mind.

DDD may cause primarily axial lumbar pain but may also be associated with nerve root compression; a detailed neurologic examination is critical.

Imaging Studies

When treating DDD surgically, all imaging studies should point to the same level or levels as the source of the pain. Imaging studies such as plain radiographs, magnetic resonance imaging (MRI) and computed tomography (CT) scans are often utilized. Lumbar diskography has been a controversial test that has been traditionally used as a confirmatory test as to the pain generator. With some studies suggesting the potential for accelerated deterioration of lumbar disks and the potential decreased usefulness of this test, diskography should be used sparingly and after patient counseling.

 Treatment

Nonoperative Treatment

Exhausting nonoperative treatment is imperative when considering surgical candidates for DDD. Extensive physical therapy, activity modification, weight control, smoking cessation, nonsteroidal anti-inflammatory drugs (NSAIDs) and possible interventional pain management modalities should all be considered. Patient selection has a significant effect on outcomes, often regardless of specific technique used.

Surgical Technique

Laparoscopic ALIF is performed with the patient supine on a radiolucent operating table to allow fluoroscopic visualization of the spine during the procedure. An endoscopic transperitoneal approach uses several portals for the endoscope and insufflators, and two or more working portals to allow for dissection, retraction, and discectomy (**Fig. 58.1**).

Lumbar laparoscopy requires an absolute understanding of the vascular anatomy around the disk. A cross-sectional review of the MRI and/or CT should be done preoperatively to make sure there are normal anatomic landmarks. A

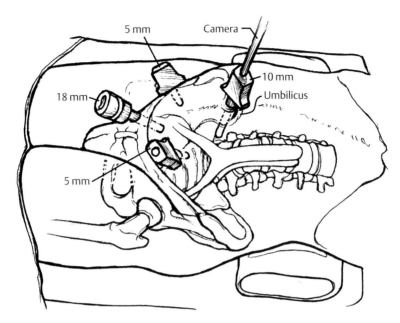

Fig. 58.1   An endoscopic transperitoneal approach is demonstrated using a portal for the endoscope, one for the insufflators, and two working portals to allow for dissection, retraction, and discectomy.

high-riding L5–S1 level may behave like an L4–L5 level in terms of dissection and make the approach more challenging. Approaching L4–L5 laparoscopically is challenging and should generally be performed only by experienced laparoscopic spinal surgeons. Vascular dissection at L4–L5 with mobilization of the common iliac vein and the iliolumbar branch requires extensive experience using the laparoscopic techniques (**Fig. 58.2**).

After the disk is exposed safely, laparoscopic instruments are used to accomplish the traditional goals of ALIF. Using laparoscopic curettes, rongeurs, and elevators, a complete discectomy and fusion preparation are required. After the discectomy and preparation are completed, the interbody fusion cage or graft is inserted, keeping in mind traditional goals of distraction and preservation of endplate integrity. Specific implant or graft selection varies and should be consistent with open ALIF (i.e., similar implant, graft choice, or bone graft substitute choice). After the interbody work is completed, intraoperative fluoroscopic visualization should be used to confirm acceptable position of the implant. At the completion of the procedure, appropriate hemostasis should be observed, and the integrity of the visceral structure should be confirmed in the surgical field. Once this has been ensured, the laparoscopic instruments can be carefully removed.

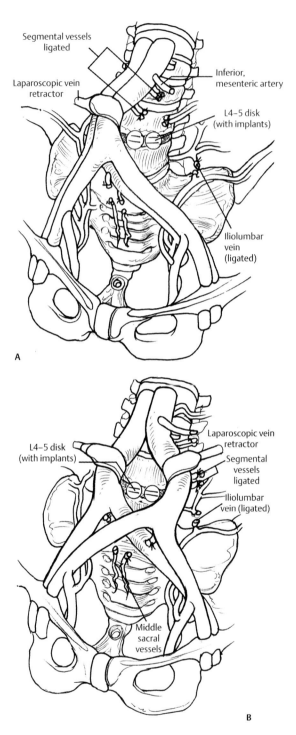

Fig. 58.2 Intraoperative exposure techniques vary depending on the patient's anatomy. An anterior exposure of L4–L5 can be accomplished by retracting the aorta and inferior vena cava to either **(A)** the ipsilateral side or **(B)** the contralateral side.

Outcome

Some early studies yielded potentially promising results with laparoscopic ALIF. Across the board, a steep learning curve was the standard. While some studies suggested a shorter hospital stay (as low as 1.4 days on average) and lower operative blood loss, several studies showed an increase in operative time and complication rates. Fusion rates varied, mostly as they related to whether the procedure was done as a stand-alone or in combination with a posterior surgery. With generally agreed-on higher complication rates with laparoscopic ALIF and given several other techniques available for achieving a solid interbody lumbar arthrodesis, ALIF via a laparoscopic technique has been used in limited numbers of patients over the last several years.

Complications

Generally, complications related to the laparoscopic approach have been related to prolonged operative time, level operated on (higher vascular injuries with L4–L5), and surgeon experience. Statistically significant increase in neurologic problems as they relate to intraoperative disk extrusion has been reported in several studies. Increased ureteral injury, vascular injury, and retrograde ejaculation have also been reported in several studies. Emergent conversions to open techniques have also been reported in the literature.

Laparoscopic ALIF today is used sparingly and should be considered mostly by experienced lumbar laparoscopists.

Suggested Readings

Burns BH. An operation for spondylolisthesis. Lancet 1933;224:1233

> *This is the first study to describe anterior lumbar interbody fusions for the treatment of spondylolisthesis and has been instrumental in the development of anterior surgical techniques.*

Inamasu J, Guiot BH. Laparoscopic anterior lumbar interbody fusion: a review of outcome studies. Minim Invasive Neurosurg 2005;48(6):340–347

> *The authors compared laparoscopic and mini-open anterior lumbar approaches. While they state there is insufficient evidence to support one technique over the other, laparoscopic approaches have been associated with higher rates of retrograde ejaculation and conversion to open surgery.*

Kleeman TJ, Michael Ahn U, Clutterbuck WB, Campbell CJ, Talbot-Kleeman A. Laparoscopic anterior lumbar interbody fusion at L4–L5: an anatomic evaluation and approach classification. Spine 2002;27(13):1390–1395

> *On the basis of operative reports and preoperative MRI or CT from 139 patients who underwent laparoscopic ALIF involving L4–L5, the authors devise a classification system that would allow prediction of the safest approach for any given vascular configuration.*

Lieberman IH, Willsher PC, Litwin DE, Salo PT, Kraetschmer BG. Transperitoneal laparoscopic exposure for lumbar interbody fusion. Spine 2000;25(4):509–514, discussion 515

This prospective clinical trial attempts to determine safety and effectiveness and to document technique and perioperative complications of a laparoscopic exposure for lumbar interbody fusion.

Mahvi DM, Zdeblick TA. A prospective study of laparoscopic spinal fusion. Technique and operative complications. Ann Surg 1996;224(1):85–90

In this study of 20 patients with discogenic back pain, the authors conclude that laparoscopic transperitoneal ALIF is safe, and the early results are encouraging.

Regan JJ, Aronoff RJ, Ohnmeiss DD, Sengupta DK. Laparoscopic approach to L4–L5 for interbody fusion using BAK cages: experience in the first 58 cases. Spine 1999;24(20):2171–2174

In this study, the authors describe variations in the approach used to address anatomical variations in the location of the great vessel bifurcation in the region of the L4–L5 intervertebral disk space when performing laparoscopic interbody fusion procedures.

Regan JJ, Yuan H, McAfee PC. Laparoscopic fusion of the lumbar spine: minimally invasive spine surgery. A prospective multicenter study evaluating open and laparoscopic lumbar fusion. Spine 1999;24(4):402–411

In a multicenter clinical trial, 240 consecutive patients who underwent laparoscopic instrumented interbody fusion were compared with 591 consecutive patients undergoing open anterior fusion. The authors conclude that once mastered, the method is effective and safe compared with open techniques of fusion.

Wood KB, Devine J, Fischer D, Dettori JR, Janssen M. Vascular injury in elective anterior lumbosacral surgery. Spine 2010;35(9, Suppl):S66–S75

The authors reviewed 40 articles relating to vascular injury following anterior lumbar surgery. They noted a higher rate of vascular injury using laparoscopic techniques.

Zucherman JF, Zdeblick TA, Bailey SA, Mahvi D, Hsu KY, Kohrs D. Instrumented laparoscopic spinal fusion. Preliminary Results. Spine 1995;20(18):2029–2034, discussion 2034–2035

Based on a study of 17 consecutive patients undergoing laparoscopic instrumented interbody fusion, the authors predict that operative time and hospital stay are expected to decrease with future instrumentation development and surgeon experience.

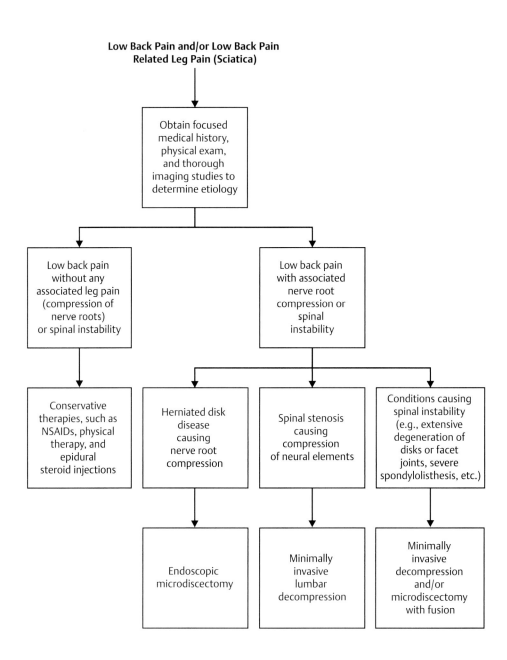

59

Posterior Lumbar Minimally Invasive Surgery

Sapan D. Gandhi and D. Greg Anderson

Only a small number of patients with low back pain are considered candidates for surgical intervention. Surgical options for the lumbar spine include lumbar decompression, microdiscectomy, and interbody fusion. These procedures are indicated only in those patients who show spinal instability, herniated disk disease, and/or spinal canal or neuroforaminal stenosis (i.e., narrowing). Typically, an associated leg pain due to compression of neural elements secondary to the previously mentioned changes is also observed. Surgical intervention is usually more successful at alleviating the associated leg pain due to nerve root compression than the low back pain. Traditionally, midline approaches to the posterior lumbar spine utilizing a large incision were used for these procedures. This technique demanded large amounts of soft-tissue dissection and prolonged use of self-retaining retractors to achieve adequate visualization, leading to long recovery times for patients undergoing the procedure. Recently, minimally invasive spine surgery has seen a surge in interest because of developments in technology that have solidified its ability to achieve similar outcomes to open spine surgery while reducing approach-related morbidities and hastening patient recovery.

Classification

Candidates for minimally invasive posterior lumbar spine surgery can be categorized into one of three categories based on the underlying etiology of their symptoms. Those patients who have neural element compression due to herniated disk disease would be good candidates for endoscopic microdiscectomy. Those patients who have nerve root compression due to spinal stenosis may be candidates for a minimally invasive decompression. Those patients who have severe degeneration of the intervetebral disk or facet joints and associated instability of the spine may require a complete discectomy or decompression and fusion of the vertebral bodies.

Workup

History and Physical Examination

A complete medical history and physical examination should be undertaken to rule out potentially serious underlying medical conditions and help identify the specific pain etiology. When planning a minimally invasive surgery, body habitus and age should be taken under consideration and planned for, as the approach can be more technically demanding for obese or elderly patients. However, neither age nor body mass index (BMI) has been shown to be a contraindication to minimally invasive spine surgery, and it can be accomplished with similar outcomes to the general population.

Spinal Imaging

Appropriate imaging studies are vital to decision making in spine surgery, particularly when planning a minimally invasive approach. Imaging studies such as magnetic resonance imaging (MRI), computed tomography (CT), and plain radiographs are needed to determine the underlying spinal pathology. Invasive diagnostic testing, such as nerve root blocks and diskography, can play a role in determining pain etiology. Noninvasive procedures like epidural steroid injections can also play a role in elucidating the specific pain source and determining whether surgery will appropriately address the spinal pathology.

Treatment

Patients with degenerative spinal conditions should first attempt conservative treatment, such as nonsteroidal anti-inflammatory drugs (NSAIDs), physical therapy, and epidural steroid injections. Surgical interventions should be undertaken only when these conservative treatments fail. In general, minimally invasive procedures may be considered as surgical approaches for treatment of herniated disk disease, spinal stenosis, or any range of spinal pathologies that cause spinal instability, such as spondylolisthesis. Minimally invasive approaches have been refined for microdiscectomy procedures, decompression surgery, and a variety of lumbar fusion procedures. Most of these procedures have been shown to be as effective as their counterpart open procedures.

Generally, minimally invasive spine surgery utilizes both a slightly lateral, paramedian approach to minimize iatrogenic soft-tissue damage, and a tubular retractor system is used to create a small surgical portal for the procedure. Serial dilators are used to create the surgical corridor gently, providing access to the vertebral column while minimizing paraspinal muscle retraction (**Fig. 59.1**). The tubular retractor is then used to maintain visualization of the surgical site (**Fig. 59.2**). Tubular retractor systems also can be "wanded" to the contralateral side, allowing the surgeon to perform bilateral decompressions from a single unilateral incision. Pedicle screws and rods can also be placed percutaneously,

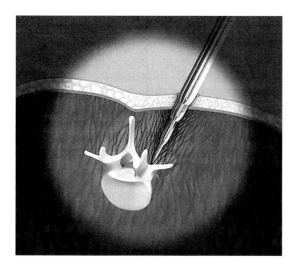

Fig. 59.1 Sequential dilators are used to prepare the surgical site for placement of a tubular retractor. (With permission of Endius Inc., Plainville, MA.)

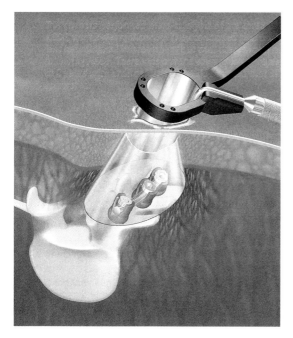

Fig. 59.2 A FlexPosure tubular retractor maintains surgical exposure, providing access for instrumentation, decompression, and bone grafting through a 1-inch surgical incision. (With permission of Endius Inc., Plainville, MA.)

further minimizing the amount of paraspinal muscle trauma during lumbar fusions. Minimally invasive versions of virtually all posterior lumbar spine surgical procedures have been refined and can be potentially utilized in the right circumstances.

Use of Computer-Assisted Spinal Surgery

```
                        Spinal surgery
                              │
                              ▼
                  Intraoperative imaging needed?
                       │              │
                       ▼              ▼
                     Yes             No
                                      │
                                      ▼
                              Planned spinal surgery

          ┌───────────────┴───────────────┐
          ▼                                ▼
  Computer-assisted spinal surgery    Standard fluoroscopy

   ┌──────────┬──────────┬──────────┐
   ▼          ▼          ▼          ▼
CT-based  Fluoroscopic Isocentric  Introperative
navigation navigation  navigation  CT navigation
```

60

Computer-Assisted Spinal Surgery

Iain H. Kalfas

The management of spinal disorders has been greatly influenced by the development and use of screw-based fixation devices. Accurate placement of these screws requires the spinal surgeon to have a precise orientation to that part of the spinal anatomy that is not exposed in the surgical field. Although conventional intraoperative imaging techniques such as fluoroscopy have proven useful, they are limited in that they provide only two-dimensional imaging of a complex three-dimensional structure. Consequently, the surgeon is required to extrapolate the third dimension based on an interpretation of the images and knowledge of the pertinent anatomy. This "dead reckoning" of the anatomy can result in varying degrees of inaccuracy when placing screws into the unexposed spinal column.

Several studies have shown the unreliability of routine radiography in assessing pedicle screw placement in the lumbosacral spine. The rate of disruption of the pedicle cortex by an inserted screw ranges from 15% to 31% in these studies.[1–4] The disadvantage of these conventional radiographic techniques in orienting the spinal surgeon to the unexposed spinal anatomy is that they display, at most, only two planar images. While the lateral view can be relatively easy to assess, the anteroposterior (AP) or oblique view can be difficult to interpret. For most screw fixation procedures, it is the position of the screw in the axial plane that is most important. This plane best demonstrates the position of the screw relative to the neural canal. Conventional intraoperative imaging cannot provide this view.

An additional concern of conventional intraoperative imaging is the radiation exposure experienced by the surgical team and the patient. Rampersaud has demonstrated that compared with other orthopedic procedures utilizing intraoperative fluoroscopy, spinal procedures potentially result in a 10–12-fold increase in radiation exposure because of such factors as backscatter radiation and the increased energy levels needed to image the lumbar spine. This creates a potentially significant hazard to those individuals who perform a high volume of complex spinal surgery.[5] Computer-assisted spinal surgery, or image-guided spinal navigation, is a computer-based surgical technology designed to improve intraoperative orientation to the nonvisualized anatomy during complex spinal procedures.[6,7] It provides the spinal surgeon with the ability to manipulate multiplanar computed tomographic (CT) or fluoroscopic images during the procedure to gain a greater degree of orientation to the surgical anatomy, optimizing the precision and accuracy of the surgery. An additional advantage is that, compared with conventional intraoperative imaging, image-guided navigation eliminates or significantly reduces radiation exposure to the surgical team.

Principles of Computer-Assisted Spinal Surgery

Computer-assisted spinal surgery facilitates surgical accuracy by matching spinal image data to the corresponding intraoperative anatomy. It is based on the principle that both the image data and the surgical anatomy represent a three-dimensional coordinate system. Each point in the image dataset and in the surgical field has a location in space defined by specific x, y, and z Cartesian coordinates. Using defined mathematical algorithms, a specific point in the image dataset can be "matched" to its corresponding point in the surgical field. After matching a limited number of these points together, any point in the surgical field can then be selected and its corresponding point in the images displayed in several planes, giving the surgeon a greater degree of orientation to the pertinent surgical anatomy.

There are currently four general types of computer-assisted spinal surgery available. *CT-based navigation* uses CT images of the patient acquired prior to the surgery. Conventional intraoperative imaging is not necessary. During navigation the surgeon is presented with reformatted CT images in multiple planes, with the selected screw entry point and trajectory superimposed on the images (**Fig. 60.1**). This information updates in real time as adjustments are made to the selected trajectory in the surgical field.

Fluoroscopic navigation uses a standard AP and lateral image of the spinal anatomy acquired just before surgery begins. No additional intraoperative imaging is needed. The selected trajectory information is superimposed on the AP and lateral images on the workstation screen (**Fig. 60.2**). In contrast to CT-based navigation, no axial image is available. The advantage of fluoroscopic navigation is that it uses less radiation than conventional fluoroscopy and does not require a preoperative CT scan, as CT-based navigation does.

Intraoperative isocentric fluoroscopic navigation is a variation of standard fluoroscopic navigation. It acquires images just prior to surgery by rotating the specialized C-arm in a 180-degree arc around the patient. These images can then be reformatted to provide images in the axial and sagittal planes, as in CT-based navigation, but without the need to acquire a preoperative CT scan. Although the images are not of the same quality as a standard CT image set, they are adequate for navigation in most cases.

Intraoperative CT navigation is the most recent advancement in computer-assisted surgery. It consists of a portable CT scanner that uses flat-panel detector technology to improve intraoperative image acquisition and quality.

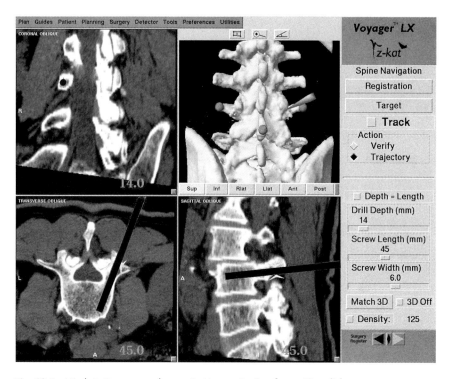

Menu bar: Plan Guides Patient Planning Surgery Detector Tools Preferences Utilities

CORONAL OBLIQUE

R

14.0

TRANSVERSE OBLIQUE

L

A

45.0

SAGITTAL OBLIQUE

A

45.0

Voyager™ *LX*

z-kat

Spine Navigation

Registration

Target

☐ **Track**

Action
◇   Verify
◆   Trajectory

Sup | Inf | Rlat | Llat | Ant | Post

☐ Depth = Length

Drill Depth (mm)
14

Screw Length (mm)
45

Screw Width (mm)
6.0

Match 3D   ☐ 3D Off

☐ Density: 125

Surgery
Register ◀ ▮ ▶

Fig. 60.1   Workstation screen demonstrating navigation for an L3 pedicle screw.

The scanner has a configuration similar to a standard C-arm fluoroscope. In addition to being able to acquire standard AP and lateral images, its C-arm configuration can be "closed" to completely encircle the patient. This allows the flat-panel detector to be swept in a 360-degree arc around the patient, significantly improving the acquired image quality. The reformatted images are similar in quality to conventional CT imaging and superior to isocentric fluoroscopic imaging. The use of automated registration makes this form of computer-assisted spinal surgery very applicable to minimally invasive surgery.

The common components of most navigation systems include an image-processing computer workstation interfaced with a two-camera optical localizer (**Fig. 60.3**). When positioned during surgery, the optical localizer emits infrared light toward the operative field. A hand-held navigational probe mounted with a fixed array of passive reflective spheres serves as the link between the surgeon and the computer workstation (**Fig. 60.4**). Passive reflectors can also be attached to standard surgical instruments. The spacing and positioning of the passive reflectors on each navigational probe or customized trackable surgical instrument is known by the computer workstation. The infrared light that is transmitted toward the operative field is reflected back to the optical localizer by the passive reflectors. This information is relayed to the computer workstation, which can then calculate the precise location of the instrument

although several discrete points in both the image dataset and in the surgical field are frequently required to improve the accuracy of surface mapping. The positional information of these points is transferred to the workstation, and a topographic map of the selected anatomy is created and "matched" to the patient's image set.[9]

Automated registration is performed when fluoroscopic navigation or intraoperative CT imaging systems are used. This technique involves attachment of a reference frame on the exposed spinal anatomy or, with lumbar surgery, the iliac crest. A second reference frame is attached to the CT imaging scanner or fluoroscope. As the intraoperative images are acquired, the two reference frames allow for registration to occur without the need for surgeon input. The CT scanner or fluoroscope can then be removed and real-time navigation of up to five separate spinal levels performed.[10]

Following accurate registration, the navigation probe can be positioned on any surface point in the surgical field. As the probe is tracked by the camera, the computer workstation will relate the corresponding image data to show the position of the probe relative to the local bony anatomy. If CT-based navigation is used, three separate reformatted CT images centered on the corresponding point in the image dataset are displayed. These images will allow the surgeon to select the appropriate screw trajectory and entry point in the sagittal, coronal, and axial planes. The appropriate screw length and diameter can also be selected. As the surgeon moves the probe into different positions and angles, the image data will update in real time to demonstrate the new selected entry point and trajectory. If fluoroscopic navigation is used, the trajectory line will be superimposed on the preoperatively acquired AP and lateral fluoroscopic images on the workstation monitor.

 ## Clinical Applications

Image-guided spinal navigation was initially evaluated by assessing its accuracy when used to place pedicle screws into the thoracic and lumbosacral spines of cadaver specimens.[7] The first study evaluating navigational accuracy in the clinical setting was performed in a series of 30 patients undergoing lumbar pedicle screw fixation. Accuracy of screw insertion was documented by plain film radiography and thin-section CT imaging of the instrumented levels. Satisfactory screw placement was noted for 149 of 150 inserted screws.[6]

Several additional studies have also demonstrated the improved accuracy of pedicle screw insertion with the assistance of image-guided navigation.[1,11–13] These studies all demonstrated a statistically significant improvement in the accuracy of pedicle screw placement in the navigation-assisted cohort.

Other applications of computer-assisted spinal surgery soon developed, directed by the complexity of the procedure and, specifically, by the need to "visualize" the unexposed spinal anatomy. In addition to thoracic and lumbar pedicle screw insertion, other applications include placement of iliac wing screws, transoral decompressive surgery, cervical screw fixation procedures, cervical corpectomy, decompression of spinal metastasis and anterior thoracolumbar decompression and fixation procedures[14–20] (**Fig. 60.5**).

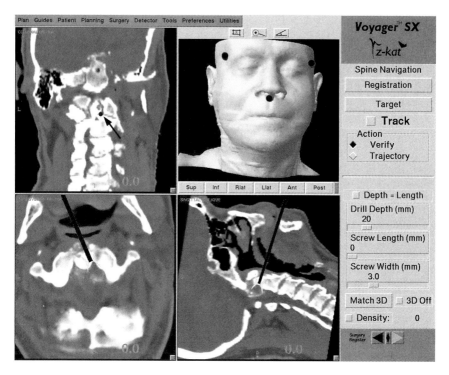

Fig. 60.5 Workstation screen demonstrating navigational information during transoral decompression. (Probe tip location highlighted by *arrow.*)

Computer-assisted surgery can be used with or without standard intraoperative imaging techniques (i.e., fluoroscopy). With CT-based navigation it can also be used for preoperative planning because of the capability for multiplanar image manipulation on the navigational workstation.

While image-guided spinal navigation is a versatile and effective technology, it is not a replacement for the surgeon's having a thorough knowledge of the pertinent spinal anatomy as well as correct surgical techniques. It merely serves as an additional source of information used by the surgeon to make selected intraoperative decisions.

 Conclusion

Computer-assisted navigation technology has been successfully applied to spinal surgery. It can be used for both conventional and minimally invasive spinal procedures. By linking digitized image data to spinal surface anatomy, computer-assisted navigation facilitates the surgeon's orientation to unexposed spinal structures, improving the precision and accuracy of the surgery and reducing or eliminating the need for conventional intraoperative imaging.

References

1. Amiot LP, Lang K, Putzier M, Zippel H, Labelle H. Comparative results between conventional and computer-assisted pedicle screw installation in the thoracic, lumbar, and sacral spine. Spine 2000;25(5):606–614
2. George DC, Krag MH, Johnson CC, Van Hal ME, Haugh LD, Grobler LJ. Hole preparation techniques for transpedicle screws. Effect on pull-out strength from human cadaveric vertebrae. Spine 1991;16(2):181–184
3. Gertzbein SD, Robbins SE. Accuracy of pedicular screw placement in vivo. Spine 1990; 15(1):11–14
4. Weinstein JN, Spratt KF, Spengler D, Brick C, Reid S. Spinal pedicle fixation: reliability and validity of roentgenogram-based assessment and surgical factors on successful screw placement. Spine 1988;13(9):1012–1018
5. Rampersaud YR, Foley KT, Shen AC, Williams S, Solomito M. Radiation exposure to the spine surgeon during fluoroscopically assisted pedicle screw insertion. Spine 2000;25(20): 2637–2645
6. Kalfas IH, Kormos DW, Murphy MA, et al. Application of frameless stereotaxy to pedicle screw fixation of the spine. J Neurosurg 1995;83(4):641–647
7. Murphy MA, McKenzie RL, Kormos DW, Kalfas IH. Frameless stereotaxis for the insertion of lumbar pedicle screws. J Clin Neurosci 1994;1(4):257–260
8. Kalfas IH. Spinal registration accuracy and error. In: Germano, IM, ed. Advanced Techniques in Image-Guided Brain and Spine Surgery. New York, NY: Thieme; 2002:37–44
9. Tamura Y, Sugano N, Sasama T, et al. Surface-based registration accuracy of CT-based image-guided spine surgery. Eur Spine J 2005;14(3):291–297
10. Wood MJ, Mannion RJ. Improving accuracy and reducing radiation exposure in minimally invasive lumbar interbody fusion. J Neurosurg Spine 2010;12(5):533–539
11. Laine T, Schlenzka D, Mäkitalo K, Tallroth K, Nolte LP, Visarius H. Improved accuracy of pedicle screw insertion with computer-assisted surgery. A prospective clinical trial of 30 patients. Spine 1997;22(11):1254–1258
12. Merloz P, Tonetti J, Eid A, et al. Computer assisted spine surgery. Clin Orthop Relat Res 1997;337(337):86–96
13. Schwarzenbach O, Berlemann U, Jost B, et al. Accuracy of computer-assisted pedicle screw placement. An in vivo computed tomography analysis. Spine 1997;22(4):452–458
14. Kalfas IH. Image-guided spinal navigation. Clin Neurosurg 2000;46:70–88
15. Assaker R, Reyns N, Vinchon M, Demondion X, Louis E. Transpedicular screw placement: image-guided versus lateral-view fluoroscopy: in vitro simulation. Spine 2001;26(19): 2160–2164
16. Kalfas IH. Image-guided spinal navigation: application to spinal metastasis. In: Maciunas RJ, ed.: Advanced Techniques in Central Nervous System Metastasis, Lebanon, NH: AANS Publications; 1998:245–254
17. Welch WC, Subach BR, Pollack IF, Jacobs GB. Frameless stereotactic guidance for surgery of the upper cervical spine. Neurosurgery 1997;40(5):958–963, discussion 963–964
18. Youkilis AS, Quint DJ, McGillicuddy JE, Papadopoulos SM. Stereotactic navigation for placement of pedicle screws in the thoracic spine. Neurosurgery 2001;48(4):771–778, discussion 778–779
19. Bolger C, Wigfield C. Image-guided surgery: applications to the cervical and thoracic spine and a review of the first 120 procedures. J Neurosurg 2000;92(2, Suppl):175–180
20. Weidner A, Wähler M, Chiu ST, Ullrich CG. Modification of C1–C2 transarticular screw fixation by image-guided surgery. Spine 2000;25(20):2668–2673, discussion 2674

Suggested Readings

Amiot LP, Lang K, Putzier M, Zippel H, Labelle H. Comparative results between conventional and computer-assisted pedicle screw installation in the thoracic, lumbar, and sacral spine. Spine 2000;25(5):606–614

   This article compares the accuracy of pedicle screw insertion between two patient groups. The control group consisted of 100 patients with 544 screws placed using conventional techniques. The computer-assisted group had 50 patients with 294 screws placed. Correct screw placement was 85% in the control group and 95% in the computer-assisted group.

Kalfas IH. Image-guided spinal navigation. In: Winn HR, ed. Youman's Neurological Surgery, 5th ed. Philadelphia, PA: WB Saunders; 2011:3088–3096

This chapter provides a comprehensive summary of the principles and clinical applications of image-guided spinal navigation.

Rampersaud YR, Foley KT, Shen AC, Williams S, Solomito M. Radiation exposure to the spine surgeon during fluoroscopically assisted pedicle screw insertion. Spine 2000;25(20):2637–2645

This paper addresses the radiation exposure that spinal surgeons are potentially exposed to during fluoroscopically assisted pedicle screw insertion. Factors such as higher radiation dosage needed to image the lumbar region and backscatter radiation ipsilateral to the beam source contribute to a 10–12-fold increase in radiation exposure for the spinal surgeon compared to a non-spine surgeon using fluoroscopy.

Sasso RC, Garrido BJ. Computer-assisted spinal navigation versus serial radiography and operative time for posterior spinal fusion at L5-S1. J Spinal Disord Tech 2007;20(2):118–122

This paper compares the use of fluoroscopic image-guided navigation to serial radiography for pedicle screw placement in 105 patients. The navigation group demonstrated statistically significant shorter operative times compared to the serial radiography group.

Youkilis AS, Quint DJ, McGillicuddy JE, Papadopoulos SM. Stereotactic navigation for placement of pedicle screws in the thoracic spine. Neurosurgery 2001;48(4):771–778, discussion 778–779

This paper reviews the use of navigation for placement of pedicle screws in the thoracic region. A total of 266 screws were placed using image-guided navigation. Thin-section CT was obtained postoperatively. Only 5 screws (2.2%) were classified as having structurally significant pedicle violations.

XIII Non-Fusion Techniques

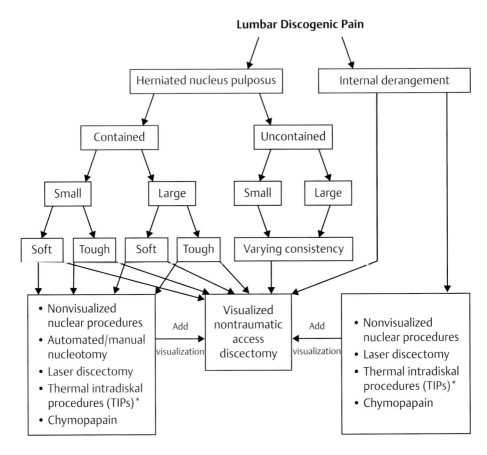

Lumbar Discogenic Pain

Herniated nucleus pulposus → Contained → Small / Large; Uncontained → Small / Large

Internal derangement

- Small / Large (Contained) → Soft / Tough / Soft / Tough
- Small / Large (Uncontained) → Varying consistency

- Nonvisualized nuclear procedures
- Automated/manual nucleotomy
- Laser discectomy
- Thermal intradiskal procedures (TIPs)*
- Chymopapain

Add visualization →

Visualized nontraumatic access discectomy

← Add visualization

- Nonvisualized nuclear procedures
- Laser discectomy
- Thermal intradiskal procedures (TIPs)*
- Chymopapain

*TIPs (thermal intradiskal procedures) that have been disapproved by CMS (The Centers for Medicare and Medicaid Services, government agency) are commonly identified as intradiskal electrothermal therapy (IDET), intradiskal thermal annuloplasty (IDTA), percutaneous intradiskal radiofrequency thermocoagulation (PIRFT), radiofrequency annuloplasty (RA), intradiskal biacuplasty (IDB), percutaneous (or plasma) disk decompression (PDD) or coblation, or targeted disk decompression (TDD)

61

Percutaneous Discogenic Pain Treatment

David A. Ditsworth, Luis A. Lombardi, and Irina G. Bogacheva

Low back pain is one of the most commonly encountered problems in a medical practice. Discogenic low back pain, or pain arising from the intervertebral disks, has been called the most common cause of chronic low back pain. Historically, surgical solutions were initially open, traumatic approaches that were associated with significant morbidity. Driven in part by the desire of patients and physicians to reduce the morbidity of spinal procedures, less-invasive approaches have grown significantly in popularity in recent years.[1] There is a growing need for clearer language that can differentiate between the various "minimally invasive" procedures. A purported advantage of percutaneous procedures is that they have low approach-related trauma, although certain techniques have yet to be proven effective.

Classification

Although no universally accepted classification system has been suggested for percutaneous techniques for discogenic pain, the following definitions are helpful. Discogenic pain is produced by complex chemical and mechanical interactions. Internal disk derangement of the nucleus pulposus (dehydration and collagen disorganization) and associated annular disruption allow nuclear material and inflammatory cytokines, such as cyclooxygenase, interleukins, and prostaglandins, to come in contact with the perineural tissue surrounding the outer layers of the disk. Axial pain is believed to be produced by a combination of outer annular chemical sensitization, whereas radicular pain is produced by a direct mass effect and chemical inflammation of the nerve roots.[2]

Disk herniations can be further subdivided into contained (within disk boundaries) and uncontained (outside of the disk boundaries and into the spinal canal; i.e., extruded and sequestered). A spectrum of herniations is seen based on location, size, and consistency.

Intradiskal procedures (both visualized and nonvisualized) are used to treat contained herniation and internal disk derangement and can be further subdivided into (a) intranuclear and (b) annular. Extradiskal procedures (visualized) are used to treat uncontained herniations.

Workup

History and Physical Examination

The workup for percutaneous procedures is similar to the workup of disk problems in general. A focused history and physical examination are performed, followed by radiologic studies.

Spinal Imaging

The most useful screening test is magnetic resonance imaging (MRI) to visualize the disk pathology directly. It is recommended that percutaneous procedures be preceded by diskography with postdiskography computed tomography (CT) scanning. The CT scan includes focal cuts through the affected levels.[2-5] Postdiskography CT helps determine the size and location of the herniation and the presence of fissures, usually with greater accuracy than the MRI alone.

This radiological study provides a route map for the guide-wire passage and defines the safe entrance zones to the disk to avoid vital structures, such as bowel or kidney, which could potentially be in the track of the guide-wire passage. Diskography may also help predict the outcome of the treatment (success rates based on positive diskograms are higher than in cases with negative results).[3-6] In some cases, diskography shows dramatic pathology not seen on MRI (**Fig. 61.1A–D**).

Treatment

Nonvisualized Nuclear Procedures

Although these procedures utilize different physical methods, the basic principle is to reduce the disk volume by removal of 10–15% of the nuclear material and thus reduce intradiskal pressure, allowing room for the herniated area to remodel gradually inward.

Remodeling may or may not occur. If it does, it would be expected to occur over many months.[2]

In general, these procedures have the highest success rates in patients with contained, wide-neck herniations with intact posterior annulus and no migration or sequestration.

Nonvisualized intranuclear procedures include chemonucleolysis, percutaneous automated nucleotomy, percutaneous laser disk decompression (PLDD), nucleoplasty, and the Dekompressor system (Stryker Interventional Spine, Allendale, NJ).

Nonvisualized annular procedures include intradiskal electrothermal therapy (IDET), annuloplasty, and bipolar biacuplasty.

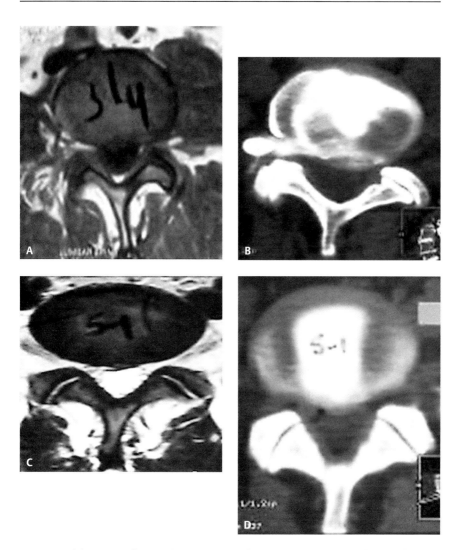

Fig. 61.1   (A) L3–L4 axial MRI with a very equivocal left far lateral herniation. **(B)** Postdiskography CT scan of the same patient, clearly showing an extruded left far lateral fragment. **(C)** Axial MRI at L5–S1 showing a "high-intensity zone" accompanied by central disk bulge (internal disk structure is not clearly demonstrated). **(D)** Postdiskography CT scan of the same patient showing a wide, full-thickness annular tear.

Chemonucleolysis

In 1963, Smith administered the enzyme chymopapain to the first chemonucleolysis patient. By 1984, 75,000 patients had been treated with this method. However, in 1999, this procedure was widely discontinued in the United States after several cases of transverse myelitis and anaphylactic deaths were reported.[7,8]

Percutaneous Automated Nucleotomy

In 1975 Hijikata introduced the percutaneous manual nucleotomy, which was expanded by Onik, a radiologist, who developed an automated device (Nucleotome, Clarus Medical, Minneapolis, MN). This consists of a small probe that is positioned into the nuclear chamber via a standard posterolateral approach. The probe contains a distal window with an internal cutter and a suction mechanism. The nuclear material is cut and suctioned to an outside reservoir. The reported success rates of this procedure by itself vary from 29% to 75%.[9,10] Success rates vary depending on the pathology, specifically, whether the herniation has a wide neck. It is a relatively simple and safe technique, and major complications are very rare.[2,9–12]

The Dekompressor probe has been recently introduced but received a very weak recommendation due to poor scientific support for its efficacy.[2,13]

Percutaneous Laser Disk Decompression (PLDD)

Since its introduction by Ascher and Choy in 1986, the utilization of laser energy to reduce the nucleus pulposus volume has gained increasing popularity because of its small size, technical simplicity, and low incidence of complications. The effectiveness of PLDD varies from 56% to 87%, with an average relief of 72% at 1-year follow-up. The incidence of complications is around 1% and includes infectious diskitis, cauda equina syndrome, bowel perforation, and nerve root damage.[2,14,15]

Nucleoplasty

In 2002 the U.S. Food and Drug Administration (FDA) approved the use of controlled ablation technology for percutaneous disk decompression. Disc Nucleoplasty (ArthroCare, Stockholm, Sweden) uses a 1-mm instrument that creates radiofrequency energy, which dissolves disk nucleus and removes such tissue at low temperatures, therefore preserving the integrity of the healthy tissue.

Evidence for the success of this approach is anecdotal at the current time. The Centers for Medicare and Medicaid Services (CMS) have disallowed this procedure.[1] Even though complications are rare, Cohen reported new onset of "neurologic" symptoms attributed to provocation of posterolateral disk nerve fibers.[2,16,17]

Annular Procedures

Intradiskal Electothermal Therapy (IDET)   The Intradiskal Electrothermal (Smith & Nephew, Memphis, TN) treatment (IDET) was introduced by physiatrists Jeffrey and Joel Saal. The mechanism of action of this procedure is a subject of controversy and is not well described in the literature. Complications are rare. Thomas et al. reported a case in which the tip of the catheter broke off into the spinal canal and migrated into the dural sac, to be removed later by a wide laminectomy.[18] Long-term data collection found that the results were less promising than previously expected. Pauza et al. (2003) reported that even though 40% of their patients achieved greater than 50% relief of their pain, ~ 50% of the patients experience no appreciable benefit.[19]

According to Assietti et al., the global clinical success rate was 78%, with a strong success correlation in highly concordant diskography findings, high-intensity zone (HIZ), and higher percentage of annulus covered by the catheter.[2,20–22] The CMS disallowed this procedure.[1]

Newer thermal annular procedures include unipolar radiofrequency annuloplasty and bipolar biacuplasty, with only anecdotal studies reported in the literature.[23–25]

Visualized Intradiskal and Extradiskal Procedures

Percutaneous Access Discectomy

Disk removal is performed through a small working channel scope, passed through a cannula. Visualization is done on a monitor. Depending on the location of the disk fragments, minimal or no tissue removal may be required to remove the herniated fragment.

For extradiskal, free fragments, the contents of the spinal canal can be well seen and fragments removed with a grasper. Access into the spinal canal can be obtained by either a transforaminal approach (**Fig. 61.2A–D**) or paramedian approach (**Fig. 61.3A–D**).[26] The success rate (excellent and good) for this type of paramedian approach fragmentectomy at L5–S1 (**Fig. 61.3A–D**) has been reported as 93% in a series of 111 patients.[27] In contrast to other procedures presented above, these procedures, removing free fragments in the spinal canal, are fundamentally different; they provide compelling visual, radiologic, and physical evidence of clear pathology, and that pathology is effectively dealt with and removed as a specimen.

Outcome

Scientifically controlled outcome studies have not been performed for most of the techniques discussed at the time of this writing.

Complications

Potential risks of all procedures include infection, neurologic injury, retained pathology, continued pain, and injury to vital structures.

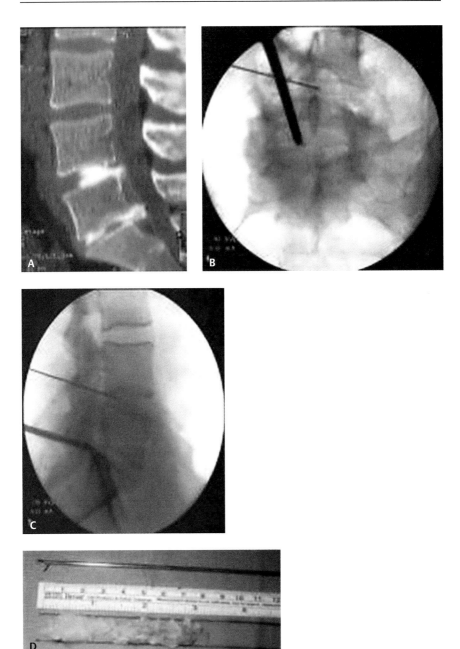

Fig. 61.2 **(A)** Sagittal postdiskography CT scan. **(B)** Intraoperative fluoroscopic AP films showing the grasper in the epidural space at L5–S1. **(C)** Intraoperative fluoroscopic lateral films showing the grasper in the epidural space at L5–S1. **(D)** Free disk fragments that have been removed from the spinal canal.

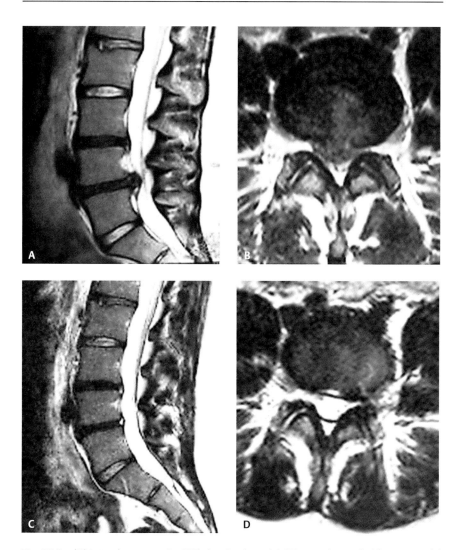

Fig. 61.3 **(A)** Lateral preoperative MRI showing large L4–L5 central extruded fragments. **(B)** Axial preoperative MRI showing large L4–L5 central extruded fragments. **(C)** The large extruded fragments were removed using the authors' Non-Traumatic Access technique. Lateral 6-month postoperative MRI. **(D)** Axial 6-month postoperative MRI showing extruded fragments gone.

References

1. Phurrough S, Salive M, O'Connor D, et al. Decision Memo for Thermal Intradiscal Procedures. U.S. Department of Health and Human Services, Centers for Medicare and Medicaid Services. www.cms.hhs.gov/mcd/viewdecisionmemo.asp?from2=viewdecisionmemo.asp&id=215&. Updated 2008 Accessed September 30, 2008.
2. Singh V, Derby R. Percutaneous lumbar disc decompression. Pain Physician 2006;9(2):139–146
3. Ditsworth DA, Lombardi LA. Enhanced discography (pre-operative mapping): a prelude to small guided lumbar endoscopic discectomy. Paper presented at: International Intradiscal Therapy Society Conference, 2005
4. Ditsworth DA. Endoscopic transforaminal disc removal and reconfiguration. Presented at: Spine Disorders 1996 annual meeting joint section (CNS/AANS) spine and peripheral nerves, 1996
5. Ditsworth DA. Endoscopic transforaminal lumbar discectomy and reconfiguration: a postero-lateral approach into the spinal canal. Surg Neurol 1998;49(6):588–597, discussion 597–598
6. Derby R, Howard MW, Grant JM, Lettice JJ, Van Peteghem PK, Ryan DP. The ability of pressure-controlled discography to predict surgical and nonsurgical outcomes. Spine 1999;24(4):364–371, discussion 371–372
7. Smith L. Enzyme dissolution of the nucleus pulposus in humans. JAMA 1964;187:137–140
8. Javid MJ. Chemonucleolysis. In: Cohen AR, Haines SJ, eds. Minimally Invasive Techniques in Neurosurgery. Concepts in Neurosurgery; vol 7. Baltimore, MD: Williams & Wilkins; 1995:240–246
9. Chatterjee, 1995
10. Onik G, Mooney V, Maroon JC, et al. Automated percutaneous discectomy: a prospective multi-institutional study. Neurosurgery 1990;26(2):228–232, discussion 232–233
11. Hijikata S. Percutaneous nucleotomy. A new concept technique and 12 years' experience. Clin Orthop Relat Res 1989;238(238):9–23
12. Hirsch JA, Singh V, Falco FJ, Benyamin RM, Manchikanti L. Automated percutaneous lumbar discectomy for the contained herniated lumbar disc: a systematic assessment of evidence. Pain Physician 2009;12(3):601–620
13. Singh V, Benyamin RM, Datta S, Falco FJ, Helm S II, Manchikanti L. Systematic review of percutaneous lumbar mechanical disc decompression utilizing Dekompressor. Pain Physician 2009;12(3):589–599
14. Davis JK. Percutaneous laser discectomy. In: Cohen AR, Haines SJ, eds. Minimally Invasive Techniques in Neurosurgery. Concepts in Neurosurgery; vol 7. Baltimore, MD: Williams & Wilkins; 1995:254–257
15. Singh V, Manchikanti L, Benyamin RM, Helm S, Hirsch JA. Percutaneous lumbar laser disc decompression: a systematic review of current evidence. Pain Physician 2009;12(3):573–588
16. Manchikanti L, Derby R, Benyamin RM, Helm S, Hirsch JA. A systematic review of mechanical lumbar disc decompression with nucleoplasty. Pain Physician 2009;12(3):561–572
17. Gerges FJ, Lipsitz SR, Nedeljkovic SS. A systematic review on the effectiveness of the Nucleoplasty procedure for discogenic pain. Pain Physician 2010;13(2):117–132
18. Thomas, et al. 2004
19. Pauza, et al. 2003
20. Ditsworth DA. IDET and PED: benefits of combination treatment. Paper presented at: Spine Disorders 2000 annual meeting joint section (CNS/AANS) spine and peripheral nerves, 2000.
21. Helm S, Hayek SM, Benyamin RM, Manchikanti L. Systematic review of the effectiveness of thermal annular procedures in treating discogenic low back pain. Pain Physician 2009;12(1):207–232
22. Assietti R, Morosi M, Block JE. Intradiscal electrothermal therapy for symptomatic internal disc disruption: 24-month results and predictors of clinical success. J Neurosurg Spine 2010;12(3):320–326
23. Finch PM, Price LM, Drummond PD. Radiofrequency heating of painful annular disruptions: one-year outcomes. J Spinal Disord Tech 2005;18(1):6–13

24. Kapural L, Ng A, Dalton J, et al. Intervertebral disc biacuplasty for the treatment of lumbar discogenic pain: results of a six-month follow-up. Pain Med 2008;9(1):60–67
25. Kapural L, Hayek S, Malak O, Arrigain S, Mekhail N. Intradiscal thermal annuloplasty versus intradiscal radiofrequency ablation for the treatment of discogenic pain: a prospective matched control trial. Pain Med 2005;6(6):425–431
26. Ditsworth DA, Lombardi LA, Bogacheva IG. Chapter title. In: Anderson DG, Vaccaro AR. Decision Making in Spinal Care. New York, NY: Thieme; 2007:415–420
27. Ditsworth DA, Lombardi LA. Non-traumatic, trans-ligamentum flavum approach for L5/S1 extruded disc herniations. Paper presented at: Spine Disorders 2010 annual meeting joint section (CNS/AANS) spine and peripheral nerves, 2010

Suggested Readings

Ditsworth DA. Endoscopic transforaminal lumbar discectomy and reconfiguration: a postero-lateral approach into the spinal canal. Surg Neurol 1998;49(6):588–597, discussion 597–598

> *This is one of the pioneer articles in percutaneous endoscopic lumbar discectomy. It expands the previous limited indications for percutaneous intranuclear techniques to become small, nontraumatic access techniques for free-fragment resection outside of the disk boundaries, especially within the spinal canal. It also provides useful safety and planning tips through the description of wide-view preoperative CT scanning.*

Singh V, Derby R. Percutaneous lumbar disc decompression. Pain Physician 2006;9(2): 139–146

> *This focused review provides useful pathophysiological considerations of degenerative disk disease as well as the evolution and clinical application of the different percutaneous lumbar nuclear decompression techniques.*

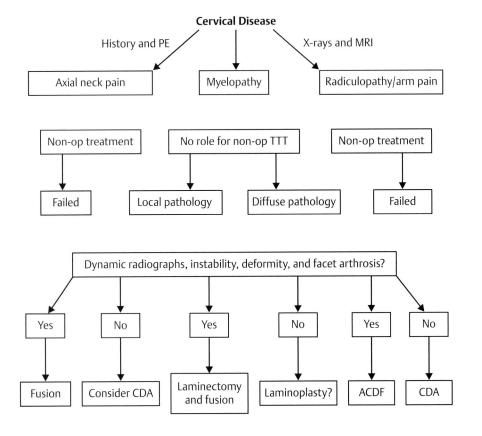

PE, physical examination; MRI, magnetic resonance imaging; Non-op, nonoperative;
TTT, treatment; CDA, cervical disk arthroplasty; ACDF, anterior cervical decompression and fusion

62

Cervical Intervertebral Disk Arthroplasty

Mostafa H. El Dafrawy and Lee H. Riley

Despite the high success rate and long-term track record of anterior cervical decompression and fusion (ACDF) for treating degenerative cervical conditions,[1] concerns persist regarding the increased biomechanical stresses at the adjacent segments.[2] These concerns have resulted in interest in motion-sparing alternatives. Cervical disk arthroplasty (CDA) attempts to replicate the native disk's kinematics, decreasing stress on adjacent vertebral levels and reducing adjacent-segment degeneration. The main theoretical advantages of disk arthroplasty are maintaining range of motion and avoiding adjacent-segment degeneration by restoring disk height and spinal alignment, and thereby the cervical spine's biomechanical characteristics. Other benefits include less surgical morbidity compared with fusion bone grafting, lack of pseudarthrosis as a complication, native avoidance of complications from instrumentation or immobilization, and early return to function.

Prosthetic Designs

Prostheses are classified as unconstrained, semiconstrained, or constrained (**Table 62.1**) based on the allowed motion relative to normal coupled motion (**Fig. 62.1A,B**).[3] Unconstrained, or physiologic, designs do not constrain the center of rotation (COR) to a fixed point so that the locus of points that define the normal COR can be replicated. They simulate the six native degrees of freedom of movement. Most[4] have a mobile polymer COR with a compressible nucleus and allow unconstrained resistance to angular motion. Semiconstrained prostheses have a mobile COR as in a ball-in-trough joint that allows five degrees of freedom of movement—three angular motions and two translations (usually in the sagittal and coronal planes)—but no compressibility. Constrained designs, with a fixed COR, have a ball-and-socket or saddle-type joint articulation and

Proper sizing of the implant involves as much coverage of the endplate as possible. A small disk will increase contact forces on the endplate, leading to subsidence. A too-large prosthesis might become extruded anteriorly.

Overdistraction of the interbody space should be avoided because it may lead to nerve root stretch, facet joint overload, and loss of motion.

Outcome

The highly predictable and favorable outcome of ACDF in cervical disease has always posed a strong argument against the need for CDA.[2] For the past two decades, many spine surgeons have compared the efficacy and safety of CDA and fusion. A recent systematic literature review[11] reported on 13 case series presenting clinical data on the effectiveness of CDA (single- and multiple-level), four randomized controlled trials comparing single-level fusion to arthroplasty, and one nonrandomized comparative study.[6–8,12,13] Three randomized controlled trials represented FDA-regulated investigational device exemption (IDE) studies that evaluated the safety and effectiveness of the Prestige ST Cervical Disk System (Medtronic, Memphis, TN),[13] Bryan Disk (Medtronic Sofamor Danek, Memphis, TN),[6] and ProDisc-C (Synthes Spine, West Chester, PA).[7] The Prestige System study concluded that it maintained physiologic segmental motion at 24 months after implantation and provided improved neurologic success, improved clinical outcomes, and a reduced rate of secondary surgeries compared with ACDF.[13] The Bryan disk study showed there was no statistical difference between the ACDF and CDA groups with regard to the rate of secondary surgical procedures performed.[6] Patients who received the artificial cervical disk returned to work nearly 2 weeks earlier than did those in the ACDF group.[6] The ProDisc-C study showed no difference in visual analog scale scores for neck and arm pain between the CDA and ACDF groups, but ProDisc-C patients achieved equal to or greater than 4 degrees of motion or maintained motion relative to preoperative baseline at the operated level.[7] There was a statistically significant difference in the number of secondary surgeries, with 8.5% of ACDF patients needing a reoperation, revision, or supplemental fixation within the 24-month postoperative period compared with 1.8% of ProDisc-C patients.[7]

In summary, there was level I evidence of significant improvement on the Neck Disability Index and neck and arm pain visual analog scale scores for the CDA and ACDF groups, similar mean angular motion values before and after surgery for the CDA group, faster return to work for the CDA group, and lower reoperation rates for the patients in the CDA group.

Complications

Approach-Related

Complications of the anterior approach to the cervical spine include dysphagia, hoarseness, and unilateral vocal fold paralysis, which are not specific to arthroplasty.[12,14]

Specific to Arthroplasty

Infection

Of more than 5500 Bryan cervical disks implanted worldwide, 11 are known to have been explanted, with four revised because of infection.[10] Three of the ~300 implanted Prestige disks were retrieved, with one disk revised because of infection.[10]

Prosthesis Migration

Extrusion, retropulsion, and subsidence are well-known complications of CDA.

Wear

Wear is affected by the type of material, duration of exposure to debris, prosthetic load and kinematics, specific joint, lubrication, host responsiveness, and particle size, shape, and concentration. The nature of fibrocartilaginous joints may mean that there is a less inflammatory response in the cervical spine than in relatively proinflammatory synovial joints. Accelerated wear and particle debris formation leading to device loosening do not appear to be an issue.[10]

Heterotopic Ossification

Motion preservation after CDA is guaranteed only if spontaneous fusion can be prevented. According to McAfee et al.,[15] heterotopic ossification (HO) after CDA can be classified as grades 0 to 4. Reports of HO are variable among different prostheses, ranging from 21% to 71.4%.[16] One study reported 49.4% of the patients with grade 2 to 3 ossification after 1 year.[17] Early HO after arthroplasty can potentially be avoided by administering nonsteroidal anti-inflammatory drugs (NSAIDs) in the immediate postoperative period.[18]

 ## Conclusion

CDA is a reasonable alternative to ACDF for one-level disease in patients with soft disk herniations and minimal bony degenerative changes. Complete discectomy and osteophyte removal, preservation of the bony endplate, and proper positioning and sizing of the implant are critical for preservation of motion. The indications and contraindications of the procedure are currently evolving with wider use and longer patient follow-up.

References

1. Kaiser MG, Haid RW Jr, Subach BR, Barnes B, Rodts GE Jr. Anterior cervical plating enhances arthrodesis after discectomy and fusion with cortical allograft. Neurosurgery 2002; 50(2):229–236, discussion 236–238

2. Hilibrand AS, Carlson GD, Palumbo MA, Jones PK, Bohlman HH. Radiculopathy and my-elopathy at segments adjacent to the site of a previous anterior cervical arthrodesis. J Bone Joint Surg Am 1999;81(4):519–528

3. Kang H, Park P, La Marca F, Hollister SJ, Lin CY. Analysis of load sharing on uncovertebral and facet joints at the C5-6 level with implantation of the Bryan, Prestige LP, or ProDisc-C cervical disc prosthesis: an in vivo image-based finite element study. Neurosurg Focus 2010;28(6):E9

4. Kouyoumdjian P, Bronsard N, Vital JM, Gille O. Centering of cervical disc replacements: useful-ness of intraoperative anteroposterior fluoroscopic guidance to center cervical disc replace-ments: study on 20 Discocerv (Scient'X prosthesis). Spine 2009;34(15):1572–1577

5. Yi S, Shin HC, Kim KN, Park HK, Jang IT, Yoon H. Modified techniques to prevent sagittal imbalance after cervical arthroplasty. Spine 2007;32(18):1986–1991

6. Heller JG, Sasso RC, Papadopoulos SM, et al. Comparison of BRYAN cervical disc arthro-plasty with anterior cervical decompression and fusion: clinical and radiographic results of a randomized, controlled, clinical trial. Spine 2009;34(2):101–107

7. Murrey D, Janssen M, Delamarter R, et al. Results of the prospective, randomized, con-trolled multicenter Food and Drug Administration investigational device exemption study of the ProDisc-C total disc replacement versus anterior discectomy and fusion for the treat-ment of 1-level symptomatic cervical disc disease. Spine J 2009;9(4):275–286

8. Nabhan A, Ahlhelm F, Pitzen T, et al. Disc replacement using Pro-Disc C versus fusion: a prospective randomised and controlled radiographic and clinical study. Eur Spine J 2007; 16(3):423–430

9. Jawahar A, Cavanaugh DA, Kerr EJ III, Birdsong EM, Nunley PD. Total disc arthroplasty does not affect the incidence of adjacent segment degeneration in cervical spine: results of 93 patients in three prospective randomized clinical trials. Spine J 2010;10(12):1043–1048

10. Anderson PA, Rouleau JP, Toth JM, Riew KD. A comparison of simulator-tested and -retrieved cervical disc prostheses. Invited submission from the Joint Section Meeting on Disorders of the Spine and Peripheral Nerves, March 2004. J Neurosurg Spine 2004;1(2):202–210

11. Cepoiu-Martin M, Faris P, Lorenzetti D, et al. Artificial Cervical Disk Arthroplasty (ACDA): a systematic review. Spine (Phila Pa 1976) 2011;25(Feb):10.1097/BRS.0b013e3182163814

12. Atkins D, Best D, Briss PA, et al. Grading quality of evidence and strength of recommenda-tions. BMJ 2004;328(7454):1490

13. Mummaneni PV, Burkus JK, Haid RW, Traynelis VC, Zdeblick TA. Clinical and radiographic analysis of cervical disc arthroplasty compared with allograft fusion: a randomized con-trolled clinical trial. J Neurosurg Spine 2007;6(3):198–209

14. Campbell PG, Yadla S, Malone J, et al. Early complications related to approach in cervical spine surgery: single-center prospective study. World Neurosurg 2010;74(2-3):363–368

15. McAfee PC, Cunningham BW, Devine J, Williams E, Yu-Yahiro J. Classification of heterotopic os-sification (HO) in artificial disk replacement. J Spinal Disord Tech 2003;16(4):384–389

16. Yi S, Kim KN, Yang MS, et al. Difference in occurrence of heterotopic ossification according to prosthesis type in the cervical artificial disc replacement. Spine 2010;35(16):1556–1561

17. Mehren C, Suchomel P, Grochulla F, et al. Heterotopic ossification in total cervical artificial disc replacement. Spine 2006;31(24):2802–2806

18. Bryan VE Jr. Cervical motion segment replacement. Eur Spine J 2002;11(Suppl 2): S92–S97

Suggested Readings

Cavanaugh DA, Nunley PD, Kerr EJ III, Werner DJ, Jawahar A. Delayed hyper-reactivity to metal ions after cervical disc arthroplasty: a case report and literature review. Spine 2009;34(7): E262–E265

> *The authors present a case of a woman who, after initially doing well after undergo-ing a CDA, developed recurrence of her symptoms. Revision surgery revealed inflam-matory tissue thought to be related to metal ions and similar to the tissue seen in metal-on-metal total hip arthroplasties. This represents a rare complication, but one of which surgeons should be aware.*

Chen J, Wang X, Bai W, Shen X, Yuan W. Prevalence of heterotopic ossification after cervical total disc arthroplasty: a meta-analysis. Eur Spine J 2011

> *The authors performed a meta-analysis to determine the incidence of HO after CDA. They found the prevalence of HO to be 44.6% at 1 year and 58.2% at 2 years. The prevalence of severe HO was 11.1% and 16.7% at 1 and 2 years, respectively. The clinical significance of HO has not been established.*

Garrido BJ, Wilhite J, Nakano M, et al. Adjacent-level cervical ossification after Bryan cervical disc arthroplasty compared with anterior cervical discectomy and fusion. J Bone Joint Surg Am 2011;93(13):1185–1189

> *The authors compared 21 patients who had undergone CDA to 25 patients who had ACDF. The ACDF group showed significantly higher rates of adjacent-segment ossification at both 2 and 4 years.*

McAfee PC, Cappuccino A, Cunningham BW, et al. Lower incidence of dysphagia with cervical arthroplasty compared with ACDF in a prospective randomized clinical trial. J Spinal Disord Tech 2010;23(1):1–8

> *The authors evaluated the incidence of dysphagia among 251 patients randomized to ACDF or CDA. CDA resulted in significantly lower rates of dysphagia at 3 and 12 months postoperatively.*

Upadhyaya CD, Wu JC, Trost G, et al. Analysis of the three United States Food and Drug Administration investigational device exemption cervical arthroplasty trials. J Neurosurg Spine 2011

> *The authors performed meta-analysis of the three IDE trials comparing CDA with ACDF, with 2-year follow up. They concluded that both techniques resulted in excellent neurological improvement but that there was a higher rate of revision surgery following ACDF. There was a trend toward lower rates of adjacent-segment disease at 2 years with arthroplasty. It should be noted that all of these studies are industry sponsored.*

Many different TDR prostheses have been created, with varying degrees of constraint. The motion across the intervertebral disk space can be classified with six degrees of freedom, with rotation and translation occurring in all three axes. The L5–S1 disk has the highest level of freedom of motion, averaging 19.6 degrees. With rostral progression, the freedom of motion decreases, with L1–L2 averaging 12.7 degrees.[6,7] The initial attempts to replicate this motion were reported in the 1960s, when Fernstrom implanted stainless steel spheres into the disk space. This implant fell out of favor because of reported high failure rates. In the 1980s the Stefee disk was introduced, consisting of metal/plastic plates with rubber interfaces. This prosthesis would eventually be discontinued secondary to catastrophic failure of the rubber core.[8] Modern TDR constructs rely on either a metal on ultra-high-molecular-weight polyethylene (UHMWPE) interface or a metal-on-metal interface. Both the Charite TDR (Depuy Spine, Raynham, MA) and Pro-Disc-L TDR (Synthes Spine, West Chester, PA) have been approved for clinical use in the United States. Both consist of two chrome-cobalt endplates interfacing with a UHMWPE core. While the Charite TDR is approved only for single-level arthroplasty (L4–L5 or L5–S1), the Pro-Disc-L is approved for one- to two-level replacements from L3 to S1. The Maverick (Medtronic, Memphis, TN) and Flexicore TDR are two metal-on-metal constructs; the Maverick has not entered the U.S. market because of ongoing patent litigation.

Patient selection for TDR is paramount, as the current indications for the TDR preclude the majority of fusion candidates. It has been estimated that anywhere from 0% to 25% of all fusion candidates meet the criteria for a TDR.[5,9] According to Bertagnoli and Kumar, the ideal candidate for a TDR is a patient with refractory low back pain of discogenic origin at a single disk level with the involved disk having a height of 4 mm or greater.[10] The patient should also have no neurologic deficits and have an intact posterior column. The use of TDR should be avoided in patients presenting with advanced facet arthrosis, degenerative scoliosis, lytic spondylolithesis, and spondylolithesis that is greater than Grade 1. Other contraindications include active systemic/local infection, poor bone stock, spinal stenosis from bony components, and component spatial incompatibility. Furthermore, a TDR will result in an increased sacrovertebral angle; this phenomenon does not occur when a lordotic interbody construct is placed in an anterior lumbar interbody fusion (ALIF).

 Workup

Physical Examination

All patients who may be considered a candidate for a TDR should undergo a thorough neurologic examination. Inspection begins with gait analysis, checking for any gait disturbance, waddling, or antalgic gait. The skin overlying the spine should be inspected for any evidence of dimpling.

Sensation should be inspected along the lumbar/sacral dermatomes, followed by testing motor function of at least one muscle group per myotome. Deep tendon reflexes, clonus, and the presence of tension signs should all be tested.

Spinal Imaging

The initial workup should include anteroposterior (AP) and lateral radiographs to evaluate for any bony abnormalities. Radiographs will give details regarding scoliosis, spondylolisthesis, lysis, facet arthrosis, pars defects, spina bifida occulta, osteophyte formation, and calcification of the disk. Magnetic resonance imaging (MRI) is excellent in evaluation of the facet joint capsule and the level of disk degeneration. A computed tomography (CT) scan will give greater detail regarding the bony anatomy if needed after review of plain radiographs. In patients over the age of 50, consideration should be given to obtaining a dual-energy X-ray absorptiometry (DEXA) scan to evaluate for osteoporosis. The role of diskogram/diskoblock is controversial, although many surgeons require a concordant diskogram at the level of a degenerated disk as a prerequisite for surgical intervention.

Operative

The surgical approach for placing a TDR is via the anterior trans/retroperitoneal approach. Both approaches have acceptable safety profiles; however, the retroperitoneal approach has been reported to be associated with a lower incidence of retrograde ejection, peritoneal adhesions, and postoperative ileus compared with the anterior approach.[11] Depending on the construct design and insertion method, implanting a TDR may require a larger incision and greater mobilization of the vessels than a comparable ALIF procedure. Insertion of the construct is often guided with AP and lateral fluoroscopy to ensure correct placement and seating of the implant. The implant should be placed flush with the posterior edge of the vertebral body to emulate the physiologic center of rotation of the lumbar segment most closely.[12]

 # Outcome

Currently, there are 16 prospective comparative cohort studies and two randomized control trials involving the safety and efficacy of lumbar TDR versus lumbar arthrodesis.[13] In 2005, Blumenthal et al. reported the 2-year results of the FDA investigational device exemption (IDE) trial of the Charite TDR. This was a randomized controlled trial with greater than 90% follow-up.[14] They found that the TDR group reported greater satisfaction at 2 years and better visual analog scale (VAS) and ODI scores at 1 year compared with the fusion cohort. The TDR group also had a shorter hospital stay and faster recovery relative to the fusion group. Complications were similar, with no significant differences.

Similarly, in 2007 Zigler et al. reported the 2-year data of the FDA IDE trial involving the ProDisc-L.[15] At 2 years the ProDisc-L cohort had higher ODI and VAS scores compared with the fusion group. The arthroplasty group also had a shorter operative time, hospital stay, and lower estimated blood loss (EBL).[15]

Guyer et al. in 2009 published the 5-year results of the Charite TDR FDA IDE trial.[16] Only 44% of the original cohort patients were included. The overall success at 5 years was 58% for the Charite group and 51% for the fusion group;

this was statistically significant. The ODI, VAS pain scores, and Short Form 36 (SF-36) scores were comparable between both groups; however, the TDR group had a substantially higher return-to-work rate compared with the fusion group (65.6% versus 46.5%).

Lamaire et al. in 2005 reported minimum 10-year follow-up results in 100 patients treated with Charite TDR.[17] He reported a greater than 90% return-to-work rate and 10% poor result rate.

Complications

Lumbar TDR complications can be categorized as related to the surgical approach, prosthesis, infection, or miscellaneous. Surgical approach–related complications include injury to the great vessels, nerve root injury, and retrograde ejaculation. Prosthesis-related complications include implant subsidence, endplate fracture, and dislocation of the prosthesis. Prosthesis dislocation is a catastrophic complication, with a reported prevalence ranging from 0% to 25%, with the risk of dislocation substantially increasing with multilevel surgery.[18–21] As with most anterior spinal surgeries, the infection risk is low; however, other complications, such as heterotopic ossification (HO), spontaneous fusion, prosthesis loosening, facet arthrosis, and osteolysis, have up to a 20% prevalence among patients.[22] In some series the prevalence of HO can be as high as 30%.[23] Interestingly, the presence of HO has not been shown to affect the overall clinical outcome: the ODI scores among patients with HO were no different from those without.[23] Revision of a TDR is a daunting task. The most feared major complication associated with revision surgery is injury to the great vessels that can occur while dissecting through scar tissue or while mobilizing the great vessels with retractors. The incidence of great vessel damage during revision surgeries has been reported to approach 17%.[24]

Although modern lumbar TDR constructs have limited long-term outcome data, the short-term data are promising. In select patients with CLBP and DDD, TDR may provide an alternative to fusion. In the two large FDA IDE TDR head-to-head inferiority studies, the TDR group reported slightly better patient satisfaction scores and higher return-to-work rates versus arthrodesis.[25] Objectively, TDR provides an operation that may result in lower blood loss, shorter intraoperative times, and shorter hospital stays compared with anterior arthrodesis.[26]

With the strict and narrow indications for TDR, only a handful of patients with lumbar DDD will be candidates. However, in this small subset patient population, a TDR represents a viable alternative to interbody fusion. Long-term outcomes will eventually shed light on the incidence of adjacent-segment disease with TDR versus fusion.

References

1. Fischgrund JS, Montgomery DM. Diagnosis and treatment of discogenic low back pain. Orthop Rev 1993;22(3):311–318
2. Schwarzer AC, Aprill CN, Derby R, Fortin J, Kine G, Bogduk N. The prevalence and clinical features of internal disc disruption in patients with chronic low back pain. Spine 1995;20(17):1878–1883

3. Fritzell B. Detection of adverse events: what are the current sensitivity limits during clinical development? Vaccine 2001;20(Suppl 1):S47–S48
4. Fernström U. Arthroplasty with intercorporal endoprothesis in herniated disc and in painful disc. Acta Chir Scand Suppl 1966;357:154–159
5. Wong DA, Annesser B, Birney T, et al. Incidence of contraindications to total disc arthroplasty: a retrospective review of 100 consecutive fusion patients with a specific analysis of facet arthrosis. Spine J 2007;7(1):5–11
6. Yoshioka T, Tsuji H, Hirano N, Sainoh S. Motion characteristic of the normal lumbar spine in young adults: instantaneous axis of rotation and vertebral center motion analyses. J Spinal Disord 1990;3(2):103–113
7. Pearcy MJ, Bogduk N. Instantaneous axes of rotation of the lumbar intervertebral joints. Spine 1988;13(9):1033–1041
8. Enker P, Steffee A, Mcmillin C, Keppler L, Biscup R, Miller S. Artificial disc replacement. Preliminary report with a 3-year minimum follow-up. Spine 1993;18(8):1061–1070
9. Huang RC, Lim MR, Girardi FP, Cammisa FP Jr. The prevalence of contraindications to total disc replacement in a cohort of lumbar surgical patients. Spine 2004;29(22):2538–2541
10. Bertagnoli R, Kumar S. Indications for full prosthetic disc arthroplasty: a correlation of clinical outcome against a variety of indications. Eur Spine J 2002;11(Suppl 2):S131–S136
11. Bendo JA, Quirno M, Errico T, Spivak JM, Goldstein J. A comparison of two retroperitoneal surgical approaches for total disc arthroplasty of the lumbar spine. Spine 2008;33(2):205–209
12. Dooris AP, Goel VK, Grosland NM, Gilbertson LG, Wilder DG. Load-sharing between anterior and posterior elements in a lumbar motion segment implanted with an artificial disc. Spine 2001;26(6):E122–E129
13. van den Eerenbeemt KD, Ostelo RW, van Royen BJ, Peul WC, van Tulder MW. Total disc replacement surgery for symptomatic degenerative lumbar disc disease: a systematic review of the literature. Eur Spine J 2010;19(8):1262–1280
14. Blumenthal S, McAfee PC, Guyer RD, et al. A prospective, randomized, multicenter Food and Drug Administration investigational device exemptions study of lumbar total disc replacement with the Charite artificial disc versus lumbar fusion: part I: evaluation of clinical outcomes. Spine 2005;30(14):1565–1575, discussion E387–E391
15. Zigler J, Delamarter R, Spivak JM, et al. Results of the prospective, randomized, multicenter Food and Drug Administration investigational device exemption study of the ProDisc-L total disc replacement versus circumferential fusion for the treatment of 1-level degenerative disc disease. Spine 2007;32(11):1155–1162, discussion 1163
16. Guyer RD, McAfee PC, Banco RJ, et al. Prospective, randomized, multicenter Food and Drug Administration investigational device exemption study of lumbar total disc replacement with the Charite artificial disc versus lumbar fusion: five-year follow-up. Spine J 2009;9(5):374–386
17. Lemaire JP, Carrier H, Sariali H, Skalli W, Lavaste F. Clinical and radiological outcomes with the Charité artificial disc: a 10-year minimum follow-up. J Spinal Disord Tech 2005;18(4):353–359
18. Guyer RD, Geisler FH, Blumenthal SL, McAfee PC, Mullin BB. Effect of age on clinical and radiographic outcomes and adverse events following 1-level lumbar arthroplasty after a minimum 2-year follow-up. J Neurosurg Spine 2008;8(2):101–107
19. Di Silvestre M, Bakaloudis G, Lolli F, Vommaro F, Parisini P. Two-level total lumbar disc replacement. Eur Spine J 2009;18(Suppl 1):64–70
20. Geisler FH, Guyer RD, Blumenthal SL, et al. Patient selection for lumbar arthroplasty and arthrodesis: the effect of revision surgery in a controlled, multicenter, randomized study. J Neurosurg Spine 2008;8(1):13–16
21. Geisler FH, Guyer RD, Blumenthal SL, et al. Effect of previous surgery on clinical outcome following 1-level lumbar arthroplasty. J Neurosurg Spine 2008;8(2):108–114
22. Park CK, Ryu KS, Jee WH. Degenerative changes of discs and facet joints in lumbar total disc replacement using ProDisc II: minimum two-year follow-up. Spine 2008;33(16):1755–1761
23. Park SJ, Kang KJ, Shin SK, Chung SS, Lee CS. Heterotopic ossification following lumbar total disc replacement. Int Orthop 2011;35(8):1197–1201
24. McAfee PC, Geisler FH, Saiedy SS, et al. Revisability of the Charite artificial disc replacement: analysis of 688 patients enrolled in the U.S. IDE study of the Charite Artificial Disc. Spine 2006;31(11):1217–1226

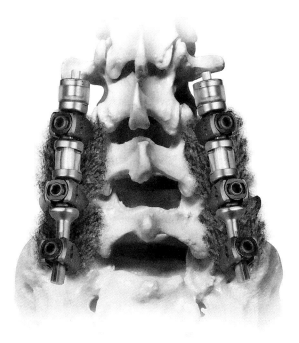

Fig. 64.2 The Transition system consists of titanium pedicle screws with elastic spacers. (Used with permission from Globus Medical, Audubon, PA.)

A second prospective study followed 19 patients to a mean of 52 months. Patients showed maintenance of pain relief and walking distance improvement with no progression of spondylolisthesis, despite three patients showing radiographic signs of screw loosening. One patient showed screw breakage and instability at 4 years. Interestingly, 47% of patients had adjacent-level degeneration on radiographs at 4 years.[9]

Both the Dynesys and Transition systems have been FDA approved for use only as adjuncts to thoracolumbar fusion. Use of either system as a non-fusion construct is considered a non-FDA-approved, off-label application. The Dynesys was rejected by an FDA panel in November of 2009 as a stand-alone non-fusion device. There are currently no available clinical data on the Transition device.

Conclusions

Posterior non-fusion lumbar devices are continuing to evolve. All of the implants mentioned in this chapter may play a role in the future of spinal surgery. To date, however, the best-studied and most frequently used implants are the interspinous process spacers. Further data on facet replacements and pedicle screw–based soft stabilization systems will be necessary to define the safety and efficacy of these devices.

References

1. Lindsey DP, Swanson KE, Fuchs P, Hsu KY, Zucherman JF, Yerby SA. The effects of an interspinous implant on the kinematics of the instrumented and adjacent levels in the lumbar spine. Spine 2003;28(19):2192–2197
2. Swanson KE, Lindsey DP, Hsu KY, Zucherman JF, Yerby SA. The effects of an interspinous implant on intervertebral disc pressures. Spine 2003;28(1):26–32
3. Zucherman JF, Hsu KY, Hartjen CA, et al. A multicenter, prospective, randomized trial evaluating the X STOP interspinous process decompression system for the treatment of neurogenic intermittent claudication: two-year follow-up results. Spine 2005;30(12): 1351–1358
4. Kuchta J, Sobottke R, Eysel P, Simons P. Two-year results of interspinous spacer (X-Stop) implantation in 175 patients with neurologic intermittent claudication due to lumbar spinal stenosis. Eur Spine J 2009;18(6):823–829
5. Zhu Q, Larson CR, Sjovold SG, et al. Biomechanical evaluation of the Total Facet Arthroplasty System: 3-dimensional kinematics. Spine 2007;32(1):55–62
6. Schulte TL, Hurschler C, Haversath M, et al. The effect of dynamic, semi-rigid implants on the range of motion of lumbar motion segments after decompression. Eur Spine J 2008;17(8):1057–1065
7. Niosi CA, Wilson DC, Zhu Q, Keynan O, Wilson DR, Oxland TR. The effect of dynamic posterior stabilization on facet joint contact forces: an in vitro investigation. Spine 2008;33(1): 19–26
8. Stoll TM, Dubois G, Schwarzenbach O. The dynamic neutralization system for the spine: a multicenter study of a novel non-fusion system. Eur Spine J 2002;11(Suppl 2):S170–S178
9. Schaeren S, Broger I, Jeanneret B. Minimum four-year follow-up of spinal stenosis with degenerative spondylolisthesis treated with decompression and dynamic stabilization. Spine 2008;33(18):E636–E642

Suggested Readings

Zucherman JF, Hsu KY, Hartjen CA, et al. A multicenter, prospective, randomized trial evaluating the X STOP interspinous process decompression system for the treatment of neurogenic intermittent claudication: two-year follow-up results. Spine 2005;30(12):1351–1358

> *This prospective randomized trial, conducted by the inventors of the X-Stop, demonstrated superior outcomes with the X-Stop compared to nonsurgical treatments.*

Stoll TM, Dubois G, Schwarzenbach O. The dynamic neutralization system for the spine: a multicenter study of a novel non-fusion system. Eur Spine J 2002;11(Suppl 2):S170–S178

> *This prospective multicenter trial from Switzerland attempted to establish the safety and efficacy of the Dynesys system for a variety of lumbar instability conditions.*

XIV Spinal Imaging

Back Pain ± Limb Symptoms

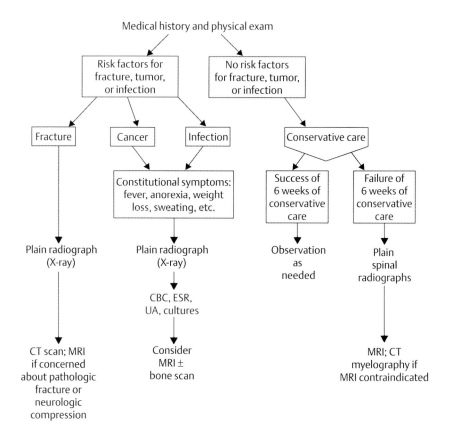

CBC, complete blood count; CT, computed tomography; ESR, erythrocyte sedimentation rate; MRI, magnetic resonance imaging; UA, urinalysis

65

Imaging for Back Pain and Spinal Infection

Gregory Gebauer, Chadi A. Tannoury, Michael A. Pahl, and D. Greg Anderson

Of the advances that have been made in recent years in spine care, none is more significant than the advances in spinal imaging. Modern imaging studies improve the diagnostic capability of the spine surgeon and allow a more targeted approach to spinal pathology. Imaging studies reviewed in conjunction with the history and physical examination play a role in establishing the diagnosis of many spinal conditions.

Classification

Although there is no specific classification for spinal imaging, the following tests are discussed: plain radiographs, computed tomography (CT) scanning, CT myelography, magnetic resonance imaging (MRI), and bone scans.

Workup

The workup of a patient with spinal complaints must begin with a thorough history and physical examination. Only then can a differential diagnosis for the patient's problem be considered and a rationale for workup be suggested. Imaging studies are an important part of that workup. However, imaging studies should never be used as the sole means for diagnosing spinal conditions, as most modern imaging modalities have the potential to reveal pathology that is not symptomatic or pertinent to the patient's complaints.

Spinal Imaging

Plain radiographs are generally the first study to be ordered for most patients. They are less expensive than MRI or CT and provide information on the spinal alignment, degenerative changes, and bone quality (**Fig. 65.1A–C**). They are helpful in excluding fractures, deformities, and destructive bony lesions. They can also show soft-tissue shadows that are helpful in some cases. Dynamic flexion-extension views are helpful in ruling out instability of the spinal segments. Plain radiographs are relatively insensitive for early infection or metastasis and do not show soft-tissue pathology, such as a disk herniation.

MRI has become the advanced imaging modality of choice for most spinal conditions requiring more than plain radiographs. MRI provides excellent detail of the hard and soft tissue and demonstrates the spinal canal, neural elements, ligaments, disks, and paravertebral tissues in addition to the skeletal structures (**Fig. 65.2**). MRI can be used to define early infections and metastasis and may demonstrate occult fractures of the vertebral body. In the postoperative setting, MRI is helpful in defining many sources of pain, including infection and retained pathology, although the early (first 3 months) MRI studies done following surgery may be difficult to interpret accurately because of postoperative edema. In this setting, MRI is often performed with gadolinium to help delineate between scar, infection, and retained disk material. MRI has limited value for defining a fracture in cortical bone (posterior element fracture) and is contraindicated in patients with pacemakers, certain metallic implants (cochlear implants), metallic fragments in the eyes, and/or aneurysm clips. MRI may demonstrate significant artifact when used around large metallic implants, particularly if the implants are made from metals other than titanium alloy.

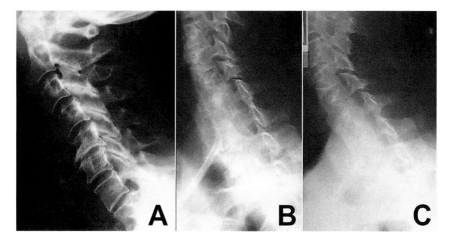

Fig. 65.1 Lateral plain radiograph **(A)** shows degenerative changes at the level of the cervical spine. The oblique views **(B,C)** help in assessing spondylosis at the neural foramen levels.

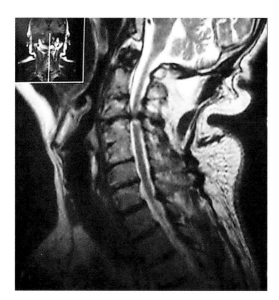

Fig. 65.2 MRI scan shows spinal canal narrowing at a single and multiple levels: the cord is compressed anteriorly by the herniated disk materials and posteriorly by the infolded ligamentum flavum and posterior element degenerative changes. Note the signal changes within the cord (myelomalacia), denoting myelopathy.

CT scans are excellent at providing information about bony structures, including osteoarthritis, ossification of posterior longitudinal ligament, bony canal stenosis, and pathologies around the lateral recess and neural foramen. When CT is used with myelographic contrast, the resulting CT myelograms are an ideal way of demonstrating stenosis of the neural elements. CT myelography is more invasive than MRI scans, so it is often used when a patient is unable to undergo MRI because of a pacemakers or other conditions.

Diskography and post-diskogram CT may be useful in defining whether pain is emanating from a particular intervertebral disk (**Fig. 65.3**). A provocative diskogram is performed on an awake patient who is instructed to grade the severity of pain and verbalize whether pain at the time of disk injection is identical to the "usual pain," indicating that the disk is a possible source of the pain. To be useful, a painless control disk level should be present. Following the diskogram, a CT scan can help to determine the morphology of the disk and may show annular disruption with dye leakage. Studies have shown that provocative diskography is prone to "false-positive" interpretations, and thus, these tests should be interpreted with caution, looking at all the available information.

Bone scanning and single-photon emission computed tomography (SPECT) imaging are useful for conditions with an increased bone turnover, such as osteoarthritis, infection, tumors, or an occult fracture. Because bone scanning is nonspecific, this test rarely provides a specific diagnosis in isolation but is useful in conjunction with other tests. Bone scans can be particularly helpful as screening tools to identify the locations of metastatic disease or for determining whether compression fractures are acute or chronic for patients who cannot undergo MRI.

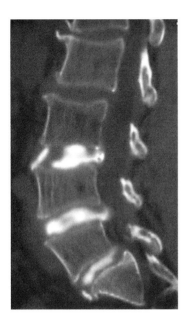

Fig. 65.3 Diskogram is used to determine whether a degenerative process is the cause of a patient's pain (discogenic low back pain). It provides an anatomical definition of the herniated disk levels. The image shows three-level disease (L3–L4, L4–L5, and L5–S1).

Outcomes

The outcome of spinal diagnosis and treatment is markedly enhanced by the use of imaging studies.

Complications

Plain radiographs, CT scanning, and bone scanning produce ionizing radiation that should be considered. MRI is generally safe, although claustrophobia and the presence of metallic objects in the body must be considered. Myelography is associated with an incidence of infection, spinal headache, neurologic deficit, arachnoiditis, and allergic reactions, although the incidence is much lower now that nonionic contrast agents are utilized. Contrast, both for CT scans and MRI, should be used with caution in patients with renal impairment because of the risk of accelerating their renal disease.

Suggested Readings

Allgayer B, Frank A, Daller D, von Einsiedel H, Trappe A. [Magnetic resonance tomography (MRT) in the diagnosis of Failed Back Surgery Syndrome (FBSS)]. Rofo 1993;158(2):160–165

> *MRI findings were compared with surgical observations. MRI had a sensitivity of 94% in diagnosing recurrent prolapse, a specificity of 100%, and accuracy of 94%.*

Coskun E, Süzer T, Topuz O, Zencir M, Pakdemirli E, Tahta K. Relationships between epidural fibrosis, pain, disability, and psychological factors after lumbar disc surgery. Eur Spine J 2000;9(3):218–223

> *The purpose of this prospective study was to evaluate the relationships among the severity of epidural fibrosis, psychological factors, back pain, and disability after lumbar disk surgery.*

Gemmel F, De Winter F, Van Laere K, Vogelaers D, Uyttendaele D, Dierckx RA. 99mTc ciprofloxacin imaging for the diagnosis of infection in the postoperative spine. Nucl Med Commun 2004;25(3):277–283

> *The low uptake of technetium-99m ciprofloxacin into normal bone marrow, combined with its claimed bacterial specificity, makes it an ideal candidate for evaluating postoperative spinal infections.*

Gundry CR, Fritts HM. Magnetic resonance imaging of the musculoskeletal system: the spine. Clin Orthop Relat Res 1998; (346):262–278

> *The most common indication for postoperative imaging is in the distinction between postoperative fibrosis and recurrent disk herniation. MRI is invaluable in the assessment of potential causes of failed back surgery syndrome, such as postoperative infection, arachnoiditis, and adjacent-segment degeneration.*

Palestro CJ. Radionuclide imaging after skeletal interventional procedures. Semin Nucl Med 1995;25(1):3–14

> *Bone scintigraphy, especially SPECT, is of considerable value in the workup of patients with persistent back pain after spinal surgery. Postoperatively, spinal fusion is characterized by diffusely increased uptake of radiotracer in the fused area, whereas focally increased uptake has been shown to be related to bony nonunion.*

Ross JS. Magnetic resonance imaging of the postoperative spine. Semin Musculoskelet Radiol 2000;4(3):281–291

> *This article reviews standard imaging protocols, the normal postoperative appearance of the spine, and the characteristic imaging findings for each of the abnormal postoperative conditions.*

Spinal Fusion

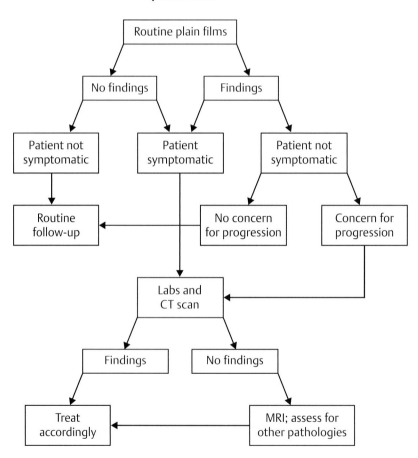

Due to the lack of an ideal imaging modality to diagnose pseudarthrosis, multiple imaging modalities are usually used when clinically indicated.[1] This algorithm can be used when deciding on an imaging strategy.

66

Spinal Imaging for Pseudarthrosis

Daniel J. Blizzard, Qusai Hammouri, Joshua William Hustedt, and Jonathan Newman Grauer

Failure of spinal arthrodesis or fusion leads to a condition called pseudarthrosis. Though the term literally means "false joint," it is commonly used in clinical practice to refer to nonunion at greater than 1 year following the index surgery.[2] Pseudarthrosis incidence rates following spinal arthrodesis reported in the literature range from 0% to 56%, varying with site, approach, fusion material, instrumentation, and year of the study.[3,4] The true incidence, however, is likely underestimated by the literature, as many patients with pseudarthrosis remain asymptomatic. More importantly, the diagnosis of pseudarthrosis in the absence of symptoms is not necessarily an indication for surgical revision.

Although many imaging techniques are available for evaluation of pseudarthrosis, none is perfect, and no universally agreed-upon imaging criterion exists. Open surgical exploration remains the "gold standard" for the diagnosis of pseudarthrosis.

Classification

Heggeness and Esses[5] classified patients with spinal pseudarthrosis according to the appearance of the fusion on imaging studies into four categories: atrophic, transverse, shingle, and complex (**Table 66.1**).

Workup

History

Pain is the most common complaint associated with pseudarthrosis. Pain may be persistent from before the procedure, but most commonly pain is noted to recur after a period of temporary relief around the time of surgery. This temporary period of improvement (often referred to as a honeymoon period) is

XV Spinal Monitoring

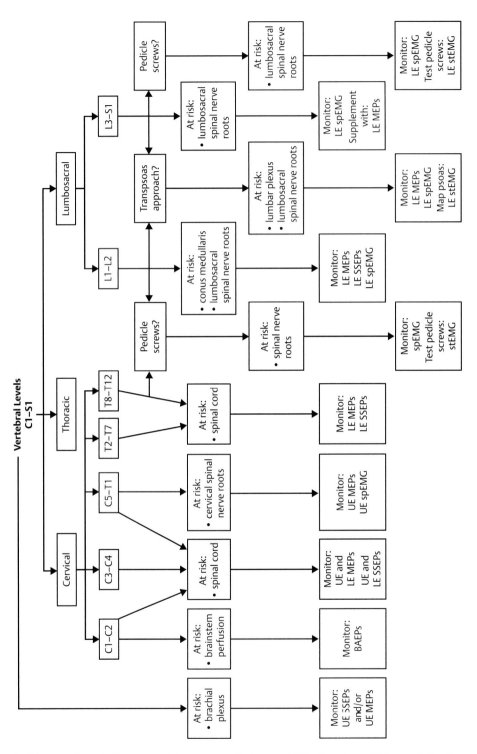

Decision tree for selecting appropriate neuromonitoring modalities based on which neural structures and pathways are at risk for iatrogenic injury as a function of vertebral level. UE, upper extremity; LE, lower extremity; BAEPs, brainstem auditory evoked potentials

67

Intraoperative Neuromonitoring During Spine Surgery

Vidya M. Bhalodia, Anthony K. Sestokas, and Daniel M. Schwartz

Intraoperative neurophysiologic monitoring (IONM) is the continuous use of electrophysiologic recording techniques to identify changes in the functional status of neural elements (spinal cord, spinal nerve roots, peripheral nerves) at risk for iatrogenic injury during the course of spinal surgery. It permits detection of changes in neural function early enough to initiate timely interventional measures, thereby minimizing the risk of postoperative neural deficit. In general, IONM is warranted whenever the cost of potential complications (e.g., medicolegal, extended hospital stay, rehabilitation, quality of life change) outweighs that of intraoperative monitoring fees.

The monitoring techniques used most commonly during spinal surgery include (1) transcranial electrical motor evoked potentials (tceMEPs), (2) mixed-nerve somatosensory evoked potentials (SSEPs), (3) spontaneous electromyography (spEMG), and (4) stimulated electromyography (stEMG). These individual modalities should be combined to form a neuromonitoring battery that provides broad-scale neurophysiologic surveillance of the spinal cord motor and sensory tracts, nerve roots, and peripheral nerves/brachial plexus, which are potentially at risk for neural injury.

Transcranial Electrical Motor Evoked Potentials

TceMEPs are myogenic responses elicited by the application of electrical stimulation to the brain. Electrical pulse trains are applied through subdermal scalp electrodes that overlie motor cortex. Following depolarization of cortical neurons, efferent neural signals course down the internal capsule to the caudal medulla, where the majority of corticospinal tract (CST) fibers decussate and descend into the spinal cord motor pathways. CST axons then enter the spinal cord gray matter, interact with spinal cord interneurons, and go on to synapse with alpha motor neurons. Alpha motor neuron axons exit through their corresponding neural foramina as spinal nerve roots that innervate skeletal muscle.

523

Somatosensory Evoked Potentials

Mixed-nerve somatosensory evoked potentials (SSEPs) are elicited by electrical stimulation applied to a peripheral nerve (e.g., ulnar, median, posterior tibial, peroneal), which initiates an afferent neural volley that enters the spinal cord via the lumbosacral plexus. The afferent volley ascends within the posterior sensory column and medial lemniscal pathways of the spinal cord and brainstem, respectively, and is relayed from the thalamus to the cortex via the internal capsule. Electrodes placed anywhere along this pathway, such as over the cervical spine (C2), and at multiple scalp locations, are used to record the volume conducted evoked potentials.

Electromyography

Intraoperative electromyography differs from that used in the electrodiagnostic laboratory in several ways. The conventional electrodiagnostic EMG is based on a quantitative and qualitative analysis of motor unit potentials recorded from an insulated, concentric needle electrode inserted into muscle at varying depths with the target muscle at rest, and again in a state of voluntary contraction. Diagnosis of neuromuscular disorders or nerve root injury is then made on the basis of pattern recognition for spontaneous motor unit activity, as well as calculation of duration, amplitude, and shape of the motor unit potential relative to a laboratory norm.

While intraoperative spontaneous electromyography also involves the recording of electrical activity produced by skeletal muscle, its purpose is not to diagnose neuromuscular disease/disorder, but to identify acute irritation of a spinal nerve root secondary to mechanical contact, direct traction, heat dispersion from electrocautery, or other such noxious stimuli that trigger nerve root depolarization. The compound muscle action potential elicited by irritation of the innervating nerve root is recorded using short, uninsulated, monopolar needle electrodes inserted subdermally into muscle prior to surgery. No attempt is made to record motor unit force or to assess alterations in spontaneous activity with muscle at rest and under voluntary contraction, as with the awake patient in the electrodiagnostic setting.

Although intraoperative monitoring of spontaneous electromyographic activity (spEMG) allows for real-time identification of spinal nerve root irritation from mechanical contact, acute tractional force, or heat dispersion, it is insensitive to nerve root ischemia, sharp dissection, or the application of slow progressive traction.

The spine surgeon should be aware that recording of spontaneous EMG activity alone cannot assess the functional integrity of the spinal nerve root. Rather, its primary use is to identify presence or absence of nerve root irritation. Consequently, it may be prudent to augment spEMG with intermittent recording of tceMEPs for surgeries in which individual nerve roots are at particular risk for mechanical or ischemic injury.

The counterpart to spEMG is stimulated electromyography (stEMG or triggered EMG). Stimulated electromyography makes use of the same recording electrodes as spEMG to detect activation of motor fibers. Instead of detecting activation of the nerve from surgical mechanical force or heat transfer, however, stEMG detects activation following direct or indirect electrical stimulation using a hand-held, sterile, monopolar probe that is insulated down to the tip. Indirect stimulation consists of an electrical stimulus applied through instrumentation such as a pedicle screw or K-wire, or stimulation through tumor tissue or muscle. The minimum amount of electrical current required to elicit a recordable compound muscle action potential from an innervated myotome represents the depolarization threshold. This threshold value can then be used to make inferences about: (1) the proximity of the neural element to the plane of surgical dissection (e.g., during trans-psoas approach to the lumbar plexus), (2) proximity of the closest nerve root, (3) functional nerve root integrity, (4) presence of medial pedicle wall violation from pedicle screw encroachment, (5) motor versus sensory neural elements, (6) distortion of normal nerve root anatomy by tumor.

One of the more time-honored applications of stEMG during lumbar spine surgery is in identification of medial pedicle wall fracture. Compound muscle action potentials triggered at screw stimulation intensities of less than 5 mA correlate highly with presence of medial cortical breach, based on the premise of decreased resistance to the flow of electrical energy to adjacent nerve through the fracture site versus intact bone. stEMG is not sensitive, however, to identifying lateral pedicle wall fracture.

It is essential that the surgeon use care when stimulating pedicle screws. Inadvertent stimulator contact with a retractor, surrounding muscle, or blood produces current shunting, thereby raising the possibility of a false threshold reading. Taking a few extra seconds to ensure that the stimulation site is free of blood, that the stimulator is touching only the hexagonal port or head of the pedicle screw, and that neuromonitoring personnel have an opportunity to record a series of responses at progressively increasing intensity levels can make the difference between an accurate assessment of pedicle wall integrity and a false-negative high-threshold reading.

In recent years, hydroxyapatite-coated pedicle screws have been introduced as a means of increasing pullout strength in dynamic stabilization systems. Unfortunately, these coated screws have high electrical resistance compared with their conventional non-coated counterparts, resulting in shunting of applied electrical current through adjacent soft tissue rather than through the screw shank. The spine surgeon should be aware that use of hydroxyapatite-coated screws will preclude reliable stEMG testing for presence of medial pedicle wall breach.

As with coated screws, questions about the reliability of stEMG also arise when placing percutaneous pedicle screws for lumbar fixation. Here, the use of an insulated sleeve can help isolate surrounding soft tissue from the monopolar stimulator, thereby minimizing the possibility of current shunting.

Recently there has been a surge of interest in the minimally invasive direct or extreme lateral trans-psoas lumbar interbody fusion. This lateral approach requires blunt dissection through the psoas muscle and proximate neural elements of the lumbar plexus. Continuous monitoring with stimulated and spontaneous EMG can help identify approximate location and distance from these neural elements, as well as induced nerve irritation, thereby facilitating safe entry to the intervertebral disk space.

It is important for the spine surgeon to appreciate that stimulated EMG does not provide assessment of lumbar plexus function and, further, cannot detect microvascular changes that may affect nerve conduction during the trans-psoas approach to the disk space. Because of the significant risks associated with mechanical impingement on the lumbar plexus and nerve roots in these cases, as well as the limited direct visualization of neural elements, it is prudent to augment spEMG and stEMG monitoring with intermittent recording of tceMEPs as a means of assessing the integrity of motor conduction. **Figures 67.1** and **67.2** provide supportive evidence for this recommendation by illustrating delayed compromise of nerve root function despite stEMG recordings indicating that nerve root elements were not in immediate proximity to the retractors. Similarly, spEMG did not demonstrate evidence of nerve root irritation as the dilators were passed through psoas muscle and retractors were placed for direct lateral interbody fusion. Despite these negative findings, there was a significant loss of tceMEP amplitude ~45 minutes following placement of psoas muscle dilators, most likely due to ischemic changes from progressive nerve compression.

This example highlights the value of having an experienced surgical neurophysiologist to guide multimodality intraoperative monitoring and emphasizes limitations of automated monitoring devices marketed by some spinal implant manufacturers. An automated monitoring device would have missed this change, placing the patient at potential risk of an unidentified neural injury.

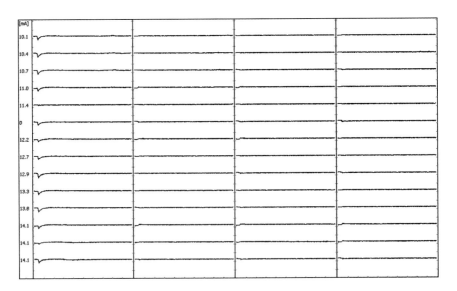

Fig. 67.1 stEMG results showing no evidence of nerve root depolarization following stimulation of retractors during a trans-psoas approach to the L4–L5 disk space.

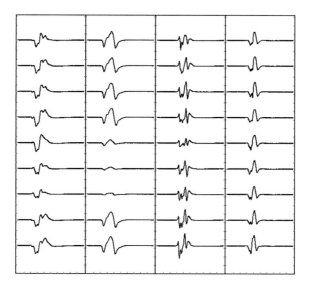

Fig. 67.2   Loss of tceMEP amplitude from right quadriceps muscle 45 minutes following place-ment of psoas muscle retractors despite negative stEMG testing for presence of nearby neural element.

Choice of IONM Modalities

The choice of monitoring modalities utilized during a particular spine surgery depends on the specific neural structures and/or pathways considered to be at risk for iatrogenic injury, as summarized in the decision tree. Prior to the introduction of tceMEPs, mixed nerve somatosensory evoked potentials were the mainstay of neurophysiologic monitoring. Despite the demonstrated high specificity of posterior tibial nerve SSEPs for monitoring of spinal cord function during scoliosis surgery, there exists a definitive risk of false-negative findings. Because SSEPs are mediated by the posterior sensory columns of the spinal cord, they provide only indirect information as to the functional integrity of the anterolateral motor tracts and spinal cord gray matter. In some patients, the vascular supply to the anterior and lateral aspects of the spinal cord may be tenuous, making motor tracts selectively susceptible to ischemic injury. In con-trast to SSEPs, tceMEPs provide a direct measure of corticospinal tract function. tceMEPs have a high specificity and sensitivity for identifying emerging cor-ticospinal tract compromise and should be considered the modality of choice when assessing spinal cord function.

Upper and lower extremity SSEP monitoring plays an important comple-mentary role to tceMEP recordings by facilitating detection of spinal cord dorsal column compromise, evolving positional plexopathy and/or peripheral nerve injury.

Spinal nerve root function has been monitored traditionally using a combination of spontaneous and stimulated electromyography. Spontaneous EMG allows for real-time and continuous assessment of nerve root irritation or traction; however, it does not provide any measure of functional root integrity. Moreover, spEMG is insensitive to slowly developing nerve root ischemic injury as well as sharp root dissection.

In those procedures where the spinal nerve root is exposed, it is possible to assess functional integrity via direct nerve root stimulation and recording of a compound muscle action potential from innervated myotomes. Alternatively, recording of tceMEPs also can provide valuable information as to the actual health of a nerve root. While some surgeons are reluctant to monitor tceMEPs during most lumbar interbody fusion surgeries, it is advisable at least to consider this type of monitoring for patients who present with preexisting lower-extremity weakness or other symptoms reflecting nerve root functional compromise. In these cases, the probability of false-negative EMG results is increased considerably.

How to Use Neuromonitoring Information

Effective use of information communicated by monitoring personnel is among the most challenging aspects of IONM during spine surgery. There is a tendency to assume that any loss of neurophysiologic signal amplitude always correlates with paralysis or paresis, without consideration of the underlying physiological causes of the sentinel event. Neurophysiologic changes can be caused by many factors, ranging from the unexpected use of inhalational agents or muscle relaxants, to systemic hypotension, to the more dangerous hypo-perfusion of the spinal cord and/or direct impingement of instrumentation on the spinal cord or nerve root. The professional neurophysiologist should have the ability to correlate and manage neurophysiologic data with anesthetic status, and surgical stage to provide the surgeon with the most accurate information and guidance.

Alterations in neurophysiologic responses during spine surgeries need to be interpreted within the context of neural structures that are presumed to be at risk, as well as the surgical stage. For example, neurophysiologic changes that occur prior to the start of surgical manipulations (e.g., during exposure of the spine) may be caused by global factors, such as hypovolemia/hypotension or anemia. These changes can be readily resolved by identification and correction of the primary cause. While they may not be immediate precursors to irreversible neural injury, these changes should not be left unaddressed, as they may predispose the patient to later neural injury or may mask significant changes later on in the surgical procedure.

Changes that occur during surgical manipulations near the spine need to be interpreted in that context. While global factors still need to be investigated, common causes of neurophysiologic changes include: (1) inadequate spinal cord perfusion due to lowered mean arterial pressure states, (2) transient disruption of spinal cord biochemistry (sodium-potassium gradient) following mechanical force, as can occur during impaction of an interbody fusion graft, or insult from a migrating surgical instrument, or (3) irritation or traction of a spinal nerve (e.g., during decompression). Frequent testing of IONM modalities during the surgical course can be beneficial in identifying which of a series of maneuvers contributed to the neurophysiologic manifestation.

If a neurophysiologic change is correlated to a particular surgical maneuver (e.g., correction of scoliosis deformity or insertion of interbody cage), it may be advisable to reverse the maneuver, increase blood pressure, and await the return of homeostasis. In many of these situations, neurophysiologic signals will begin to improve within 15–20 minutes, with the anticipation that the patient will emerge from surgery with no new-onset neurologic deficit.

On the very rare occasions that neurophysiologic changes do not resolve despite intervention, the decision to continue, alter, or terminate the procedure should not be taken without careful consideration of all potential consequences for the patient's well-being, including the possibility of postoperative neural deficits.

This tempered approach will help alleviate surgeon anxiety, avoid overreaction to signal change, and foster better communication between the surgeon and neuromonitoring personnel. To be sure, vascular etiologies for evoked potential amplitude changes, such as those attributable to application of distractive forces to correct a spinal deformity or changes secondary to direct penetrating trauma, such as migration of a pedicle screw in the thoracic canal, are the most serious neuromonitoring events that deserve the surgeon's undivided attention.

Conclusion

Neuromonitoring during spine surgery has become "standard of care" in most hospitals. As with any specialty, the reliability and validity of neuromonitoring for detecting alterations in spinal cord or nerve root function are related directly to the skills of the neuromonitoring specialist, his/her ability to interpret the data within the context of surgery, anesthesia, and hemodynamics, and effectiveness of communication with the surgeon and/or anesthesiologist as to the meaning of neurophysiologic change and need for rescue intervention. Failure on the part of the neuromonitoring specialist to help guide the surgeon's thoughts in this regard can result in a loss of confidence and reduced effectiveness of monitoring. To the contrary, in the proper hands, neuromonitoring has proven highly valuable in minimizing the incidence of neurologic complication during spine surgery.

Suggested Readings

Alemo S, Sayadipour A. Role of intraoperative neurophysiologic monitoring in lumbosacral spine fusion and instrumentation: a retrospective study. World Neurosurg 2010;73(1):72–76, discussion e7

> *This study determined the efficacy of stEMG versus CT for identifying pedicle cortex fracture during instrumented lumbar spine surgery. Results demonstrated that intraoperative stEMG testing of pedicle cortex integrity is a highly effective, accurate, simple, and cost-effective method for detecting pedicle cortex breach during bone screw insertion.*

Bhalodia VM, Sestokas AK, Tomak PR, Schwartz DM. Transcranial electric motor evoked potential detection of compressional peroneal nerve injury in the lateral decubitus position. J Clin Monit Comput 2008;22(4):319–326

> *This case series discuss the application of tceMEPs in identifying position-induced peroneal nerve compression injury during lumbar spine surgery. The authors concluded that whenever there is risk or concern for position-related peripheral nerve injury during spine surgery, tceMEP monitoring should be considered.*

Bose B, Sestokas AK, Schwartz DM. Neurophysiological detection of iatrogenic C-5 nerve deficit during anterior cervical spinal surgery. J Neurosurg Spine 2007;6(5):381–385

> *This retrospective study compared the efficacy of spEMG and tceMEPs in identifying acute-onset C5 nerve root injuries during anterior cervical spine surgery. Results suggested that tceMEPs represented an excellent modality for identifying developing C5 nerve root injury during decompression as compared to conventional neuromonitoring of spEMG activity alone.*

Devlin VJ, Anderson PA, Schwartz DM, Vaughan R. Intraoperative neurophysiologic monitoring: focus on cervical myelopathy and related issues. Spine J 2006;6(6, Suppl):212S–224S

> *This literature review focused on the role of SSEPs, tceMEPs, and EMG in spinal cord and nerve root monitoring during cervical spine surgery. The authors argue for a multimodality approach to neuromonitoring to improve injury detection accuracy.*

Devlin VJ, Schwartz DM. Intraoperative neurophysiologic monitoring during spinal surgery. J Am Acad Orthop Surg 2007;15(9):549–560

> *This article provides an excellent review for spine surgeons as to current multimodality monitoring techniques for intraoperative assessment of spinal cord and nerve during spine surgery. Also discussed are possible mechanisms of neuromonitoring changes, the role of anesthesia, and a description of professional and technical credentials for personnel providing neuromonitoring services.*

Hilibrand AS, Schwartz DM, Sethuraman V, Vaccaro AR, Albert TJ. Comparison of transcranial electric motor and somatosensory evoked potential monitoring during cervical spine surgery. J Bone Joint Surg Am 2004;86-A(6):1248–1253

> *This large series retrospective study compared sensitivity and specificity of tceMEPs and conventional SSEP for detecting impending spinal cord injury during cervical spine surgery. Also investigated was the temporal relationship between intraoperative changes in signal amplitudes for either or both of these neuromonitoring modalities. Results demonstrated that tceMEPs were remarkably more sensitive (100%) for cervical spinal cord injury detection than was SSEP monitoring (25%).*

Schwartz DM, Sestokas AK. A systems-based approach to intraoperative neurophysiological monitoring during spinal surgery. Semin Spine Surg 2002;14:136–145

> *The authors described an algorithmic approach to developing an intraoperative neuromonitoring plan during spine surgery based on predetermination of: (1) the neural structures, pathways, or vascular supplies at risk for iatrogenic injury, (2) the neuromonitoring modalities that can provide continuous surveillance of functional neural integrity of at-risk neural elements, and (3) possible interventional strategies to help reverse emerging injury as shown by altered neural signals on one or more neuromonitoring modalities. Also discussed are the selection of an appropriate anesthetic technique to optimize neurophysiological signal amplitudes, the role of hemodynamics, and criteria for interpretation of neurophysiologic change.*

Schwartz DM, Auerbach JD, Dormans JP, et al. Neurophysiological detection of impending spinal cord injury during scoliosis surgery. J Bone Joint Surg Am 2007;89(11):2440–2449

> *This large series (N = 1121) retrospective study evaluated the differential sensitivities of tceMEPs versus SSEPs in identifying evolving spinal cord injury during surgical correction of adolescent idiopathic scoliosis. Results showed overwhelming evidence in favor of tceMEP monitoring for detection of spinal cord injury, with sensitivity and specificity at 100% versus 45% and 100%, respectively, for SSEPs.*

XVI Miscellaneous Topics

Spinal Cord Stimulation for Failed Back Surgery Syndrome

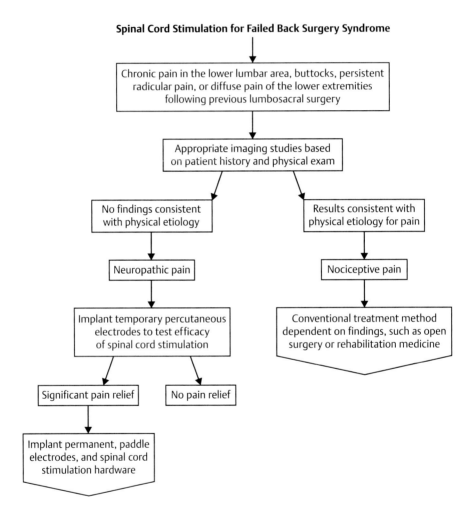

68

Spinal Cord Stimulators for Back Pain

David L. Penn, Chengyuan Wu, Steven M. Falowski, and Ashwini Sharan

Spinal cord stimulation (SCS) is a highly versatile method of treating neuropathic pain that involves delivering therapeutic doses of electrical current from the epidural space into the spinal column to several spinal cord structures, including the dorsal column–medial lemniscal afferent pathway. Electrical stimulation of the large myelinated Aβ afferent fibers involved in the dorsal column system results in ipsilateral tingling paresthesia and causes decreased discomfort and pain sensations. While the mechanisms of SCS are still unclear, leading theories involve the generation of complex electric fields in the epidural space affecting the activity of a large number of structures, including both descending and ascending pathways, which may increase central pain modulation from higher-order central nervous system (CNS) structures. Although SCS may be used to treat many forms of intractable pain, it is most commonly indicated to treat postlaminectomy syndrome, otherwise known as failed back surgery syndrome (FBSS), and complex regional pain syndrome. This chapter focuses on the techniques and issues involved in treating back pain, particularly FBSS, using SCS.

Classification

FBSS is a vaguely defined syndrome that has been used to classify chronic pain localized to the lower lumbar area, pain in the buttocks, persistent radicular pain, or diffuse pain of the lower extremities that occurs after one or more lumbosacral surgeries. Because FBSS is classified by back and leg pain, current literature on SCS efficacy has started to distinguish the locations of pain. While SCS is commonly used to treat low back pain, it has been shown to be more effective in relieving pain in the lower limbs.

Common problems that FBSS may be indicative of are broad and include arachnoiditis, epidural fibrosis, radiculitis, microinstability, recurrent disk herniations, and infection. SCS is best used for neuropathic pain, as opposed to nociceptive pain being induced by physical findings within the spinal column.

Workup

History

Patients suspected of having FBSS present with chronic back pain of neuropathic origin, require analgesics, and are unable to return to work following at least one prior spinal surgery. Obtaining detailed information about the patient's current symptoms is vital to determining the method of treatment that can be used for FBSS. During the history, the examiner should ask specific questions to assess for mechanically induced symptoms. Are the symptoms different or worse with sitting versus standing and relieved with lying down? Do symptoms improve with traction, stretch, or the buoyancy of a pool? Is there a particular sensitivity to pain, implying neuropathic symptoms over nociceptive or mechanical stresses?

Understanding the exact distribution of the back pain is paramount. Many patients may describe the gluteal region as the "back." "Sacroiliac joint pain," "hip pain," and "mid and low back pain" are descriptions in the back, and the response to stimulation varies. SCS therapy is dependent on producing a paresthesia sensation over the painful area. Typically, it is possible to deliver this paresthesia in the gluteal region; however, delivery of the stimulation in the sacroiliac region or to the mid-back above the iliac crest is often difficult.

Other valuable diagnostic information includes the extent of pain relief achieved by surgery and the length of postoperative time in which the patient was pain free. In some patients, careful questioning will reveal that the preoperative symptoms were never relieved with surgery, and this may implicate neuropathic pain from the onset.

Careful psychological screening is important in determining candidacy for SCS, because mood disorders can alter pain perception and reporting; in addition, other psychiatric diseases, major depression, anger, or unrealistic expectations can make patients inappropriate candidates for treatment. If patients receive appropriate treatment for such psychiatric disorders, they may subsequently become candidates for SCS.

Physical Examination

A thorough neurological exam should be conducted to identify any neurological deficits that may be present, which may be attributable to a structural lesion and, therefore, could be otherwise addressed with surgical decompression. As with the evaluation of any patient with low back pain, these symptoms should be correlated to imaging studies before making a clinical decision. Gait, spinal alignment, range of motion, sensation, and strength must all be examined.

Imaging Studies

As mentioned previously, complete and appropriate imaging studies, including a computed tomography (CT) scan or magnetic resonance imaging (MRI), may be performed to rule out a structural etiology of the patient's pain. Specifically, an MRI with and without intravenous gadolinium should be obtained.

Treatment

Equipment

Currently, there are two basic types of electrodes used for SCS stimulation: percutaneous leads and paddle electrodes. Percutaneous electrodes or wire electrodes are advantageous because they require less dissection for implantation. These electrodes are available with four (quadripolar) or eight (octopolar) contacts of various spacing and length. Percutaneous electrodes are appropriate for testing candidacy for permanent implantation, as they can be advanced over several segments of the spinal cord to determine optimal electrode positioning. Use of electrodes with more contacts and greater spacing allows testing of a broader range of spinal cord segments, while using electrodes with fewer contacts and smaller spacing allows better targeting of segments and electric field shaping. Present strategies involve using one or two quadripolar electrodes for limb pain and one or two octopolar electrodes for axial pain. The efficacy of placing a third electrode to create better steering of electric fields is still unclear, but this strategy has definite theoretical advantages.[1,2]

Disadvantages to percutaneous electrodes include their tendency to migrate after implantation, given their cylindrical shape and flexibility. Another drawback is decreased energy efficiency of percutaneous leads because the current is distributed circumferentially around the lead, including areas that do not contact the spinal cord. However, there have been recent studies that have indicated that the rate of percutaneous electrode migration may be slightly less than the rate of paddle electrode migration.[3] In addition, the same studies have indicated that the rate of breakage of percutaneous electrodes is almost half the rate of breakage of paddle electrodes.[3]

Paddle electrodes are offered in many sizes, shapes, lengths, spacings, and configurations of electrodes. Currently, single, dual, and three-column configurations are readily available. Recently, one manufacturer has released a five-column paddle. The more complex electrode arrays provide surgeons increased control for shaping the electric field; however, at the same time, increasing the number of contacts on a given array significantly increases power consumption by the system and complexity of programming. In 2005, it was estimated that ~3% of implanted SCS paddle leads were three- or five-column leads; however, in 2009 it was estimated that ~60% are three- or five-column leads (personal communication from St. Jude Medical Marketing, November 30, 2010) **(Table 68.1)**.

Paddle electrodes are advantageous because they are more energy efficient and should be the primary choice in patients who have had previous spinal surgery at the intended level of implantation or surgery below the intended target, preventing access by percutaneous leads. The accumulation of scar tissue following previous spinal surgeries makes it more difficult to place percutaneous electrodes properly with the Touhy needle. In addition, patients with previous laminectomies can have paddle electrodes implanted more readily because the major portion of the procedure has already been performed.

Furthermore, some patients do note significant positional and postural changes with percutaneous leads. These patients may benefit from a complex

The PROCESS Trial randomized 100 patients with FBSS to receive SCS and conventional medical management (CMM) or CMM alone.[7] Of the 52 patients initially assigned to the SCS and CMM group, 42 patients continued with treatment through the end of the trial. These patients experienced significantly less leg pain, superior functional capacity, enhanced quality of life, and greater satisfaction with treatment after 24 months of treatment.

Complications

When electrodes are implanted and treatment is managed with proper technique and expertise, patients with FBSS being treated with SCS rarely experience significant complications. The most severe complications, as with any type of spine surgery, are paralysis and other serious neurologic deficits, but these are rare. Another severe but rare complication is the occurrence of an epidural hematoma caused by rupture of the venous plexus upon insertion of the electrode. Less severe complications, but more common, are migration of the electrode, hardware complications, device malfunction, infection, cerebrospinal fluid (CSF) leakage, persistent pain at the implant site, and poor paresthesia coverage.[8]

References

1. Holsheimer J, Nuttin B, King GW, Wesselink WA, Gybels JM, de Sutter P. Clinical evaluation of paresthesia steering with a new system for spinal cord stimulation. Neurosurgery 1998;42(3):541–547, discussion 547–549
2. North RB, Kidd DH, Olin J, et al. Spinal cord stimulation for axial low back pain: a prospective, controlled trial comparing dual with single percutaneous electrodes. Spine 2005;30(12):1412–1418
3. Rosenow JM, Stanton-Hicks M, Rezai AR, Henderson JM. Failure modes of spinal cord stimulation hardware. J Neurosurg Spine 2006;5(3):183–190
4. Taylor RS, Ryan J, O'Donnell R, Eldabe S, Kumar K, North RB. The cost-effectiveness of spinal cord stimulation in the treatment of failed back surgery syndrome. Clin J Pain 2010; 26(6):463–469
5. North RB, Ewend MG, Lawton MT, Kidd DH, Piantadosi S. Failed back surgery syndrome: 5-year follow-up after spinal cord stimulator implantation. Neurosurgery 1991; 28(5):692–699
6. North RB, Kidd DH, Piantadosi S. Spinal cord stimulation versus reoperation for failed back surgery syndrome: a prospective, randomized study design. Acta Neurochir Suppl (Wien) 1995;64:106–108
7. Kumar K, Taylor RS, Jacques L, et al. The effects of spinal cord stimulation in neuropathic pain are sustained: a 24-month follow-up of the prospective randomized controlled multicenter trial of the effectiveness of spinal cord stimulation. Neurosurgery 2008;63(4):762–770, discussion 770
8. Cameron T. Safety and efficacy of spinal cord stimulation for the treatment of chronic pain: a 20-year literature review. J Neurosurg 2004;100:254–267

Suggested Readings

Cameron T. Safety and efficacy of spinal cord stimulation for the treatment of chronic pain: a 20-year literature review. J Neurosurg 2004;100(3, Suppl Spine):254–267

This literature review documents the types and frequency of complications associated with SCS treatment to show the safety and efficacy of this modality in pain management.

Holsheimer J, Nuttin B, King GW, Wesselink WA, Gybels JM, de Sutter P. Clinical evaluation of paresthesia steering with a new system for spinal cord stimulation. Neurosurgery 1998; 42(3):541–547, discussion 547–549

This study evaluates the efficacy of a transverse tripolar electrode for treating chronic neuropathic back pain, enabling finer current steering compared to conventional systems.

Kreis PG, Fishman SM, Chau K. Impact to spinal cord stimulator lead integrity with direct suture loop ties. Pain Med 2009;10(3):495–500

The authors examined microscopic damage and impedance that occurred to SCS leads from applying suture ties directly to the hardware.

Kumar K, Taylor RS, Jacques L, et al. The effects of spinal cord stimulation in neuropathic pain are sustained: a 24-month follow-up of the prospective randomized controlled multicenter trial of the effectiveness of spinal cord stimulation. Neurosurgery 2008;63(4):762–770, discussion 770

This randomized clinical trial demonstrates that patients undergoing SCS and conventional medical management typically have better outcomes over 24 months than with conventional medical management alone.

North RB, Kidd DH, Olin J, et al. Spinal cord stimulation for axial low back pain: a prospective, controlled trial comparing dual with single percutaneous electrodes. Spine 2005;30(12):1412–1418

This prospective randomized controlled trial offers data that can help guide technical decision making when implanting percutaneous electrodes to treat back pain with SCS.

North RB, Ewend MG, Lawton MT, Kidd DH, Piantadosi S. Failed back surgery syndrome: 5-year follow-up after spinal cord stimulator implantation. Neurosurgery 1991;28(5):692–699

This study demonstrates the long-term success of SCS for the treatment of FBSS using measures such as pain relief, returning to work, improvements in activities of daily living, and analgesic usage.

North RB, Kidd DH, Piantadosi S. Spinal cord stimulation versus reoperation for failed back surgery syndrome: a prospective, randomized study design. Acta Neurochir Suppl (Wien) 1995;64:106–108

This prospective randomized clinical trial demonstrates both the success of, and patient satisfaction with, SCS over reoperation in treating FBSS.

Rosenow JM, Stanton-Hicks M, Rezai AR, Henderson JM. Failure modes of spinal cord stimulation hardware. J Neurosurg Spine 2006;5(3):183–190

This retrospective study illustrates the type and frequency of various hardware-related complications experienced by patients undergoing SCS.

Taylor RS, Ryan J, O'Donnell R, Eldabe S, Kumar K, North RB. The cost-effectiveness of spinal cord stimulation in the treatment of failed back surgery syndrome. Clin J Pain 2010;26(6):463–469

This publication examines the cost-effectiveness of SCS as a treatment for FBSS and the impact of rechargeable IPGs on the cost of treatment.

Turner JA, Hollingworth W, Comstock BA, Deyo RA. Spinal cord stimulation for failed back surgery syndrome: outcomes in a workers' compensation setting. Pain 2010;148(1):14–25

This prospective, population-based controlled cohort study demonstrated that SCS does not offer significantly better results compared to alternate treatments after 6 months.

Turner JA, Loeser JD, Bell KG. Spinal cord stimulation for chronic low back pain: a systematic literature synthesis. Neurosurgery 1995;37(6):1088–1095, discussion 1095–1096

The authors performed an extensive meta-analysis of the existing literature to examine the efficacy of using SCS to treat back pain. This publication demonstrates that SCS is an effective treatment for chronic low back pain and exhibits the need for prospective randomized clinical trials to support the use of this technique further.

Spinal Cord Stimulation for Extremity Pain

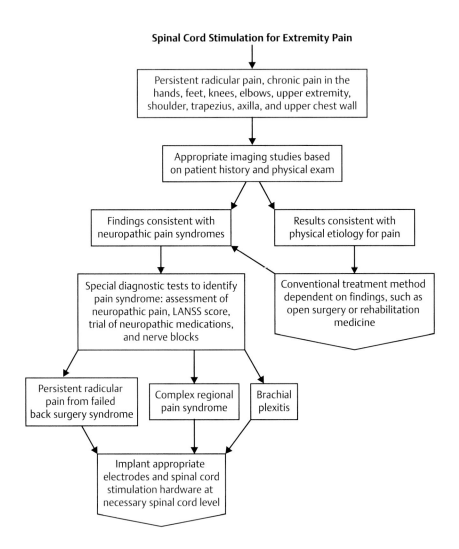

69

Spinal Cord Stimulators for Extremity Pain

David L. Penn, Chengyuan Wu, Steven M. Falowski, and Ashwini Sharan

Spinal cord stimulation (SCS) is a method of treating neuropathic pain involving implantation of electrodes, which deliver electrical current onto several spinal cord structures, including the dorsal columns. This electrical stimulation activates afferent pathways that inhibit pain perception. While SCS has been commonly used to treat failed back surgery syndrome (see Chapter 68), it also has applications for several other types of neuropathic pain affecting the extremities, such as complex regional pain syndrome (CRPS) and brachial plexitis or neurogenic thoracic outlet syndrome. This chapter focuses specifically on the use of SCS to treat pain syndromes involving the extremities. For more details on the mechanisms of function of SCS and techniques of treatment, refer to Chapter 68.

Classification

Patients with failed back surgery syndrome can experience persistent or multidistribution radicular pain in the extremities originating from the spine, indicating treatment with SCS. Radicular pain is characterized by a distribution of pain that radiates along somatosensory dermatomes. This type of pain may be precipitated by inflammation or irritation of the nerve root, known as radiculitis; however, radicular pain may be caused by other mechanisms as well, such as fibrosis.

There are several pain syndromes that originate in the spinal cord but primarily affect the extremities. CRPS, previously known as reflex sympathetic dystrophy (RSD), is a pain syndrome that occurs with unknown etiology (Type I) or secondary to injury (Type II). It is characterized by progressive severe pain, swelling, and skin color changes occurring in the hands, feet, knees, or elbows. Another pain syndrome of the extremities is brachial plexitis, which is defined as a pain affecting the upper extremities, the shoulder, the trapezius, the axilla, and/or the upper chest wall. This may result from viral influence, anatomical deformity, or even traumatic injury.

Workup

History

Potential candidates for SCS are patients with severe neuropathic pain syndromes who have failed to achieve successful pain reduction through more conservative methods, do not have a serious untreated drug habituation, and are free of confounding comorbidities that may indicate nociceptive or mechanically correctable origins of pain. Persistent radicular pain following one or more failed lumbosacral surgeries can present with a variety of described pain experiences ranging from sharp, dull, piercing, and throbbing, to burning. In some cases, the pain can change or be relieved with mechanically altered body position, such as lying down versus standing or bending forward. These may sometime be amenable to spinal surgery.

The dermatomal distribution of pain is indicative of the spinal cord or nerve level involved; however, individual variations exist, and pain distribution does not always fit expected dermatomal patterns. When paresthesia accompanies pain, the distribution of paresthesia is more characteristic, and localization of the affected spinal cord level is more precise than with pain alone.

Recently, Bennet et al. reported on and validated the use of a neuropathic pain scale. On this scale, there are a total of 24 points, and greater than 12 points is typically suggestive of neuropathic pain. Interestingly, the most significant descriptors of pain suggestive of neuropathic pain included the presence of abnormal sensations in the pain region, color changes in the pain region, and different feeling in the pain region with finger rubbing when compared with nonpainful regions. Other characteristics observed included abnormal sensitivity, pressing-associated pain, and bursting pain, with burning being the least significant. This scale is useful in giving an overall impression that a component of the limb pain may be neuropathic in origin.

Patients with CRPS typically present with burning pain and allodynia that is most prevalent in a limb but can affect any part of the body. The patient's description of the pain is often the most helpful in the diagnosis of this disease. In Type II CRPS, the onset of pain most often occurs ~24 hours from the injury; however, if the injury initially causes anesthesia, the pain symptoms may have a much later onset. The most commonly involved nerves in CRPS are the median, ulnar, and sciatic nerves, but specific nerve involvement often cannot be determined.

Brachial neuritis typically presents with acute onset of intense pain and sometimes muscle weakness, which can occur simultaneously with the onset of pain or after a variable period. This pain syndrome is characterized as a constant sharp, stabbing, throbbing, or aching that can last for several weeks.

Finally, it should be recognized that many patients may have mixed pain etiologies. Patients might easily have both a nociceptive component as well as a neuropathic component of pain. For example, a patient with a traumatic herniated lumbar disk may have both a simple radiculopathy, resulting in leg/limb pain from mechanical injury to the nerve root, and chemical irritation from the nucleus pulposus. However, identification of multidermatomal pain distribution with altered sensory patterns and hyperpathia would suggest an overlying neuropathic injury. This patient might require a planned, staged spinal intervention and neurostimulation intervention if other less invasive and conservative efforts fail. Upfront discussion with the patient on this treatment plan is, of course, very helpful.

Physical Examination

The most important tests of the physical exam to help diagnose the cause of lumbosacral radicular pain is the straight leg-raising test, or Lasègue's test, and the crossed straight leg-raising test. A positive test result, or Lasègue sign, is radicular pain elicited at an angle of less than 60 degrees when the leg is raised from the exam table. Although never proven, Lasègue sign has been considered an indication of nerve compression and may indicate that a patient is not a good candidate for SCS. Another strong indication that a patient is not a good candidate for SCS would be a positive test result when performing the crossed straight leg-raising test, which occurs when the contralateral leg is raised and pain is elicited on the ipsilateral side. In addition, some neurological signs, such as decreased patellar and Achilles tendon reflexes, can indicate a physical etiology at the nerve root. Other indications for SCS are a Leeds Assessment of Neuropathic Pain Symptoms and Signs score greater than 12, demonstrating pain of neuropathic origin, and opiate and neuropathic pain medication usage.

Examining a patient with CRPS is often difficult because of the pain experience of the patient—often the patient will not allow touch to the affected limb. Additional physical findings consist of vascular changes that can alter the appearance of affected areas of the body. The results of these changes include vasodilation or vasoconstriction, anhidrosis or hyperhidrosis, dry and scaly skin, stiff joints, tapering fingers, ridges in fingernails, and long and coarse hair or alopecia.

Finally, patients with brachial plexitis present with weakness or paralysis of the shoulder girdle muscles and mixed loss of sensory modalities in the affected arm. Some of these patients will experience extreme tenderness to palpation in the supraclavicular region or in the subclavicular region.

Imaging Studies

For any of the pain syndromes just described, the appropriate imaging studies, especially computed tomography (CT) and magnetic resonance imaging (MRI), should be conducted to rule out physical etiologies of pain that can be treated with more conventional methods or surgical procedures. In particular, patients with suspected persistent radicular pain following previous lumbosacral procedures and brachial plexitis should have an MRI at the suspected level of spinal cord involvement. These imaging studies should be conducted after the pain is expected to resolve on its own. For radicular pain associated with failed back surgery, the pain sometimes resolves after 6 to 12 weeks. Idiopathic brachial plexitis can begin to resolve ~4 weeks after the onset of pain. If patients with these pain syndromes have not experienced a decrease in pain during these time periods, imaging studies can help identify nociceptive causes.

Currently, for the diagnosis of CRPS, there is no gold standard imaging technique, and numerous tests that have been used in attempts to aid diagnosis of this disease have been eventually refuted.

Special Diagnostic Considerations

Diagnosis of radicular pain can also be aided by performing a diagnostic nerve root block, which is particularly helpful in determining the level of spinal cord involvement; however, the specificity and sensitivity of this test are undetermined. Some tests that may be useful in confirming diagnosis of CRPS include thermography, three-phase bone scan, radiographic examination for osteoporosis, response to sympathetic block, and autonomic tests, such as sweat output and skin temperature at rest and quantitative sudomotor axon reflex test.

There are a few unique issues to also consider prior to implantation of a permanent neurostimulator system. The implantation of a neurostimulator does preclude future MRI scans. Therefore, the physician and patient may consider MRI of other body regions prior to implantation and should try to also assess what the necessity of MRI may be in the future. For example, if a patient has a brain tumor and is being monitored for recurrence, that patient would need to be evaluated with CT scans instead of MRI. If this is not feasible, then a neurostimulation system may be contraindicated. Additionally, many patients may elect to have a paddle electrode inserted as their permanent implant system. Given the size of a paddle lead and considerations of having adequate space for insertion in the epidural space in the cervical or thoracic regions, it may often be desirable to obtain MRI of either the cervical or thoracic spine, prior to permanent implantation to assess for relative stenosis and to ensure that there is adequate room for paddle placement.

Treatment

Equipment

In treating extremity pain with SCS, percutaneous and paddle electrodes can be used. As mentioned in Chapter 68, percutaneous electrodes require less invasive procedures for implantation; however, they are perceived to have a greater tendency to migrate from the desired site and break. Other studies have indicated that this may not be true. The rate of percutaneous electrode migration has been demonstrated to be slightly less than the rate of paddle electrode migration. In addition, the rate of percutaneous electrode breakage has been demonstrated to be almost half the rate of breakage of paddle electrodes. Conversely, paddle electrodes require surgery for implantation and are believed to deliver current to the dorsal columns more efficiently than percutaneous electrodes. Radiofrequency generators and implantable pulse generators can be used to deliver current through the electrodes to the dorsal columns.

There are four different regions where surgeons can achieve stimulation of the large, myelinated afferents resulting in ipsilateral tingling paresthesia: the dorsal root, the dorsal root entry zone (DREZ), the dorsal horn, and the dorsal columns. It is important to note the difference in activation of the dorsal root, the DREZ, and the dorsal horn from activation of the dorsal columns because activation of the dorsal root aspects of these afferents results in radicular paresthesia of the dermatome at the level of the electrode, while activation of the dorsal columns cause paresthesia of areas of the body caudal to the level of the electrode.

Furthermore, It can be extremely difficult to differentiate between stimulation occurring at the dorsal root, DREZ, or dorsal horn. Dorsal root stimulation occurs with laterally placed electrodes, while stimulation of the DREZ and dorsal horn occurs with electrodes placed closer to the midline. Stimulation of the DREZ and dorsal horn causes segmentary paresthesia that is subsequently followed by rapid activation of the dorsal columns with a small voltage increment. Minute changes in the mediolateral positioning of electrodes have been demonstrated to cause movement of paresthesia patterns in a two-dimensional "W" pattern (**Fig. 69.1**).

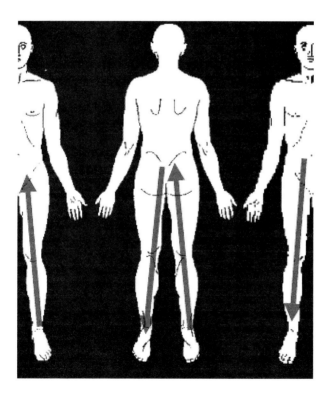

Fig. 69.1   Depiction of the two-dimensional "W" pattern of paresthesia observed with variations in mediolateral positioning of SCS electrodes on the dorsal root, DREZ, dorsal horn, and dorsal columns. (From Oakley JC, Espinosa F, Bothe H *et al*. Transverse Tripolar Spinal Cord Stimulation: Results of an International Multicenter Study. Neuromodulation. 2006;9(3):192–203. Reprinted with permission.)

Patient Management/Evaluation

For long-term successful pain relief, health care providers must carefully follow up with patients to ensure proper use and maintenance of implanted SCS equipment. Discomfort at implantation sites, electrode breakage and migration, and infection are events that can occur over the years following implantation. Patients must also be properly educated in the use of SCS equipment to achieve optimal results. Additionally, multiple programming sessions are typically required to determine the right paresthesia coverage, frequency, and pulse widths necessary for successful pain relief. Often patients will not inquire regarding these changes, and it becomes the physician's responsibility to suggest as such.

Outcome

As mentioned in the previous chapter, patients with failed back surgery syndrome often achieve greater than 50% pain reduction, with a high level of satisfaction. More specifically, other studies have demonstrated success with SCS compared with reoperation and compared with conventional medical management (CMM) in treating persistent radiculopathy and radicular pain associated with failed back surgery syndrome at ~3-year outcome. The majority of patients undergoing SCS for treatment of CRPS achieve pain reduction. Patients do not usually experience complete pain reduction but do indicate definitive decreases in their pain experience. The data regarding long-term outcomes are mixed, with some studies reporting near-complete pain relief and others reporting no differences between SCS groups and comparable controls. Trials examining the long-term efficacy of the use of SCS to treat brachial plexitis have yet to be conducted. Case studies have indicated promise in its application.

Complications

Permanent complications associated with SCS procedures are rare. As with any surgical spinal procedure, paralysis and other neurological deficits are among the most severe complications, as well as epidural hematomas from rupture of the venous plexus. Other complications are migration of electrodes, hardware complications, infections, cerebrospinal fluid (CSF) leakage, and persistent pain at the implantation site. Finally, following implantation of SCS systems, patients will be unable to undergo MRI.

Suggested Readings

Barolat G, Massaro F, He J, Zeme S, Ketcik B. Mapping of sensory responses to epidural stimulation of the intraspinal neural structures in man. J Neurosurg 1993;78(2):233–239

The authors conducted an extensive study to map the regions of the spinal cord, detailing the specific levels of the spinal cord that must be stimulated to achieve certain paresthesia patterns.

Bennett MI, Smith BH, Torrance N, Potter J. The S-LANSS score for identifying pain of predominantly neuropathic origin: validation for use in clinical and postal research. J Pain 2005; 6(3):149–158

This article describes the Leeds Assessment of Neuropathic Symptoms and Signs (S-LANSS) pain scale and compares it to the Neuropathic Pain Scale. This scale helps clinicians differentiate pain of neuropathic origin from pain of nociceptive origin. Results support the validity and reliability of S-LANSS, demonstrating this scale's utility for comparisons with other investigational measures.

Cameron T. Safety and efficacy of spinal cord stimulation for the treatment of chronic pain: a 20-year literature review. J Neurosurg 2004;100(3, Suppl Spine):254–267

This publication represents a comprehensive review of the clinical work and literature available regarding the treatment of chronic pain using SCS.

Falowski SM, Celii A, Sestokas AK, Schwartz DM, Matsumoto C, Sharan A. Awake vs. asleep placement of spinal cord stimulators: a cohort analysis of complications associated with placement. Neuromodulation 2011;14(2):130–134, discussion 134–135

This restrospecitve review compares the efficacy of placing SCS electrodes under awake conditions with the placement of similar electrodes under general anesthesia to determine which method is more desirable. Results demonstrated that procedures performed under general anesthesia are associated with fewer failure rates.

Kemler MA, Barendse GA, van Kleef M, et al. Spinal cord stimulation in patients with chronic reflex sympathetic dystrophy. N Engl J Med 2000;343(9):618–624

This is a prospective randomized clinical trial demonstrating the improved outcome when treating CRPS, with both SCS and physical therapy, as opposed to physical therapy alone.

Kemler MA, de Vet HC, Barendse GA, van den Wildenberg FA, van Kleef M. Spinal cord stimulation for chronic reflex sympathetic dystrophy—five-year follow-up. N Engl J Med 2006;354(22): 2394–2396

This study demonstrates the long-term efficacy of SCS in combination with physical training in treating CRPS as compared to physical training alone.

Kumar K, Taylor RS, Jacques L, et al. Spinal cord stimulation versus conventional medical management for neuropathic pain: a multicentre randomised controlled trial in patients with failed back surgery syndrome. Pain 2007;132(1-2):179–188

This multicenter randomized clinical trial demonstrates increased efficacy of SCS compared to conventional medical management in treating persistent radicular pain associated with failed back surgery syndrome.

Rosenow JM, Stanton-Hicks M, Rezai AR, Henderson JM. Failure modes of spinal cord stimulation hardware. J Neurosurg Spine 2006;5(3):183–190

This retrospective study illustrates the type and frequency of various hardware-related complications experienced by patients undergoing SCS.

70

Bone Graft Substitutes/Biologics

Alex Gitelman, Rahul Basho, Brandon J. Rebholz, Beck D. McAllister, and Jeffrey C. Wang

Bone grafts have been used in orthopedic surgery since the 1800s. Early techniques were only modestly successful and were applied primarily toward the treatment of fractures. Many of the current bone grafting methodologies began to be developed in the 1940s by the U.S. military. Over the next few decades, techniques like freeze-drying, fresh freezing, and irradiation continued to develop, and their use became more widespread. Still, it was not until the last few decades that advanced techniques, such as bone marrow aspirate, bone morphogenic protein (BMP), and autologous platelet concentrate, came into wide use.

The use of bone grafts and bone graft substitutes in spine surgery has been steadily increasing for several reasons. Successful fusion of separate spine segments requires the formation of bridging bone as well as maintenance of correct alignment. While good results have been obtained with the current gold standard (iliac crest autograft), there has been a general trend in the spine community to decrease its use because of significant long-term graft harvest site pain. Furthermore, advances in medical care have permitted older patients as well as patients with significant comorbidities to undergo more complex spinal surgical procedures. These factors have led to increased use of the more advanced bone grafting techniques, occasionally without good data to support their use.

Selection of appropriate bone graft options is based on several factors. The osteogenicity of a bone graft is its ability to directly contribute bone-forming cells and directly induce new bone formation. Osteoconductive bone grafts provide a scaffold for new bone formation. Osteoinductive bone grafts induce differentiation of osteoprogenitor cells into osteoblasts. Structural bone grafts and extenders provide a rigid support to the construct.

Bone Graft Substitute Options

Tricortical iliac crest autograft is widely considered to be the gold standard, as it is osteogenic, osteoconductive, and osteoinductive, and provides structural support. However, its use is limited by its finite supply, and there is significant morbidity associated with the harvesting procedure, including the potential for infection, nerve injury and donor site pain. These problems have led to the development of various bone grafting options.

Allografts

Cadaver bone is available as both structural and nonstructural allografts. The cadaver bone is processed after harvesting to decrease its antigenicity as well as the risk of disease transmission. This causes the allograft to lose its osteogenic, and most of its osteoinductive, properties.

While some studies have demonstrated the superiority of structural autograft over allograft with regard to fusion rates, overall success rates, and maintenance of interspace height in anterior cervical fusions, there is also good evidence suggesting the noninferiority of allograft structural bone in single-level instrumented and uninstrumented anterior cervical fusions. The evidence is less ambiguous in posterior lumbar spine fusions; autografts result in higher fusion rates and higher density of fusion mass than allografts.

Demineralized Bone Matrix

Demineralized bone matrix (DBM) is obtained by demineralization of bone allograft, leaving behind collagen and other noncollagenous proteins and growth factors. This process results in loss of structural support but retains the osteoconductive and weakly osteoinductive properties of autograft. It is available in several forms, including sheets, putties, and injectable gels. There is minimal oversight by the U.S. Food and Drug Administration (FDA) regarding the minimum quality and testing requirements, leading to wide variability in osteoinductive qualities of products produced by different vendors and even between individual lots of the same product.

The lack of any structural strength in DBM limits its use in anterior lumbar and cervical interbody fusions. DBM use in anterior cervical discectomy and fusion procedures with structural allografts has been associated with a greater rate of pseudarthrosis and collapse than autograft. Still, results of DBM used in conjunction with a cage or structural bone graft and internal fixation have shown high fusion rates and good clinical outcomes.

The evidence for DBM use in posterior lumbar fusion surgeries is much stronger. Several studies have demonstrated that DBM use in conjunction with autograft leads to fusion rates similar to when larger amounts of autograft without DBM are used. Prior to use of any DBM product it is advisable to investigate the individual DBM product's testing data to make sure that it has effective osteoinductive properties.

Autologous Growth Factor Concentrate

Several growth factors, such as transforming growth factor-beta (TGF-beta) and platelet-derived growth factor (PDGF), have been noted to promote bone and tendon healing following injury via promotion of mesenchymal cell differentiation and proliferation. Improved outcomes have been noted with local injection of autologous growth factor concentrate in some sports injuries, such as lateral epicondylitis and Achilles tendon injuries. Applications of these techniques in spine surgery, though, have not been as successful. Several studies demonstrated faster time to fusion with such autologous growth factor concentrates, but there was no effect on overall fusion rates. At this time, convincing evidence for use of autologous platelet products in spine fusion surgery is lacking.

Ceramics

Ceramics, such as calcium carbonate and beta-tricalcium phosphate, provide an osteoconductive scaffold for new bone formation but lack osteoinductive and structural support qualities. Some ceramic bone graft substitutes may be coated with hydroxyapatite, which may improve bone ingrowth. While ceramics can be manufactured in different shapes and sizes, they are brittle and require internal fixation when used as a structural bone graft substitute.

Ceramics require large surface areas of decorticated bone for optimal fusion in the lumbar spine. This limits their use in intertransverse posterolateral fusions, even in conjunction with bone marrow aspirate or local bone graft. However, some data show that good fusion rates can be achieved when ceramics are combined with autograft and large, bleeding bone surface areas are available. Good results have also been obtained when ceramics were combined with BMP.

The use of ceramics in anterior spine surgery appears to have better results than in posterior spine procedures. Good fusion rates have been obtained when ceramics are used in anterior cervical interbody fusions in conjunction with rigid plating. While there is little evidence to support the use of ceramics in stand-alone anterior lumbar interbody fusions (ALIFs), good results have been obtained when they have been used as part of circumferential instrumented fusions.

Bone Marrow Aspirate

Mesenchymal stem cells have a significant osteogenic potential owing to their ability to differentiate into an osteoprogenitor cell lineage. Bone marrow aspiration can provide a large number of mesenchymal stem cells without the morbidity associated with iliac crest harvest. Stem cells can be obtained via both iliac crest aspirations and transpedicular vertebral body aspiration, with some data demonstrating higher numbers of progenitor cells obtained using the latter.

Bone marrow aspirate needs to be combined with an osteoconductive carrier for optimal fusion mass formation. Equivalent clinical outcomes and radiographic fusion rates have been achieved when bone marrow aspirate with a collagen/hydroxyapatite matrix was compared with iliac crest autograft in posterolateral fusions. Similarly, bone marrow aspirate with a collagen carrier and allograft may be a good and cost-effective alternative to BMP with a collagen carrier in revision single-level posterior spine fusions. On the other hand, bone marrow aspirate appears to be less effective than autograft in anterior lumbar procedures. Still, at this time there are limited data available on the efficacy of bone marrow aspirate in spine fusion procedures.

Bone Morphogenic Protein

Although BMP was identified in 1965, it became widely commercially available since about 2000. This protein has significant osteogenic potential, but it lacks structural and osteoconductive properties. The two currently commercially available BMP products are rhBMP-2 and rhBMP-7. Both BMPs must be used with a carrier matrix to prevent rapid dissolution from the operative site.

BMP-2 is currently FDA approved for use in ALIF procedures. Level 1 evidence suggests that BMP-2 produces better clinical results and fusion rates than allograft alone, and the clinical and radiographic results are equivalent to autograft. Cost analysis studies have also demonstrated that while the initial cost of BMP-2 use is higher than that of iliac crest autograft, long-term costs may be similar because of avoidance of the morbidity associated with autograft harvest.

Excellent results have also been noted with BMP-2 use in posterior lumbar spine fusions. Several studies have demonstrated equivalent or better clinical outcomes and fusion rates with use of BMP compared with iliac crest autograft, both with and without pedicle screw instrumentation. BMP-2 use in posterior lumbar spine fusions is currently physician-directed, as it is not FDA-approved for these procedures.

Similarly, BMP-2 use in the anterior cervical spine has been reported to result in improved fusion rates. This may be particularly important in multilevel procedures, where it may obviate the need for posterior supplemental fixation. Still, significant complications such as dysphagia and increased prevertebral swelling due to local inflammation have been associated with BMP-2 use. Although these appear to be dose-dependent, the FDA put out a public health notification in June 2008 regarding possible life-threatening complications associated with rhBMP use in the anterior cervical spine.

Several other complications have also been noted with BMP-2 use. A small percentage of patients have had aggressive early resorption of bone graft as well as surrounding host bone following BMP use. Ectopic bone formation around nearby neural structures has also been reported. The use of BMP-2 for posterior and transforaminal interbody fusions has been associated with increased rates of postoperative radiculitis. Accordingly, while BMP is a very strong bone-forming adjuvant, its potential side effects and significant cost should be considered prior to its use.

Decision Making

Despite the multiple bone graft and bone graft substitute options currently available, good evidence as to which option is better or may be more appropriate for a given indication is lacking. In general, anterior lumbar procedures require structural support, and good results have been obtained with both structural allograft as well as a cage with demineralized bone matrix. Concomitant use of bone morphogenic protein has led to increased fusion rates in these procedures. Similarly, anterior cervical procedures require structural support, and good fusion rates have been achieved with structural allograft or cages with demineralized bone matrix when used with anterior plate fixation.

Multiple graft options are reasonable for posterior lumbar and cervical procedures. DBM with local autograft, as well as bone marrow aspirate with a collagen sponge, typically result in good fusion rates. When a large decorticated area is available for fusion, ceramics with local autograft have also led to good clinical and radiographic results. Still, further research is necessary to clearly delineate appropriate indications for each bone grafting option.

Suggested Readings

Bishop RC, Moore KA, Hadley MN. Anterior cervical interbody fusion using autogeneic and allogeneic bone graft substrate: a prospective comparative analysis. J Neurosurg 1996;85(2): 206–210

> *This excellent study compares the outcomes of allograft versus autograft in anterior cervical interbody fusions. This study also noted the detrimental effect of smoking, particularly in the allograft group.*

Cammisa FP Jr, Lowery G, Garfin SR, et al. Two-year fusion rate equivalency between Grafton DBM gel and autograft in posterolateral spine fusion: a prospective controlled trial employing a side-by-side comparison in the same patient. Spine 2004;29(6):660–666

> *This study compared iliac crest autograft and DBM with a smaller amount of autograft side by side in the same patients. Authors noted that the use of DBM can produce equivalent fusion results while decreasing the amount of autograft needed, thus possibly reducing the risk and severity of donor site morbidity.*

Chen WJ, Tsai TT, Chen LH, et al. The fusion rate of calcium sulfate with local autograft bone compared with autologous iliac bone graft for instrumented short-segment spinal fusion. Spine 2005;30(20):2293–2297

> *Iliac crest bone graft on one side was compared with local autograft with calcium sulfate on the other side in the same patient undergoing instrumented one- or two-level lumbar spine fusion. The authors noted that the fusion rates were equivalent among the two groups.*

Dimar JR, Glassman SD, Burkus KJ, Carreon LY. Clinical outcomes and fusion success at 2 years of single-level instrumented posterolateral fusions with recombinant human bone morphogenetic protein-2/compression resistant matrix versus iliac crest bone graft. Spine 2006;31(22):2534–2539, discussion 2540

> *This is a prospective, randomized study comparing autograft to BMP with compression-resistant matrix in posterolateral spine fusions. The authors noted higher fusion rates and lower operative time and blood loss in the BMP group.*

Lewandrowski KU, Nanson C, Calderon R. Vertebral osteolysis after posterior interbody lumbar fusion with recombinant human bone morphogenetic protein 2: a report of five cases. Spine J 2007;7(5):609–614

> *This report of five cases draws attention to the possible complication of vertebral osteolysis following transforaminal lumbar interbody fusion with BMP. Although all cases resolved with nonoperative care, the possibility of this complication should be considered.*

Neen D, Noyes D, Shaw M, Gwilym S, Fairlie N, Birch N. Healos and bone marrow aspirate used for lumbar spine fusion: a case controlled study comparing Healos with autograft. Spine 2006;31(18):E636–E640

The authors compare the fusion rates of bone marrow aspirate with a collagen sponge versus iliac crest autograft in both anterior and posterior lumbar spine fusions. They note equivalent fusion rates in the posterior procedures among the two options. The fusion rates of the iliac crest autograft were noted to be superior to those of the bone marrow aspirate/collagen sponge group in the ALIFs.

Samartzis D, Shen FH, Goldberg EJ, An HS. Is autograft the gold standard in achieving radiographic fusion in one-level anterior cervical discectomy and fusion with rigid anterior plate fixation? Spine 2005;30(15):1756–1761

This very good study demonstrates equivalent and excellent results of one-level anterior cervical interbody fusion with rigid plate fixation comparing autograft and allograft. Smoking was not noted to affect fusion rates significantly. This study demonstrates the advantage of rigid plate fixation when compared to the Bishop et al. 1996 study noted previously.

Taghavi CE, Lee KB, Keorochana G, Tzeng ST, Yoo JH, Wang JC. Bone morphogenetic protein-2 and bone marrow aspirate with allograft as alternatives to autograft in instrumented revision posterolateral lumbar spinal fusion: a minimum two-year follow-up study. Spine 2010; 35(11):1144–1150

This retrospective cohort study compares autograft, BMP, and bone marrow aspirate in revision instrumented posterolateral lumbar fusions. The authors noted that BMP may be a reasonable alternative to autograft in both single and multilevel revision surgeries, while bone marrow aspirate may produce equivalent results at a lower cost and morbidity than either of the other options in single-level procedures.

Vaidya R, Carp J, Sethi A, Bartol S, Craig J, Les CM. Complications of anterior cervical discectomy and fusion using recombinant human bone morphogenetic protein-2. Eur Spine J 2007;16(8):1257–1265

This retrospective study evaluates the safety and cost of BMP use in anterior cervical discectomy and fusion. The authors noted that the use of BMP resulted in significantly higher rates of prevertebral swelling and dysphagia than in the allograft/ DBM group, while the cost of the allograft/DBM group was much lower.

Wang JC, Alanay A, Mark D, et al. A comparison of commercially available demineralized bone matrix for spinal fusion. Eur Spine J 2007;16(8):1233–1240

This study demonstrates that there are significant differences between different commercially available DBM products. Prior to the use of a DBM product, its data should be thoroughly examined, as the osteogenic potential may vary significantly.

Bracing and Orthoses

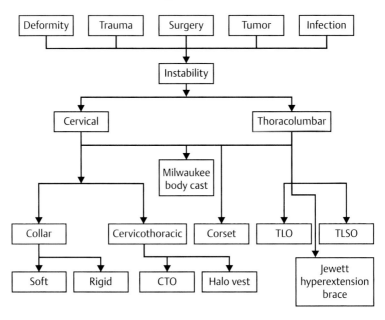

71

Bracing and Orthoses

Peter Lewkonia and Charles G. Fisher

External immobilization of the spine has been used for centuries to treat spinal conditions from acute trauma to chronic deformity. Current use is controversial and remains variable in clinical practice, as good-quality evidence is often lacking. The goal of bracing is to eliminate or to neutralize the forces acting on the spine to provide stability when normal physiologic stability has been compromised by a pathologic process. This situation arises in acute trauma, tumor, or infection as well as in idiopathic scoliosis and degenerative conditions of the spine. It is important that there should be a foreseeable endpoint to brace treatment. If no such end to bracing can be predicted, surgery or an alternate treatment must be strongly considered.

To immobilize the spine effectively, a brace must overcome both intrinsic forces, such as muscle pull or imbalance, and external forces, such as gravity. Unlike braces and orthoses used in the extremities, a spine brace is limited by the difficulty in obtaining fixation points, particularly in the upper and lower extremes of the spine. It is also limited by the distance between the brace itself and the bony spinal column, a space which is filled with soft tissue, including the visceral organs and large muscle groups. Many braces overcome this difficulty by extending beyond the area of pathology to fix on very proximal or distal points. In the cervical spine, some orthoses capture fixation on the skull, mandible, or the occiput, while in the lumbar spine, these devices fix to the bony prominences of the pelvis or the thigh.

Braces should be fitted by a qualified orthotist working closely with the spine team. Because of the risk of complications, close surveillance is required, and brace adjustments should be made if necessary. Patient factors, including body size and habitus, as well as concurrent injury, must all be considered before the choice to use an orthosis is made. Patients and their caregivers should also be aware of the considerable cost of many customized braces and need to be taught the appropriate techniques for donning and removing the device. Without proper use, a patient may use a brace inappropriately or ineffectively, leading to treatment failure and potential morbidity. Patient preference must be strongly considered when deciding on a brace for treatment, as a brace that is not worn through poor compliance will fail to be of any use to the patient or physician.

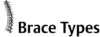

Brace Types

Cervical Spine

A broad range of cervical and cervicothoracic orthoses are available. These vary from soft collars that have very limited effect on spinal motion to rigid external devices that fix the position of the skull relative to the shoulders and chest. The different devices vary both in the material of construction and the points of fixation. Those with poor proximal and distal fit suffer from so-called parallelogram motion as the head extends and the spine flexes, particularly when the collar lacks an anterior buttress. Another shared problem with all cervical and cervicothoracic orthoses is "snaking," or segmental motion in the sagittal plane with no overall change in position of the most proximal and distal points. This most frequently occurs in the mid-cervical region, which must be considered when a brace is used to treat instability in this region.

The simplest cervical orthosis is a soft collar. This device has limited usefulness because it does little to restrict cervical motion. It has virtually no points of fixation proximally or distally and allows motion in all degrees of freedom. There are a variety of hard cervical collars or high cervicothoracic orthoses, including the Miami J (Jerome Medical, Moorestown, NJ), the Philadelphia collar (Philadelphia Cervical Collar Co., Thorofare, NJ), and the Aspen collar (Aspen Medical Products, Irvine, CA) (**Fig. 71.1**). These devices all share similar characteristics, with proximal fit onto either the occiput posteriorly or the mandible anteriorly, and extension over the base of the neck and medial shoulder girdle distally. Biomechanical and radiographic in vivo studies have shown the effectiveness of these devices to be very similar. All are more effective in the upper cervical spine and are particularly poor at controlling motion below the C6 level. Collars are generally uncomfortable, so patient preference should be considered in light of their similar effectiveness.

Cervicothoracic orthoses (CTOs) obtain fixation to the chest and lateral shoulder girdle, which provides enhanced stability to the lower cervical spine and cervicothoracic junction. The larger working distance from the face or skull to the chest also improves immobilization in the upper spine, particularly at the occiput to C2 levels, where fractures often occur. A variety of CTOs are available, including the SOMI (sternal-occipital-mandibular immobilizer) brace, the Lerman Minerva brace (United States Manufacturing Company, Pasadena, CA), and the two- or four-post Aspen CTOs, which include the Aspen collar as a component (Aspen Medical Products, Irvine, CA) (**Fig. 71.2**). Probably the gold standard is the halo vest, a commonly used cervicothoracic orthosis with direct fixation of the skull. It consists of pins inserted around the skull at its widest point, connected with a ring and rigid bars to a tightly fitting vest (**Fig. 71.3**). Contraindications to using a halo vest include skull

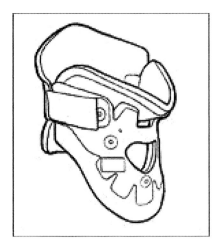

Fig. 71.1   Aspen collar.

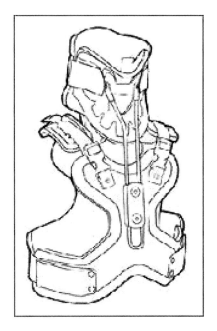

Fig. 71.2   Aspen cervicothoracic orthosis (CTO).

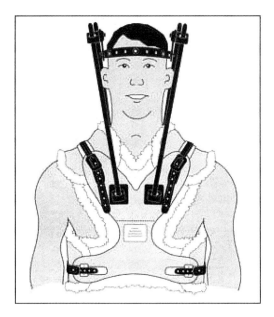

Fig. 71.3   Halo vest.

fracture, sepsis, head injury, and chest injury. It maintains excellent immobilization of the cervical spine, particularly at the cervicothoracic junction and upper cervical spine. It allows some snaking motion of the mid-cervical spine, however, limiting its use for treating injuries at these levels. Other CTOs, such as the Minerva brace, are less effective in controlling rotation and motion at the cervicooccipital junction, but they can be more effective in preventing snaking. The Milwaukee body cast, which is no longer commonly used except in deformity treatment, has the best control of the spine in all areas. In choosing a cervical or cervicothoracic orthosis, one needs to consider the amount of immobilization required, as well as the spinal levels of most importance, while limiting patient discomfort and inconvenience.

Thoracic and Lumbar Spine

A variety of orthoses are used to immobilize the thoracic and lumbar spine, ranging from a soft lumbar corset to rigid plastic thoracolumbosacral orthoses (TLSOs). The thoracic spine has inherent stability because of its attachment to the rib cage from T1 to T10. The same stability does not apply to T11 and T12, which have floating ribs. Distally, lumbar braces must have some point of fixation four to five levels below the level of pathology. This often mandates the tight fit of a rigid orthosis onto the iliac crest, sacrum, or a thigh extension. Because of the increased soft-tissue thickness between the brace and the spine as well as the large forces generated by the paraspinal muscles, complete immobilization of the lumbar spine is particularly difficult.

The simplest brace is a lumbar corset. These devices have been used to treat back pain and postsurgical instability, although there is minimal evidence for their effectiveness. Although it lacks a rigid external structure, the corset adds stability by increasing intraabdominal pressure. Several more rigid devices exist, including off-the-shelf orthoses and custom thermoplastic body casts. Noncustomized braces employ a three-point bending strategy with a metal frame to control either flexion (Jewett brace) (**Fig. 71.4**) or extension (Williams brace). These braces do not control rotation or lateral flexion well. They have the advantage of being easy to fit and cheaper, and are less intrusive than plastic body casts. TLSO braces are typically made from a custom mold using thermoplastic, rigid materials. They may be one piece (e.g., Boston brace) or clamshell style with strong attachments from front to back (**Fig. 71.5**). Any motion or slide between the clamshell halves reduces the overall function of the orthosis. TLSOs are effective only as high as T6 without the use of a neck extension, and lose their effect dramatically below L3–L4. A thigh extension may be extended distally to immobilize the L4–L5 and L5–S1 levels. The extension is typically added to the stronger leg. For the thoracolumbar region, off-the-shelf hyperextension braces as well as both one-piece and two-piece clamshell braces all have reasonable effectiveness in immobilizing the spine in extension, which is the most common goal.

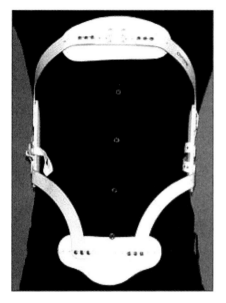

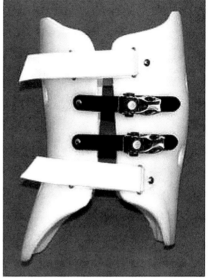

Fig. 71.4   Front view of Jewett extension brace.

Fig. 71.5   Side view of clamshell thoraco-lumbosacral orthosis (TLSO).

Spinal Conditions

Trauma

Most physicians are familiar with the use of spinal braces for treating fractures and other injuries of the spine. The goals of treatment are to prevent deformity, manage pain from instability, enable early mobilization, and promote healing. The use of an orthosis to treat any fracture or spinal injury mandates close clinical and radiographic follow-up. The development of worsening deformity (i.e., loss of reduction), neurologic symptoms, or brace complications are all indications for changes in treatment. Standing radiographs are an essential part of the evaluation of the adequacy of an orthosis in any part of the spine and should be obtained early in the treatment protocol and frequently until stability has been restored. This surveillance may require multiple imaging studies, which add significantly to the overall cost and burden of nonoperative treatment.

In the cervical spine, rigid collars may be used for injuries such as unilateral facet fractures, spinous process avulsions, isolated lateral mass fractures, and some odontoid fractures, particularly in the elderly. Often, however, more robust immobilization is required with a CTO or halo vest. The use of a halo vest allows the treating physician to use traction for an initial reduction, which is preferred to traction followed by transfer into a CTO such as a Minerva brace. Fractures treated with this strategy include C1, C2 and subaxial burst fractures, hangman's fractures of C2, some flexion teardrop or flexion compression injuries, and unilateral facet dislocations. It is critical that traction be reduced or removed before applying the vest to ensure that fracture fragments are not distracted. The choice of orthosis also depends on the level of pathology and patient comfort. The halo vest is invasive and allows snaking, but it provides excellent immobilization of the upper cervical spine and cervicothoracic junction. Rigid collars are less invasive and generally more comfortable, but they lack control of the lower cervical spine and allow more motion at other cervical levels.

Brace treatment of thoracolumbar injuries, particularly burst fractures, remains a matter of great debate. Historically, treatment mandated long periods of bedrest with or without traction and hyperextension positioning. This remains the primary treatment modality in many developing nations, where operative treatment and modern braces are unavailable. The popularity of spinal instrumentation in developed countries, however, has caused a shift to the use of operative treatment more frequently in the management of spinal injuries. For many patients, brace treatment with TLSOs has remained a useful intermediate, allowing early mobilization without surgical intervention. Without reduction (which requires a cooperative patient), the brace is thought to prevent deformity rather than correct it. Despite its popularity, a number of recent meta-analyses and randomized trials have shown results of brace treatment to be similar to early mobilization without a brace. No difference was found in back pain, the development of segmental kyphosis, or return to work and activity. TLSO brace treatment, therefore, remains a reasonable treatment option, but may not truly alter the natural history of the injury. Most authors agree that acute segmental kyphosis in excess of 30 degrees, associated neurologic injury, or burst fractures outside of the thoracolumbar (T11 to L2) segment require special consideration.

Flexion-distraction injuries may be treated with a brace, particularly if the injury is bony and is likely to heal satisfactorily without surgical intervention. In this case, an off-the-shelf extension brace (e.g., Jewett) is required. Patients with multiple injuries or associated abdominal trauma, however, are often better served with early surgery and internal fixation to allow quicker mobilization and avoid complications such as ileus or pulmonary restriction. The role of brace treatment of other fractures is often controversial. In cases where stability or deformity progression is unlikely, less rigid and more comfortable orthoses may be used to control pain as long as a specific goal or well-defined endpoint is established. Refractory pain in osteoporotic vertebral compression fractures of the thoracic spine is an example of this situation.

Deformity

The use of braces and external supports to correct deformity in adults and children has a long history. In current practice, braces are most commonly used for the treatment of idiopathic scoliosis in infants and adolescents to prevent curve progression. In the mid 20th century, the Milwaukee brace was used most frequently, but practice has now evolved toward the use of rigid plastic TLSOs and Boston body jackets. In the case of adolescent idiopathic scoliosis, most surgeons now use a brace in skeletally immature patients with thoracic curves exceeding 25 to 30 degrees and demonstrating ongoing progression. The curve is partially corrected with the use of carefully placed pads over the convexity and cutouts on the concavity. Considerable debate persists in the literature regarding the overall effectiveness of any brace treatment, but it is generally agreed that full-time brace wear has been shown to improve the chance of the success of nonsurgical treatment. There is a paucity of literature on using orthoses for deformity correction in skeletally mature adults, but most surgeons agree that braces are not effective for the primary treatment of adult scoliosis. Orthoses do play a role in postoperative management of fusion for correction of scoliosis, and they may be used as a short-term treatment for painful exacerbations.

Spinal orthoses including halo vests and Minerva CTLOs are used to treat kyphotic deformities of both the cervical and thoracic spine in pathologies such as ankylosing spondylitis (AS) and Scheuermann kyphosis, respectively. In AS, the halo vest may be used during or after surgical correction or to treat acute undisplaced fractures. Other cervical collars are generally not useful because of the significant underlying deformity. Long periods of rigid immobilization are required to achieve healing and stability. Kyphosis resulting from vertebral wedging in Scheuermann disease can be treated in skeletally immature patients with a cervicothoracolumbosacral (CTLS) orthosis, such as a TLSO brace with neck extension or an extended Minerva brace. The brace must direct a force anteriorly over the apex of the curve and a posterior counterforce both above and below the apex. This pattern creates a three-point bending effect. Indications for brace treatment and surgery continue to evolve, and the decision to institute any treatment must be made on an individual basis.

Postsurgical

Bracing of the cervical, thoracic, and lumbar spine after an operation for deformity correction, fusion, or treatment of fractures may help increase union rate, limit pain, and in some cases obviate the need for further procedures in complex reconstructive surgery. Although a brace can lead to muscular atrophy of the paraspinal and core muscles groups, it can also improve patient confidence in the early postoperative period and encourage early mobilization. It is important to remember that postsurgical patients, however, are particularly prone to the potential complications of braces, including ileus and abdominal distension, decreased pulmonary capacity, and skin breakdown or ulceration. In addition, the development and increased use of pedicle screw constructs has improved the biomechanics of spine fixation and reduced the need for postoperative bracing. Decisions regarding postoperative bracing should be considered on an individual case-by-case basis, but overall their use is diminishing as a result of improved surgery and limited supporting evidence.

Neck Pain, Back Pain, Tumor, and Infection

Small amounts of mechanical instability, or so called microinstability, can result in significant pain. In degenerative processes, as well as some cases of tumor and infection of the spine, this instability may be the primary cause of symptoms. Patients with pain relieved by recumbency are good candidates for stabilization with either surgery or bracing. The goals of the orthosis are to limit gross motion and provide trunk support; however, the use of an orthosis must be measured against the potential complications. Pathology must also be well localized, so that an appropriate device can be prescribed. Patients with long-standing degenerative disease of the spine, with pain that is poorly localized and not primarily mechanical in nature, are not well served by a brace, which may ultimately lead to further loss of motion and weakness of the paraspinal muscles.

Patients undergoing medical treatment for tumors or infection of the spine are another group who may benefit from the use of an orthosis. Collapse of the anterior spinal elements is a common event that can lead to progressive pain and disability even if medical or radiotherapy is successful. In the cervical spine, protection with a CTO is more useful than a rigid cervical collar, and in the lumbar spine, a well-fitted TLSO provides triplanar support to prevent anterior or lateral collapse. Brace control of micromotion or gross instability is also helpful in controlling pain and allowing ongoing mobilization during treatment. It is critical to recognize, however, that surgical stabilization with modern implants and techniques is often a more practical solution that avoids the need for prolonged external immobilization. Minimal access techniques for internal fixation are particularly useful for patients with high perioperative risk or soft-tissue compromise, and these techniques are often used in place of bracing. A thorough assessment of the relative risks and benefits of both options should be made for each patient.

Complications

The prescribing physician and entire team must be aware of several potential complications. All external braces may cause skin breakdown or ulceration. This problem is particularly common in patients with sensory deficits secondary to neurologic injury (such as spinal cord injury) and patients with a reduced level of consciousness. Cervical orthoses such as collars may cause skin breakdown over the chin, occiput, or chest. Thoracolumbar braces like TLSO body jackets can cause injury to the limited soft tissue over the lower ribs, iliac crest, and sacrum.

Spinal orthoses will cause paraspinal muscle weakening and may also impair underlying organ function. In the neck, swallowing difficulties or increased work of breathing has been found with rigid collars. Access to tracheostomy tubes can also be a problem. Braces covering the chest impair pulmonary function, decrease vital capacity, and may slow weaning from ventilators. In some cases, these external devices can also result in a tachycardic response, presumably related to decreased lung function and impaired venous return. Thoracolumbar orthoses need to be tight-fitting. In the case of abdominal distension from trauma or ileus, a brace may be difficult or impossible to fit and can slow recovery from abdominal injury.

Acknowledgment

The authors wish to thank Ken Moghadam, CO, for the use of the figures displayed in this chapter.

Suggested Readings

Bailey CS, Dvorak MF, Thomas KC, et al. Comparison of thoracolumbosacral orthosis and no orthosis for the treatment of thoracolumbar burst fractures: interim analysis of a multicenter randomized clinical equivalence trial. J Neurosurg Spine 2009;11(3):295–303

> *This landmark randomized study assessed the short- and medium-term outcomes of burst fractures treated without bracing.*

Benzel EC, Hadden TA, Saulsbery CM. A comparison of the Minerva and halo jackets for stabilization of the cervical spine. J Neurosurg 1989;70(3):411–414

> *This study compared the control of the cervical spine by two common braces.*

Bono CM. The halo fixator. J Am Acad Orthop Surg 2007;15(12):728–737

> *This is a recent review of the halo fixator, including biomechanics and complications.*

Dickson RA, Weinstein SL. Bracing (and screening)—yes or no? J Bone Joint Surg Br 1999; 81(2):193–198

> *This is a review of idiopathic scoliosis epidemiology and treatment principles, including a review of the current evidence for and against bracing.*

Hsu JD, Michael JW, Fisk JR. American Academy of Orthopaedic Surgeons. AAOS Atlas of Orthoses and Assistive Devices. 4th ed. Philadelphia, PA: Mosby/Elsevier; 2008

> *This is a thorough review of the spectrum of spinal orthotics and their biomechanical properties.*

McLain RF. Cancer in the Spine: Comprehensive Care. Totowa, NJ: Humana Press; 2006

> *This book includes a discussion of the use of bracing in metastatic spinal disease.*

Schneider AM, Hipp JA, Nguyen L, Reitman CA. Reduction in head and intervertebral motion provided by 7 contemporary cervical orthoses in 45 individuals. Spine 2007;32(1):E1–E6

> *This study compares a variety of cervical collars, demonstrating similar effectiveness in different models.*

Tator CH, Benzel EC. AANS Publications Committee. Contemporary Management of Spinal Cord Injury: From Impact to Rehabilitation. Park Ridge, IL: American Association of Neurological Surgeons; 2000

> *This book addresses bracing in trauma and rehabilitation.*

Penetrating Injuries to the Spine

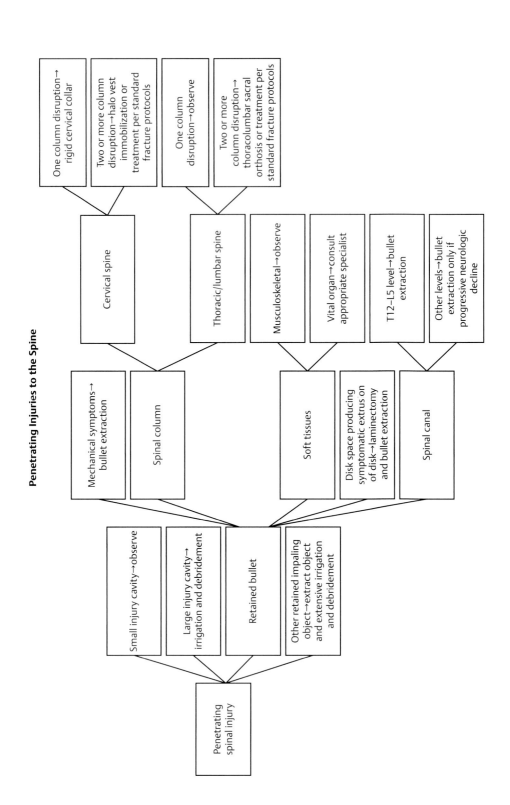

72

Penetrating Injuries to the Spine

Ashvin K. Dewan and A. Jay Khanna

In a cohort of more than 24,000 patients studied by the National Spinal Cord Injury Statistical Center, violence was found to be the third most common cause of spinal cord injury (SCI) and was responsible for 18.2% of admissions.[1] Gunshot wounds (GSWs) and knife injuries account for most violence-related SCIs. Accidents and work-related impalement injuries of the spine are relatively uncommon and constitute the remaining penetrating injuries of the spine seen in practice.[2]

Classification

To our knowledge, no formal classification scheme for penetrating SCI exists. It is convenient, however, to divide penetrating SCI treatment into two broad categories based on the mechanism of injury: impaling/stabbing injuries and ballistic injuries.

Evaluation

History

Acute penetrating SCI not only affects the spinal cord; it also puts many neighboring vital structures at risk for injury. Therefore, it is important to follow Advanced Trauma Life Support protocols[3] and involve general surgery trauma specialists and emergency department physicians as appropriate.

Once the patient is appropriately stabilized, initial evaluation of penetrating SCI involves the same detailed history and physical examination as that of patients with other suspected spine injuries. For penetrating injuries, information regarding the penetrating object helps guide appropriate management. Recovery of the actual object provides the most useful information; otherwise, a careful history, including a general description of the weapon or object, is helpful. It is also important to determine whether any neurologic symptoms occurred immediately after the injury and to document the progression, or lack thereof, of any of these symptoms.

Physical Examination

In addition to comprehensive neurologic and spine examinations, a thorough inspection of all entrance and exit wounds should be performed. Palpation of the tissue for the presence of crepitus and general turgor is important for gauging the extent of underlying tissue necrosis.[4] If an object remains impaled in the wound, it is important that it *not* be removed in the emergency department, particularly if a viscus has been perforated. Withdrawing an impaling object without appropriate surgical irrigation and débridement can result in bowel content contamination of surrounding tissues and eventual sepsis.[5]

Spinal Imaging

Standard radiographic views of the involved spinal region should always be obtained, even in the absence of neurologic deficits. Klein and colleagues[6] retrospectively analyzed 244 patients with substantial spinal injuries secondary to GSWs and found that 13% presented with no neurologic symptoms. They concluded that complete radiographic spine evaluation was mandatory after a GSW to the face, neck, or trunk, even without neurologic deficit.[6]

Spine fractures should be characterized by type and classified morphologically or through the use of one of the commonly accepted fracture classification systems, such as the subaxial injury classification score (SLIC) or the Thoracolumbar Injury Classification and Severity Score (TLICS).

Imaging modalities are chosen to visualize various aspects of the injury, including the location of foreign debris, extent of osseous involvement, and soft-tissue integrity. Radiographs should be scrutinized for residual fragments and/or foreign debris from the impaling object/projectile. Approximately one-third of the neurologic deficits secondary to GSWs are associated with retained bullet fragments in the spinal canal.[7] Computed tomography can help determine the extent of spine injury and evaluate the degree of spinal canal encroachment by bone or bullet fragments (**Fig. 72.1**). Magnetic resonance imaging provides excellent information regarding spinal neural elements and surrounding soft-tissue integrity (**Fig. 72.2**), but, in the setting of retained metallic fragments, its use is controversial, particularly if retained fragments are near vital and susceptible anatomic structures, such as the spinal cord.[1,8] An alternative study, such as a myelogram followed by immediate computed tomography, can assess the spinal neural elements after SCI secondary to GSWs.[1]

 Treatment

Initial Care

The initial care of patients with penetrating SCI begins with local wound care, most of which can occur in the emergency department. The exception is injuries with large exit wounds and physical and radiographic findings that suggest

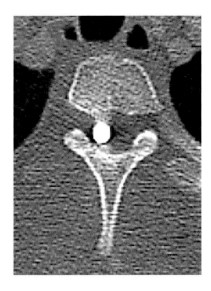

Fig. 72.1 This 21-year-old man had an incomplete SCI after a GSW to the thoracic spine. A bullet is seen in the spinal canal at the T4 level.

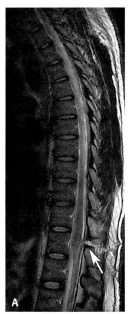
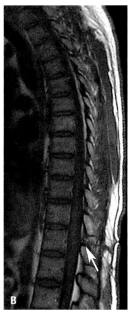
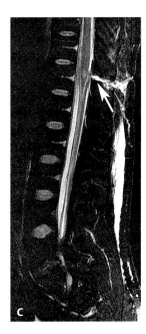

Fig. 72.2 A spinal cord injury from a stab injury to the conus medullaris. **(A)** A sagittal T2-weighted image of the thoracic spine showing a linear track (*arrow*) from the skin to the conus medullaris with an associated region of increased signal within the conus medullaris, compatible with edema. **(B)** A sagittal T1-weighted image of the thoracic spine also showing the track (*arrow*) but not showing the edema within the conus medullaris. **(C)** A sagittal STIR image of the lumbar spine accentuates the edema along the track (*arrow*) and also that within the conus medullaris. (From Okubadejo GO, Daftary AR, Buchowski JM, Carrino JA, Khanna AJ. The lumbar and thoracic spine. In: Khanna AJ, ed. MRI for Orthopaedic Surgeons. New York, NY: Thieme; 2010:269–315; Figure 11.6. Reprinted with permission.)

the presence of a large cavity at the injury site. If the wound has been contaminated by passage of an object through the pharynx, esophagus, or colon, or if the wound has been contaminated after injury, it is essential that wound cultures be taken from the injury tract. If the impaling object has been retained, it is important not to manipulate the object before surgery. Identification of its track and the organs violated along that path is essential for appropriate treatment.[5] Premature removal of the impaling object can contaminate the entire tract (e.g., with intestinal bacteria). Every effort should be made to débride and irrigate contaminated areas before the impaled object is removed in the operating room.[5] The clinician should remember to administer tetanus prophylaxis, especially if the immunization status is unknown.

Steroids are not recommended for SCI related to penetrating spine injuries. The Second National Acute Spinal Cord Injury Study did not include GSWs.[9] Three retrospective studies examining steroids in the setting of penetrating SCI suggested that steroids provide no benefit and may be associated with a higher risk of infectious complications.[10–12] In the absence of any reported efficacy of such treatment, steroids are not recommended for penetrating SCI.[1,10–13]

Impalement/Stabbing Injuries

Most impalement/stabbing SCIs are limited to soft-tissue damage, with minimal disruption of the osseous architecture (**Fig. 72.3**). Exceptions include high-energy industrial accidents involving heavy machinery, which can produce large soft-tissue and bony defects.[5] For impalement/stabbing injuries or injuries with large cavities at the injury site, patients should undergo urgent spine débridement. Preoperative coordination with the trauma team is critical in the setting of collateral or multiple injuries. Intraoperatively, it is extremely important to search for and evacuate any foreign bodies (e.g., clothing) in the wounds and to obtain wound cultures. Such injuries require a minimum of 3 weeks of parenteral antibiotics with coverage specific to the organisms found at débridement.[1] It is important to remember that spine infections after penetrating injury can be insidious and that at least 6 months of follow-up is necessary to declare a patient free of spinal infection.[1] Associated fractures of the spine identified on imaging should be treated via standard treatment algorithms.

Gunshot Wounds

With few exceptions, most GSWs to the spine can be treated with little to no surgery.[1,14,15] Previously, radical spine débridement with bullet extraction was favored in such situations, but the best results have been reported with minimal spine débridement and protection with 1 to 2 weeks of parenteral antibiotics.[15] SCIs secondary to GSWs are relatively uncontaminated, with the exception of GSWs that first penetrate the pharynx, esophagus, or colon, which require a tailored broad-spectrum antibiotic regimen of variable duration depending on the extent of visceral injury.[1,15]

Most GSWs to the spine are stable.[1,14] For the cervical spine, the use of immobilization depends on the degree of bony ligamentous disruption: with no bony

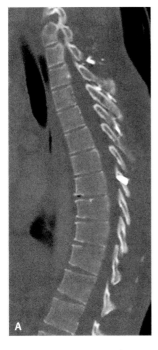
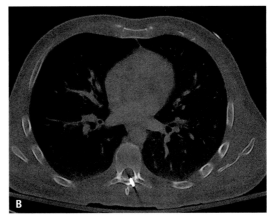

Fig. 72.3   CT images showing a knife blade that broke off in the spinal lamina in the mid-thoracic spine. **(A)** Sagittal reconstructed view. **(B)** Axial view.

involvement, no immobilization is necessary; with the anterior vertebral body fractured or posterior bony elements, a rigid cervical collar can be considered; with both the anterior vertebral body and posterior elements disrupted, halo vest immobilization is recommended.[1] For the thoracic/lumbar spine, the use of immobilization also depends on the degree of bony and ligamentous disruption: if none or only the anterior or posterior bony elements, no immobilization is needed; if both the anterior and posterior bony and ligamentous structures, a thoracolumbosacral orthosis is recommended when the patient is out of bed.[1] After 6 to 8 weeks of immobilization, flexion and extension conventional radiographs of the affected region are obtained to evaluate healing.[1] In contrast to closed SCIs, operative intervention to establish stability after a GSW of the spine is rarely necessary.[1,14]

Extraction of a retained bullet is performed only in certain circumstances. If a bullet is lodged in the disk space, three factors determine whether surgery is indicated: risk of lead poisoning, disruption of the motion segment producing mechanical symptoms, and disk extrusion that compresses neural elements. When a lodged bullet is bathed in synovial or cerebrospinal fluid (CSF), lead can leach from the bullet and predispose the patient to plumbism; the clinician should also be aware that the onset of lead poisoning secondary to a retained bullet can be delayed.[1,16] The second consideration includes the mechanical disruption of the motion segment by a bullet within the disk space. If new mechanical-type symptoms develop that worsen with upright posture and activity and decrease in recumbency, then removal of the bullet, combined with fusion, can be considered.[1,14] Finally, although it is exceedingly rare, disk extrusion due to a GSW causing symptomatic neural compression is an indication for neural decompression.

The literature provides limited information regarding the treatment of bullets lodged within the spinal canal. Some advocate extraction of all bullets in the spinal canal to minimize risks of CSF leak, meningitis, lead toxicity, chronic fibrosis, and neurologic decline.[1,14,17] Others believe a nonoperative approach is more prudent, given the morbidity of surgical extraction, unless there is documented progressive neurologic decline.[14,18] One retrospective review of 90 patients with SCI secondary to a GSW between T12 and L5 showed that bullet extraction provided significant improvement of neurologic motor function but no improvement in pain or sensation.[17] For bullets within the spinal canal between T1 and T11, however, the authors found no benefit to bullet extraction. Not enough data relating to the cervical spine were available to draw a conclusion.[17] Although cervical level bullet extraction does not improve or reverse SCI,[17] Eismont et al.[18] and Eismont and Roper[1] found that the removal of bullets in the cervical spinal canal improved adjacent nerve root function. Most clinicians agree, however, that surgery is indicated for patients with bullets in the spinal canal that produce documented compression of the neural elements with progressive, not static, neurologic deterioration.

Outcomes

Penetrating wounds of the spine result in a substantially larger number of complete injuries than do other SCIs, and the risk of complete injury is much higher for those in the thoracic spine region than those in the cervical or lumbar spine.[2] Complete and incomplete SCIs secondary to GSWs can show statistically significant neurologic improvements even at 6 months, although open SCIs tend to improve slightly later than do closed SCIs.[1] Stab wounds often produce a Brown-Sequard pattern of partial spinal cord injury when hemisection of the cord occurs from anterior to posterior, but they also have the best prognosis for recovery of all incomplete spinal injuries. Compared with patients with SCI secondary to GSW and a similar extent of paralysis, the prognosis is better for patients with stab wounds.

Complications

Penetrating SCIs create communicating tracts between the spine and neighboring structures. Consequently, the most common complications of penetrating SCI involve fistula formation and spinal infection resulting from bacterial contamination.

CSF cutaneous fistulas have been described most commonly in patients with GSWs of the spine.[19] Most often, CSF fistulas are seen after acute surgical treatment for bullet removal with laminectomy and spinal débridement. The incidence is reported to be as high as 6%.[1,19] Given that most CSF fistulas are seen after acute treatment, if bullet removal is necessary, some suggest delaying removal for 7 to 10 days.[1,19]

Most spinal infections occur in the setting of associated injuries to the pharynx, esophagus, or colon. Infection secondary to injury to other organs, such as the stomach or small bowel, is less common[1,15] Recurrent spinal infections and spontaneous drainage from sinus tracts are more common with impalement injuries.[1] The spinal infection rate after penetration of a hollow viscus and appropriate treatment has been reported to be 5% to 15%.[1,15] Infection occurs infrequently after GSWs of the spine.[1,14,18]

Excluding associated injuries to surrounding structures after penetrating SCI, other reported complications include plumbism, meningitis, late neurologic sequelae from a chronic epidural inflammatory response, hematoma, dural tears, and chronic severe deafferent pain.[1]

References

1. Eismont F, Roper JG. Gunshot wounds of the spine. In: Browner BD, Jupiter JB, Levine AM, Trafton PG, Krettek C, eds. Skeletal Trauma: Basic Science, Management, and Reconstruction. Philadelphia: WB Saunders; 2008:1019–1042
2. Young JS, Burns PE, Bowen AM, McCutchen J. Spinal Cord Injury Statistics: Experience of the Regional Spinal Cord Injury Systems. Phoenix, AZ: Good Samaritan Medical Center; 1982.
3. American College of Surgeons Committee on T. ATLS Advanced Trauma Life Support Program for Doctors. Chicago, IL: American College of Surgeons; 2004
4. Fackler ML, Bellamy RF, Malinowski JA. The wound profile: illustration of the missile-tissue interaction. J Trauma 1988;28(1, Suppl):S21–S29
5. Tokushige JI, Inokuchi A, Kawaguchi H. Impalement injuries involving the spinal canal. J Orthop Sci 2000;5(6):614–617
6. Klein Y, Cohn SM, Soffer D, Lynn M, Shaw CM, Hasharoni A. Spine injuries are common among asymptomatic patients after gunshot wounds. J Trauma 2005;58(4):833–836
7. Williams DT, Chang DL, DeClerck MP. Penetrating spinal cord injuries with retained canal fragments. CJEM 2009;11(2):172–173
8. Finitsis SN, Falcone S, Green BA. MR of the spine in the presence of metallic bullet fragments: is the benefit worth the risk? AJNR Am J Neuroradiol 1999;20(2):354
9. Bracken MB, Shepard MJ, Collins WF, et al. A randomized, controlled trial of methylprednisolone or naloxone in the treatment of acute spinal-cord injury. Results of the Second National Acute Spinal Cord Injury Study. N Engl J Med 1990;322(20):1405–1411
10. Heary RF, Vaccaro AR, Mesa JJ, et al. Steroids and gunshot wounds to the spine. Neurosurgery 1997;41(3):576–583, discussion 583–584
11. Levy ML, Gans W, Wijesinghe HS, SooHoo WE, Adkins RH, Stillerman CB. Use of methylprednisolone as an adjunct in the management of patients with penetrating spinal cord injury: outcome analysis. Neurosurgery 1996;39(6):1141–1148, discussion 1148–1149
12. Prendergast MR, Saxe JM, Ledgerwood AM, Lucas CE, Lucas WF. Massive steroids do not reduce the zone of injury after penetrating spinal cord injury. J Trauma 1994;37(4):576–579, discussion 579–580
13. Thompson EC, Porter JM, Fernandez LG. Penetrating neck trauma: an overview of management. J Oral Maxillofac Surg 2002;60(8):918–923
14. Moon E, Kondrashov D, Hannibal M, Hsu K, Zucherman J. Gunshot wounds to the spine: literature review and report on a migratory intrathecal bullet. Am J Orthop (Belle Mead, NJ) 2008;37(3):E47–E51

15. Roffi RP, Waters RL, Adkins RH. Gunshot wounds to the spine associated with a perforated viscus. Spine (Phila, PA 1976) 1989;14(8):808–811
16. Scuderi GJ, Vaccaro AR, Fitzhenry LN, Greenberg S, Eismont F. Long-term clinical manifestations of retained bullet fragments within the intervertebral disk space. J Spinal Disord Tech 2004;17(2):108–111
17. Waters RL, Adkins RH. The effects of removal of bullet fragments retained in the spinal canal. A collaborative study by the National Spinal Cord Injury Model Systems. Spine 1991;16(8):934–939
18. Eismont FJ, Currier BL, McGuire RA Jr. Cervical spine and spinal cord injuries: recognition and treatment. Instr Course Lect 2004;53:341–358
19. Stauffer ES, Wood RW, Kelly EG. Gunshot wounds of the spine: the effects of laminectomy. J Bone Joint Surg Am 1979;61(3):389–392

Suggested Readings

Eismont F, Roper JG. Gunshot wounds of the spine. In: Browner BD, Jupiter JB, Levine AM, Trafton PG, Krettek C, eds. Skeletal Trauma: Basic Science, Management, and Reconstruction. Philadelphia: WB Saunders; 2008:1019–1042

> *This chapter is a comprehensive review of the epidemiology, pathophysiology, and management of GSWs to the spine.*

Bracken MB, Shepard MJ, Collins WF, et al. A randomized, controlled trial of methylprednisolone or naloxone in the treatment of acute spinal-cord injury. Results of the Second National Acute Spinal Cord Injury Study. N Engl J Med 1990;322(20):1405–1411

> *This is a well-publicized study about the role of steroid administration after acute SCI. Although the study involves acute blunt SCI, it is important to recognize that GSW victims were not included in the study.*

Heary RF, Vaccaro AR, Mesa JJ, et al. Steroids and gunshot wounds to the spine. Neurosurgery 1997;41(3):576–583, discussion 583–584

> *This is one of the largest retrospective reviews of the role of steroids in GSWs to the spine. The authors retrospectively reviewed 254 GSW victims given methylprednisolone (NASCIS 2 protocol), dexamethasone (initial dose, 10–100 mg), or no steroids. The use of steroids was not associated with a statistically significant neurologic benefit, but there was a trend toward increased infectious complications.*

Roffi RP, Waters RL, Adkins RH. Gunshot wounds to the spine associated with a perforated viscus. Spine 1989;14(8):808–811

> *This is one of only a few reviews examining infection with GSWs to the spine associated with a perforated viscus. In 42 patients treated with minimal spine débridement and 1 to 2 weeks of parenteral antibiotics, the incidence of spinal infection was decreased to 5% to 15% for severe injuries involving the pharynx, esophagus, or colon.*

Waters RL, Adkins RH. The effects of removal of bullet fragments retained in the spinal canal. A collaborative study by the National Spinal Cord Injury Model Systems. Spine 1991;16(8):934–939

> *There is limited information regarding the treatment of bullets lodged within the spinal canal. This retrospective review examined 90 patients with SCI from a bullet lodged in the spinal canal. Gunshot spinal cord injury between T12 and L5 showed significant improvement of neurologic motor function but no improvement in pain or sensation with bullet extraction. However, no benefit was observed with the extraction of a bullet between T1 and T11.*

73

Spine Emergencies

Kris Radcliff and Christopher K. Kepler

This chapter describes identification and management of situations that may require urgent or emergent decision making and possibly surgical intervention to prevent permanent neurologic injury. This chapter discusses the diagnosis, workup, and treatment of cauda equina syndrome, epidural hematoma, epidural abscess, incomplete neurologic deficit after traumatic injury, and progressive neurologic symptoms of spinal cord compression due to tumor.

Cauda Equina Syndrome (CES)

Cauda equina syndrome is characterized by a constellation of lower-extremity pain, motor weakness, radiculopathy, saddle anesthesia, and urinary/fecal dysfunction. The presentation is variable. Patients may complain of unilateral or bilateral symptoms. The most common cause of CES is a lumbar disk herniation. CES most frequently presents in the fourth or fifth decade of life. It can also occur in patients with a baseline stenotic spinal canal, resulting in chronic CES (**Fig. 73.1A,B**). Other causes of CES include epidural abscess, tumors, fractures, or hematomas. On examination, patients with CES may have variable sensory deficit, although classically CES has been associated with saddle anesthesia (numbness in the perineum and inner thighs in the area where one might sit on a saddle). Additional symptoms may include distal-extremity weakness, depressed lower extremity reflexes, and decreased sphincter tone. Patients should also have a postvoid residual volume check after urination as urinary retention can be the presenting symptom. A postvoid residual greater than 500 mL has been demonstrated to be associated with CES.

The difficulty with a diagnosis of CES is the absence of absolute clinical diagnostic criteria. Therefore, patients presenting with complaints of any of the symptoms just discussed should undergo a careful neurologic examination to identify other signs and symptoms consistent with a diagnosis of CES. Any pa-

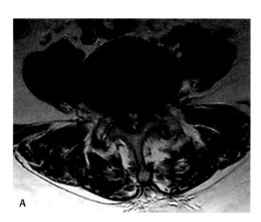
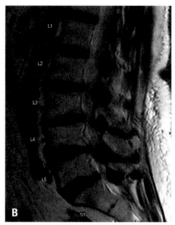

Fig. 73.1 MRI images demonstrating chronic multilevel lumbar stenosis in a patient who experienced waxing/waning symptoms consistent with chronic CES. Ultimately, the patient underwent decompression from L3 to S1 with resolution of her symptoms of saddle anesthesia and lower-extremity motor weakness and partial resolution of associated urinary symptoms. **(A)** Axial (at L4–L5). **(B)** Sagittal.

tients with symptoms suggestive of CES should undergo urgent magnetic resonance imaging (MRI) to identify the possible neural element in compression (**Fig. 73.2A,B**).

Although little debate exists regarding the need for urgent decompression, controversy remains regarding the timing of surgery. The prognosis of CES is

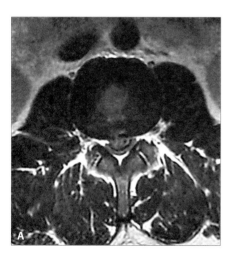
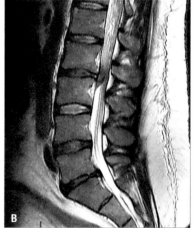

Fig. 73.2 MRI images demonstrating massive L2–L3 disk herniation in a patient who presented with urinary incontinence and bilateral lower extremity weakness. The patient underwent decompressive laminectomy with complete resolution of symptoms postoperatively. **(A)** Axial. **(B)** Sagittal.

generally poor, and a significant number of patients report long-term sphincter and sexual dysfunction. The best results have been reported with early surgery (within 24–48 hours of onset). Additionally, patients with incomplete symptoms, such as partially preserved continence or progressive motor loss, may have improved prognosis compared with patients with complete symptoms. The prognosis of patients with complete motor loss is generally poor. Regardless, decompression should be performed as soon as medically feasible.

Epidural Hematoma

Epidural hematoma similarly presents with progressive neurologic symptoms referable to the level of involvement, which can be any spinal level (**Fig. 73.3A,B**). Patients often report sharp pain localized to the spine at the level where the hematoma forms, which is followed by progressive neurologic signs and symptoms. Epidural hematomas can be postsurgical, postprocedural (after epidural injection or spinal anesthesia), or spontaneous. A thorough history is essential to identify potential contributing factors, such as recent procedures, but also should include the use of anticoagulants or history of coagulopathy. Approximately one-half of patients with spontaneous epidural hematomas will have no obvious risk factors, although men in their sixth or seventh decade of life are most commonly affected. Additionally, patients with ankylosing spondylitis can develop epidural hematomas after relatively minor trauma. Patients presenting with a progressive neurologic deficit should undergo emergent imaging. Hematoma most commonly affects the dorsal aspect of the spinal canal. Multilevel surgery and preoperative coagulopathy have been identified as risk

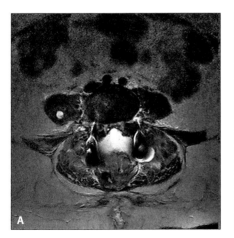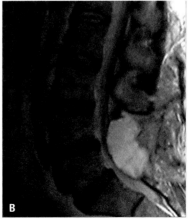

Fig. 73.3 MRI images after L4–L5 posterior spinal decompression and fusion demonstrating large dorsal hematoma. The patient complained of postoperative tingling and weakness in the L5 distribution, which resolved with decompression. **(A)** Axial. **(B)** Sagittal.

factors, while the use of postoperative drains does not seem to affect the incidence of postoperative epidural hematoma.

Patients with significant or progressive symptoms and epidural hematoma should undergo urgent or emergent decompression, with timing dictated by the degree of neurologic deficit and progression of symptoms. The need for post-decompression stabilization will depend on the level of decompression, alignment (especially in the cervical spine), presence of adjacent fusion, and degree of decompression necessary to evacuate the hematoma completely. Recovery of function after decompression is dependent on the preoperative deficit and timing of compression, with poor results when patients develop complete paralysis prior to decompression.

Epidural Abscess

Diskitis and osteomyelitis cause nonspecific axial pain and often can be present for several months prior to diagnosis. Epidural abscess may occur spontaneously after untreated diskitis/osteomyelitis, although it can also occur iatrogenically after percutaneous spinal procedures. The clinical presentation of epidural abscess is dependent on the resultant spinal canal stenosis. Patients with mild stenosis may be asymptomatic, but patients with severe stenosis may develop symptoms of radiculopathy, myelopathy, numbness, weakness, or incontinence. The key factor in identifying epidural abscess is distinguishing nonmechanical back pain (worse at night, not activity related) and/or constitutional symptoms. In the worst-case scenario, patients may have meningitis due to the infection. Patients at risk for epidural abscess, diskitis, or osteomyelitis should have blood work to facilitate diagnosis of the infection (complete blood count, erythrocyte sedimentation rate, C-reactive protein) as well as blood cultures. Radiographs will demonstrate disk space narrowing in the early phases of diskitis/osteomyelitis. MRI should be performed with gadolinium, which will show rim-enhancement of the abscess (**Fig. 73.4A,B**).

Epidural abscesses may result as a direct extension of osteomyelitis or diskitis or adjacent postsurgical infection. Alternatively, infection can be caused by epidural injections or catheter placement or through hematogenous seeding. Risk factors for epidural abscess (besides having recently undergone spinal surgery or another procedure) are those that predispose to infection in general, including diabetes mellitus, intravenous drug use, alcoholism, and immunocompromised states. *Staphylococcus aureus* is the most common pathogen, followed by *Streptococcus* species and *Staphylococcus epidermidis*. More rare pathogens may be common in at-risk populations, such as the association of *Pseudomonas* with intravenous drug use.

Untreated epidural abscesses will result in progressive neurologic deficits, sepsis, and possibly death.. Nonoperative, medical management may be considered for lumbar epidural abscesses in patients who are neurologically intact. However, extremely close follow-up is necessary to identify progression of disease and/or signs of sepsis. Cervical and thoracic epidural abscesses should be managed surgically on diagnosis because of the high incidence of permanent neurologic deficit and death. The standard treatment is decompression, with

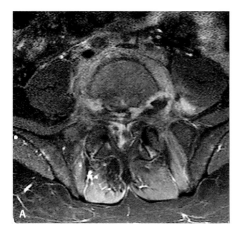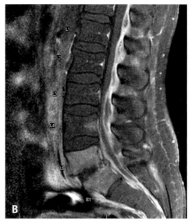

Fig. 73.4 T1 MRI images after injection of gadolinium demonstrate a multilevel epidural collection compressing the cauda equina, with involvement of the L5 and S1 vertebral bodies and the L5–S1 disk. Cultures confirmed infection. **(A)** Axial (L5–S1). **(B)** Sagittal.

the approach guided by abscess location, closure over drains, and antibiotic therapy. Instrumented fusion should be utilized when osteomyelitis presents a risk of spinal instability. The use of autograft should be considered, as it may carry a lower risk of becoming a nidus for continued infection compared with allograft, metallic implants, or bone substitutes. As with epidural hematoma, decompression should be considered emergent when symptoms are severe or the patient demonstrates progressive neurologic decline.

Incomplete Neurologic Injury After Trauma

Neurologic injury after spinal trauma can occur after many different injuries. While patients with unstable injuries often require surgical stabilization regardless of neurological status to facilitate rehabilitation, those with incomplete injuries should be treated as surgical emergencies to reduce displaced fractures, decompress neural elements, and prevent secondary injury associated with spinal instability. After adequate imaging, as by MRI or computed tomography (CT), has identified the nature of the injury (**Fig. 73.5A,B**), initial treatment may involve temporary in-situ stabilization with a halo vest; fracture reduction using traction followed by halo or cervical collar immobilization; or surgical reduction, decompression, and/or stabilization.

The presence of spinal shock may often cloud the clinical distinction between complete and incomplete injury. Spinal cord shock is defined by the absence of a bulbospongiosus reflex. For this reason, patients with apparently complete injuries who present before spinal shock has ended should be treated as though they have incomplete injuries so as to provide the best chance of neurologic recovery if spinal shock is masking an incomplete injury.

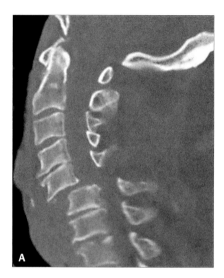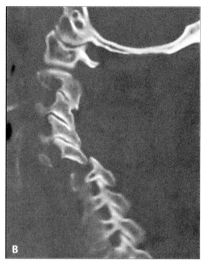

Fig. 73.5 CT scan images demonstrating patient with bilaterally jumped facets at C5–C6. The patient presented with an incomplete injury, demonstrating diminished upper and lower extremity strength, which improved after reduction. **(A)** Midline. **(B)** Parasagittal.

Neurologic Deficits Due to Tumor

Rapid tumor growth in patients with either primary or metastatic tumors compressing the spinal cord may lead to acute, progressive neurologic decline, with metastatic disease constituting the vast majority of cases (**Fig. 73.6A,B**). Although compressive tumors can theoretically be treated either with noninvasive methods, including radiation and corticosteroids, or with a combination of surgery and radiation, significant benefit from surgical decompression in the setting of metastatic disease has been demonstrated with regard to preservation of the ability to walk . A prospective, randomized study demonstrated an improvement in ambulation and outcome in patients with epidural spinal cord compression due to solid tumors who underwent surgery followed by radiation versus those treated with radiation alone. For this reason, patients with rapidly progressive neurologic decline due to spinal cord compression by a tumor should be treated with surgical decompression with or without stabilization, provided they are healthy enough to undergo surgery and have a reasonable life expectancy. Hematopoietic tumors were excluded from the study and are generally responsive to nonsurgical treatment, including radiation or chemotherapy. Surgery before these patients lose the ability to walk provides the greatest chance of preserving independent postoperative ambulation, although patients treated with surgery after losing the ability to walk have a substantially better chance of ambulating again than patients treated with radiation alone.

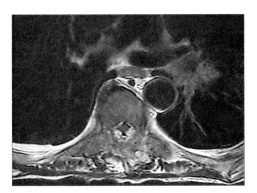 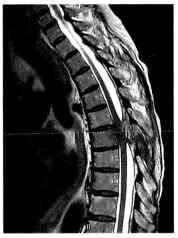

Fig. 73.6   MRI images demonstrating metastatic lesion at T9. The patient had a history of breast cancer and presented with leg weakness and difficulty ambulating. **(A)** Axial. **(B)** Sagittal.

Posterior surgery is most commonly performed in patients with neurologic deficit due to epidural compression, since the posterior approach is more utilitarian, and anterior debulking or corpectomy may be performed from a far lateral or transpedicular approach. The goal of surgery for rapid neurologic decline due to epidural compression is "separation surgery" or establishment of a physical distance between the tumor and the spinal cord to optimize radiation delivery. The timing of surgery with metastatic epidural compression is less well defined, although most authors would agree that surgery is optimal if performed within 48 hours after the patient loses ambulation potential. Finally, consideration of tumor vascularity and the need for embolization is mandatory prior to debulking.

Suggested Readings

Ahn UM, Ahn NU, Buchowski JM, Garrett ES, Sieber AN, Kostuik JP. Cauda equina syndrome secondary to lumbar disc herniation: a meta-analysis of surgical outcomes. Spine 2000;25(12): 1515–1522

> *This meta-analysis included a total of 322 patients and demonstrated no benefit in patients who underwent surgery within 24 hours of presentation compared with more than 24 hours, but it did show improved results in patients who were decompressed within 48 hours compared to more than 48 hours.*

Awad JN, Kebaish KM, Donigan J, Cohen DB, Kostuik JP. Analysis of the risk factors for the development of post-operative spinal epidural haematoma. J Bone Joint Surg Br 2005;87(9): 1248–1252

> *This retrospective study identified risk factors associated with the development of epidural hematoma: age older than 60 years, the use of preoperative nonsteroidal anti-inflammatory drugs (NSAIDs), and Rh-positive blood type. The use of drains was associated with decreased risk.*

Fehlings MG, Perrin RG. The timing of surgical intervention in the treatment of spinal cord injury: a systematic review of recent clinical evidence. Spine 2006;31(11, Suppl):S28–S35, discussion S36

> *Several studies have suggested that early decompression may improve outcome and reduce length of hospital stay and associated hospital-related complications.*

Hadjipavlou AG, Mader JT, Necessary JT, Muffoletto AJ. Hematogenous pyogenic spinal infections and their surgical management. Spine 2000;25(13):1668–1679

> *This retrospective study of 101 noniatrogenic epidural abscesses identifies patterns of clinical presentation and outcome after surgical decompression.*

Kostuik JP, Harrington I, Alexander D, Rand W, Evans D. Cauda equina syndrome and lumbar disc herniation. J Bone Joint Surg Am 1986;68(3):386–391

> *This retrospective review identifed patients with either acute or gradual symptom onset. No correlation was found between timing of decompression and return of function. Motor deficits tended to improve, while less success was seen for return of bladder function.*

Kreppel D, Antoniadis G, Seeling W. Spinal hematoma: a literature survey with meta-analysis of 613 patients. Neurosurg Rev 2003;26(1):1–49

> *A meta-analysis identifies factors associated with epidural hematoma and common presentation signs and symptoms, and it reports outcomes after treatment.*

Reihsaus E, Waldbaur H, Seeling W. Spinal epidural abscess: a meta-analysis of 915 patients. Neurosurg Rev 2000;23(4):175–204, discussion 205

> *This meta-analysis describes demographic patterns associated with development of epidural abscesses and identifies risk factors that influence incidence and outcome.*

Patchell RA, Tibbs PA, Regine WF, et al. Direct decompressive surgical resection in the treatment of spinal cord compression caused by metastatic cancer: a randomised trial. Lancet 2005;366(9486):643–648

> *A randomized controlled trial demonstrated significant advantage to surgical decompression followed by radiation compared to treatment with radiation alone in patients with progressive deficits from compressive metastatic tumors.*

Pollard ME, Apple DF. Factors associated with improved neurologic outcomes in patients with incomplete tetraplegia. Spine 2003;28(1):33–39

> *Despite the recommendations provided previously, this study showed no benefit to early surgery in patients with incomplete neurologic injury but identified younger age and the presence of either Brown-Sequard or central cord syndrome as factors associated with improved outcome.*

Index

Note: Page numbers followed by *f* and *t* indicate figures and tables, respectively.

workup for, 371–373
Spine, three-column model (Denis), 77, 78*f*, 85–86, 104
Spinolaminar line, 22, 23*f*
Spinous process(es), 85
SPO. *See* Smith-Peterson osteotomy
Spondylitis
  fungal, 391–393
  tuberculous, 391–393
Spondylolisthesis
  classification, 349, 350*t*
  definition, 349
  degenerative
    lumbar, 225–232
      algorithm for, 224*f*
    with lumbar spinal stenosis, 220
  grading, 349, 350*f*
  high-grade, 349–353
    algorithm for, 348*f*
    anatomic sites, 349
    complications, 352
    definition, 349
    epidemiology, 349
    imaging, 351
    outcomes with, 352
    physical examination, 349–351
    risk factors for, 349
    slip angle in, 351, 351*f*
    treatment, 351–352, 352*f*
    workup for, 349–351
  isthmic
    adult. *See* Adult isthmic spondylolisthesis
    definition, 243
    pediatric, 244
  workup for, 349–351
Spondylolysis, in athletes, 243
Spondyloptosis, 349, 350*f*
Spurling test, 124, 130
SSEPs. *See* Somatosensory evoked potentials
Stab injury(ies), 567
  imaging, 568, 569*f*, 570, 571*f*
  management, 570, 571*f*
  outcomes with, 572
stEMG. *See* Electromyography (EMG), stimulated
Steroid(s). *See* Corticosteroid(s)

Stiffness
  in ankylosing spondylitis, 180–181
  cervical
    after atlanto-axial injury, 24
    with disk disease, 124
    in whiplash injury, 166
  in diffuse idiopathic skeletal hyperostosis, 192
Straight leg-raising test, 545
Subaxial Injury Classification, 42, 43*t*, 44, 45*f*, 61, 62*t*, 68
Subaxial subluxation, in rheumatoid arthritis, 395–396, 398, 399*f*, 401, 402
Sulfasalazine
  for ankylosing spondylitis, 183
  for rheumatoid arthritis, 400
Superficial abdominal reflex, 198

T
Targeted disk decompression, 472*f*
tceMEPs. *See* Transcranial electrical motor evoked potentials
TDA. *See* Total disk arthroplasty
Teriparatide, for osteoporosis, 412
TFAS. *See* Total Facet Arthroplasty System
Thermal intradiskal procedures, 472*f*
Thoracic disk herniation, 197–200
  algorithm for, 196*f*
  centrolateral, 197
  classification, 197
  clinical presentation, 197–198
  hard, 197
  imaging, 198, 199*f*
  lateral, 197
  outcomes with, 200
  physical examination, 198
  soft, 197
  treatment, 199–200
  workup for, 197–198
Thoracic spine
  anterior pathology, *algorithm for,* 436*f*
  braces/orthoses for, 560, 561*f*
  kyphosis
    abnormal, 323
    normal, 323